Clinical Endocrinology of Dogs and Cats

Clinical Endocrinology
of
Dogs and Cats

An Illustrated Text

Edited by
A. RIJNBERK

Kluwer Academic Publishers
DORDRECHT – BOSTON – LONDON

Library of Congress Cataloging-in-Publication Data

Clinical endocrinology of dogs and cats : an illustrated text / edited
by A. Rijnberk ; coauthors, H.A.W. Hazewinkel ... [et al.] ; with
contributions from M.M. Bevers ... [et al.].
       p.   cm.
    Includes bibliographical references (p.   ) and index.
    ISBN-13: 978-0-7923-3416-3   e-ISBN-13: 978-94-009-0105-6
    DOI: 10.1007/978-94-009-0105-6

    1. Dogs--Diseases. 2. Cats--Diseases. 3. Veterinary
endocrinology.   I. Rijnberk, Adam. II. Hazewinkel, H. A. W.
SF992.E53C58 1995
636.7'0896--dc20   95-7371

ISBN-13: 978-0-7923-3416-3   e-ISBN-13: 978-94-009-0105-6
DOI: 10.1007/978-94-009-0105-6

Published by Kluwer Academic Publishers.
P.O. Box 17, 3300 AA Dordrecht, The Netherlands.

Kluwer Academic Publishers incorporates
the publishing programmes of
D. Reidel, Martinus Nijhoff, Dr W. Junk and MTP Press.

Sold and distributed in the U.S.A. and Canada
by Kluwer Academic Publishers,
101 Philip Drive, Norwell MA 02061, U.S.A.

In all other countries, sold and distributed
by Kluwer Academic Publishers Group,
P.O. Box 322, 3300 AH Dordrecht, The Netherlands.

The information contained in this publication is intended to supplement the knowledge of veterinary professionals regarding clinical endocrinology. This information is advisory only and is not intended to replace sound clinical judgment or individualized patient care. Kluwer Academic Publishers, editor and authors disclaim all warranties, whether expressed or implied, including any warranty as to the quality, accuracy or suitability of this information for any particular purpose.

Printed on acid-free paper

Table of Contents

Preface

Endocrinology is one of the disciplines concerned with communications and controls within the organism by means of chemical messengers. The whole of intercellular communication is covered in large part by three systems: (1) the nervous system, (2) the endocrine system, and (3) the immune system. Over the past few decades it has become apparent that the separation of these systems is artificial, in that they share many common features. The nervous system elaborates compounds that can act as local mediators or true circulating hormones, while several hormones can act as neurogenic mediators within the central nervous system. Moreover, at the level of the hypothalamus and pituitary there is an intimate link between the nervous system and the endocrine system, thereby integrating the two into one control unit. The immune system is now also recognized as a regulatory system subject to endocrine control. It in turn exerts a reciprocal controlling effect on neuroendocrine systems.

Within this wide spectrum of communication in the living animal there are messenger substances which conform to the classic characteristics of hormones, i.e., products of endocrine glands which are transported by the blood to some distant site of action. Most of the endocrine diseases known to occur in dogs and cats are the result of dysfunction of one or more of these glands and hence this book concentrates on the disorders of these glands.

Most of the chapters deal with separate endocrine glands. For each gland there is an introductory section on the relevant morphology and physiology, followed by descriptions of the disorders of the gland. Because the clinician's suspicion of the presence of an endocrine disease is largely based upon pattern recognition, in which the physical changes play an important role, many illustrations have been included. The features of some endocrine diseases differ in the dog and the cat to such an extent that separate descriptions are needed. Chapters on diagnostic and therapeutic protocols are included at the end of the book to provide a quick reference for both students and practitioners. These will suffice in many cases, but at some time the help of a specialist may be required.

Clinical endocrinology has at least four fascinating characteristics. First, hormones and thus endocrine glands are involved in the regulation of the function of almost every organ system. Therefore the study of this discipline requires the challenging combination of broad pathophysiological interest and specific expertise in the field of endocrinology. Second, endocrinology itself occupies a common ground between biochemistry, physiology, and clinical medicine. Third, in part because of the first two features, clinical endocrinology is a discipline of contemplation, reflection, and stimulating discussion. Fourth, it is very fortunate that many endocrine disorders are amenable to treatment.

The authors hope that this book will serve as a helpful guide to veterinary clinicians in this fascinating field.

Utrecht, May 1995   *Ad Rijnberk*

Acknowledgements

I wish to express my deep appreciation to the many people who have helped in the preparation of this book. First there are the co-authors and contributors. Their expertise was vital in many respects, including their constructive criticism on the chapters written by myself. Their enthusiasm and helpful suggestions were very encouraging.

I am particularly grateful to Dr. Bruce E. Belshaw, with whom I have had the pleasure of working in endocrinology for many years. Some of his approaches to endocrine diseases have been included and he has assisted with the editing of the English text.

I am also very grateful to Mrs. Yvonne W.E.A. Pollak. Her enthusiasm for endocrinology dates back to the 1960s, when she first assisted in the studies on iodine metabolism and thyroid disease in the dog. And today with the same dedication, accuracy and skill she has also made the drawings for this book. During the entire process of producing the book, authors and contributors were also greatly assisted by the very well-organized way in which she took care of all proposals for illustrations and did not lose track of the many amendments.

The high quality photographs made over the years by Mr. Hans F. Haafkens and Mr. Joop Fama have become a very essential part in this illustrated text. Their input is highly appreciated.

On several occasions during the writing of the book Dr. Hans S. Kooistra took care of my endocrine clinics. His help and our stimulating discussions are highly appreciated. My thanks also go to Dr. Joris H. Robben and Dr. Wim J. Vaartjes for critical reading of parts of chapter 5 and those who generously gave permission to use illustrations and whose names are given in the legends to these illustrations.

Thanks are also due to Mrs. Anke Henny for secretarial services and help with literature retrieval. Last but not least I thank Mr. Boudewijn Commandeur and Mrs. Nynke Coutinho of Kluwer Academic Publishers, for carrying out with experienced professionalism the task of formatting, editing and assembling the book.

My deep appreciation to all of you. I hope that you will like the book and I hope that your contributions to it will give you much satisfaction.

List of Contributors

Authors   **Dr. H.A.W. Hazewinkel**
Dr. Med. Vet. R.F. Nickel
Prof. Dr. A. Rijnberk
Dr. A.C. Schaefers-Okkens
Prof. Dr. F.J. van Sluijs
Department of Clinical Sciences of Companion Animals

Contributions   **Dr. M.M. Bevers**, Reproductive Biochemistry
Department of Reproduction and Herd Health
Dr. Ir. J.A. Mol, Endocrine Biochemistry
Department of Clinical Sciences of Companion Animals
Dr. T.S.G.A.M. van den Ingh, Pathology
Department of Pathology
Dr. G. Voorhout, Diagnostic Imaging
Department of Radiology

Illustrations   **Yvonne W.E.A. Pollak**
Department of Clinical Sciences of Companion Animals

Photography   **J.F. Haafkens**
J. Fama
Department of Clinical Sciences of Companion Animals

Faculty of Veterinary Medicine
Utrecht University, Utrecht, The Netherlands

1. Introduction

1.1 Hormones

The traditional and still major part of clinical endocrinology deals with the glands that produce hormones and in particular with the plasma concentrations of hormones to which cells expressing receptors are exposed. Glandular biosynthesis and secretion, the means of transport of hormone to target cells, and metabolic inactivation determine the effective hormone concentration. However, the capacity to form hormones is not limited to endocrine glands. Hormones may be activated by nonendocrine organs through proteolytic cleavage of protein prohormones (for example, in the vascular bed). Others, such as dihydrotestosterone, triiodothyronine, and estradiol, are in part secreted by endocrine glands and in part formed in peripheral tissues from circulating precursors. Some messengers circulate only in restricted compartments such as the hypothalamic-pituitary portal system and do not reach the systemic circulation in appreciable quantities. Many hormones, of which insulin and dihydrotestosterone are examples, have both paracrine actions in the tissues in which they are formed and classic endocrine actions at peripheral sites.

An overview of the systems of hormone synthesis and action is presented in Fig. 1–1. Other forms of intercellular communication such as neurotransmission and neurosecretion, exocrine secretions (e.g., in milk and semen), and the release of pheromones (in air or water) have been included.

Biochemistry. Two broad groups of hormones can be distinguished (Table 1–1)[1]. The hormones of group I are lipophilic and, with the exception of the iodothyronines, are cholesterol derivatives of two types: those with an intact steroid nucleus

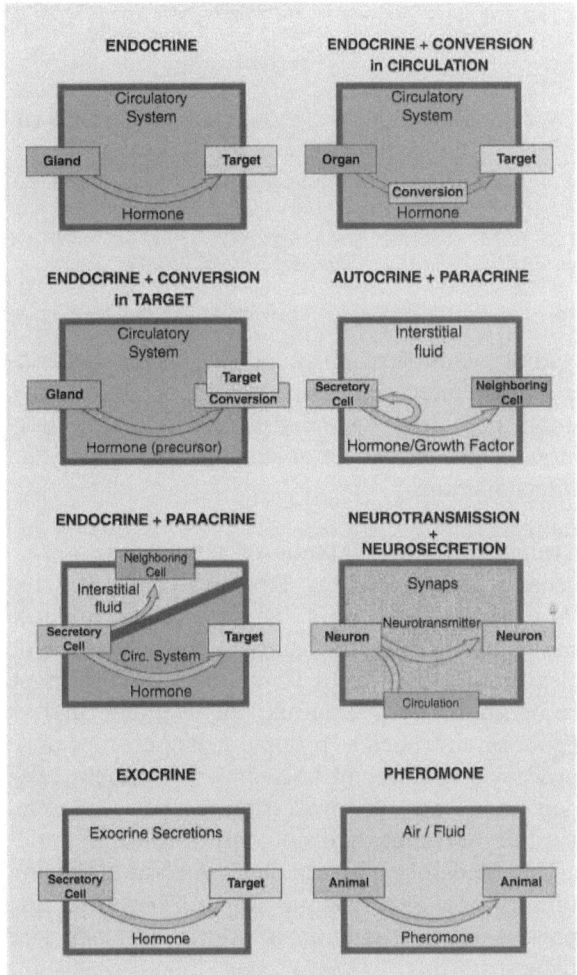

Fig. 1-1. Schematic representation of systems of intercellular communication. (Modified from LeRoith et al., 1988.[2])

(adrenal and gonadal steroids) and those in which the B ring is open (vitamin D and its various metabolites (Fig. 1–2).

The second major group consists of water-soluble hormones. The majority are peptides, in-

1

A. Rijnberk (ed.), *Clinical Endocrinology of Dogs and Cats*, 1–9.
© 1996 *Kluwer Academic Publishers.*

Table 1-1 Hormone groups.

	Group 1 Steroids Iodothyronines Calcitriol	Group 2 Polypeptides (Glyco)proteins Catecholamines
Solubility	Lipophylic	Hydrophylic
Transport proteins	Yes	Mostly not
Plasma half-life	Long (hours)	Short (minutes)
Receptor	Intracellular	Plasma membrane
Mediator	Receptor-hormone complex	cAMP and other second messengers

cluding complex polypeptides (e.g., gonadotrophins), intermediate-size peptides (e.g., insulin), small peptides (e.g., thyrotropin-releasing hormone), and derivatives of single amino acids (e.g., catecholamines).

Synthesis. In the synthesis of peptide hormones, genes code for messenger RNA which is translated into protein precursors. These proteins undergo posttranslational processing, such as proteolytic cleavage (Fig. 1–3), to form the active hormone recognized by receptors of target tissues. Prohormones such as proopiomelanocortin can be processed to different hormones in different cells, depending on the processing enzymes present. Peptide hormones are not only formed in endocrine glands but may also be formed in malignant tumors not of endocrine origin. They are also present in small amounts in normal nonendocrine tissues.

For the transformation of the precursor of steroid hormones, cholesterol, to estradiol, at least six enzymes and consequently at least six genes are needed. Probably because of the number of enzymes required, the synthesis of steroids is unusual in malignancies of nonendocrine tissues.

Storage and release. Most endocrine cells have a limited capacity to store the final product. Even in tissues with well-developed organelles for storing

hormone, such as the Golgi apparatus, the amount of hormone stored is usually limited. The major exceptions are the storage of the precursor as prohormone thyroglobulin in the thyroid follicles and the storage of intermediate forms of vitamin D in fat.

The release process may involve freeing soluble derivatives from precursor by proteolysis (thyroid hormones from thyroglobulin), exocytosis of storage granules (peptide hormones), or passive diffusion of newly synthesized molecules (steroid hormones). In many instances the rate of hormone release fluctuates, synthesis and release being tightly linked. Some pituitary hormones, such as growth hormone and luteinizing hormone, are released in a pulsatile fashion, in repetitive bursts. The release of others varies during a 24-hour cycle, mostly with superimposed small fluctuations.

Transport. Water-soluble hormones (Table 1–1) are in general transported in plasma without binding to specific proteins. This explains the half-lives of only a few minutes in plasma of most of the nonglycosylated peptide hormones. The more insoluble a hormone in water, the more important the role of transport proteins. Thyroid and steroid hormones are largely transported in protein-bound form. Protein-bound hormone cannot enter cells and serves as a reservoir from which free hormone is liberated for uptake into intracellular

TRH

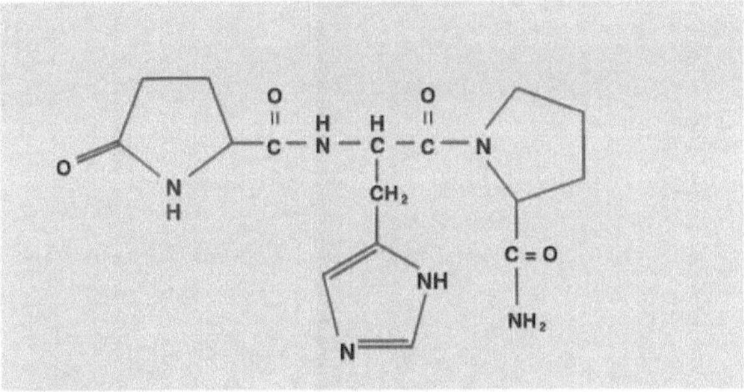

CORTISOL

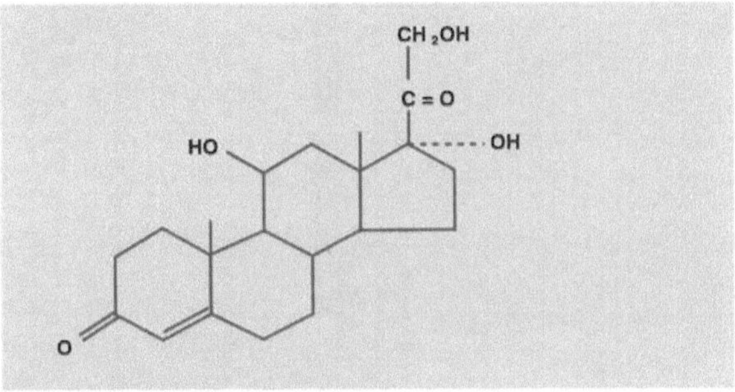

CHOLECALCIFEROL

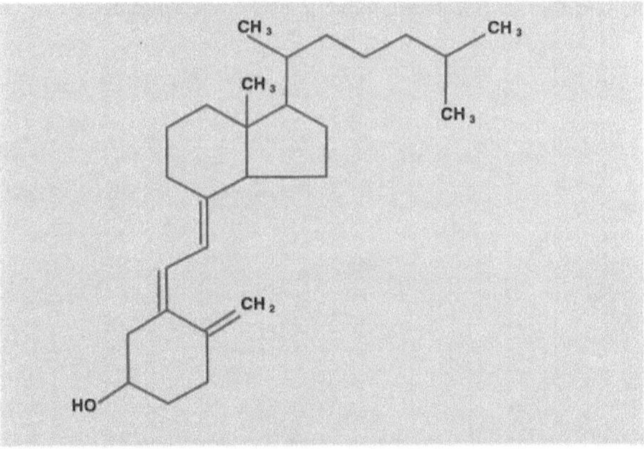

Fig. 1-2. Examples of different types of hormones. The tripeptide thyrotrophin-releasing hormone (TRH), the adrenocortical steroid cortisol, and cholecalciferol (vitamin D3).

compartments.

The distribution of bound and free hormone in plasma is determined by the amount of hormone and the amount and affinity of the binding proteins for the hormone. Only the free hormone interacts with receptors in target cells and participates in the regulatory feedback mechanisms. Hence changes in the amount of transport protein

can cause considerable changes in hormone levels in plasma without causing clinical signs of hormone deficiency or excess. If the regulatory feedback mechanisms that control hormone synthesis are intact, they will keep the level of free hormone within the normal range.

Degradation and turnover. Degradation and inactivation of hormone can occur in target tissues and also in nontarget tissues such as liver and kidney. Peptide hormones are mostly inactivated in target tissues by proteases. Steroid and thyroid hormones are metabolized and mostly conjugated for solubilization and subsequent excretion via the urine and bile.

A change in the rate of hormone degradation will not influence the steady state, provided that the feedback control of synthesis is intact. However, if the control mechanism is defective, changes in rates of hormone degradation may have clinical consequences. For example, in hyperthyroidism the degradation of glucocorticoids is enhanced and glucocorticoid insufficiency could occur if there is an inadequate adrenocortical reserve capacity.

Action. The two classes of hormones (Table 1–1) act through two different types of receptors. Peptide hormones operate via receptors located in the cell membrane with the recognition/binding site exposed on the cell surface. Activated cell surface receptors use a variety of strategies to transduce signal information, thereby activating second messengers (Fig. 1–4), which amplify and pass on the molecular information. Many peptide hormones ultimately signal via regulation of protein phosphorylation. In this most common process, through which proteins are covalently modified, a phosphate group is donated to the protein by nucleotide triphosphates. This allows peptide hormones to rapidly change the conformation and thus the function of existing cell enzymes [enzyme (in)activation]. It also allows somewhat slower changes involving transcription of genes encoding for enzyme proteins and thus influencing the concentration of cell enzymes [enzyme induction].

Steroid hormones and thyroid hormones act via structurally related intracellular receptors. These hormones are transported in plasma mainly bound

4

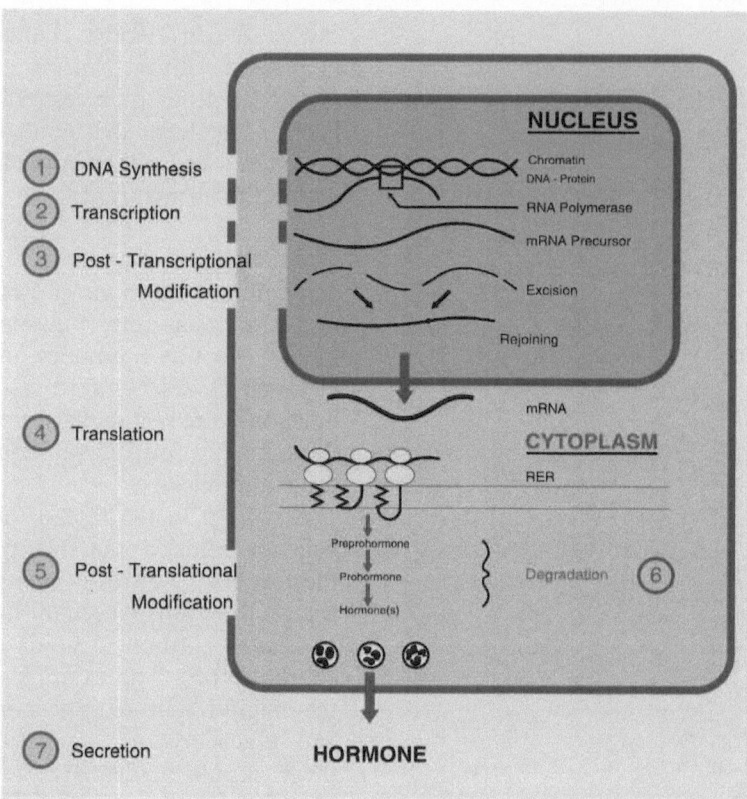

Fig. 1-3. Schematic pathway in a peptide hormone-secreting cell. The control points are indicated by circled numbers.

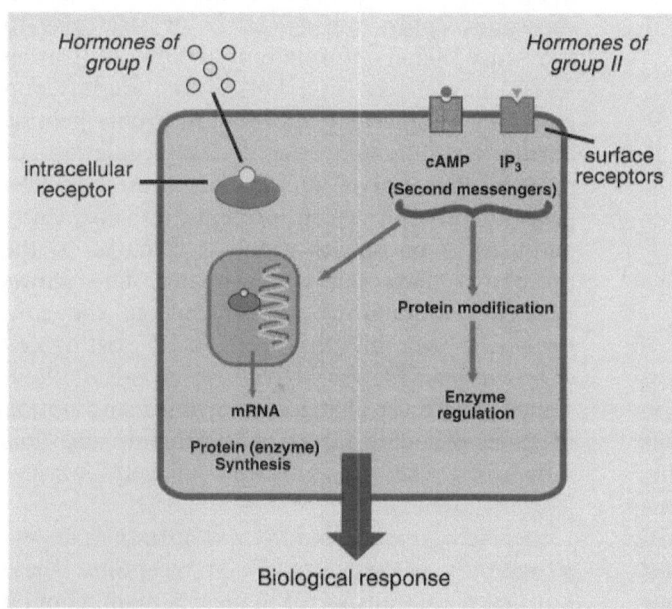

Fig. 1-4. Schematic model of hormonal action. The hormones of group I bind to cytoplasmic or nuclear receptors. The hormone-receptor complex then binds to specific regions of the DNA, resulting in activation or repression of a restricted number of genes. Hormones of group II bind to specific receptors in the cell membrane. This ligand-receptor interaction causes the generation of a second messenger. Many of the actions of the second messengers (e.g., on gluconeogenesis and lipolysis) occur outside the nucleus, but they also influence gene transcription.

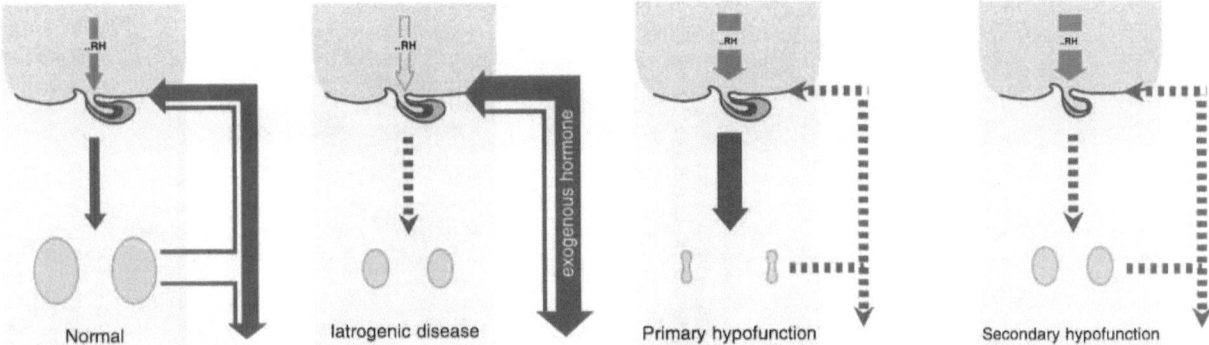

Fig. 1-5. Left: Generalized hypothalamus-pituitary system and a related endocrine gland under normal conditions and as influenced by administration of a hormone produced by the peripheral gland. The hormone secreted by the peripheral gland is distributed in the circulation between a small free fraction (open parts of arrows) and a large fraction bound to carrier proteins (dark parts of arrows). The differences in hormone production are indicated by differences in the thickness and continuity of lines and arrows. Right: Illustration of primary and secondary (pituitary) hormone deficiency states.

to carrier proteins. The small amounts of free hormones are transported into the cells and bind to specific receptor proteins to form a hormone-receptor complex. This complex can bind to specific regulatory sequences in DNA (positive and negative response elements) and thus acts as a regulator of transcription. As a result, the formation of messenger RNA is increased or decreased and thus the synthesis and secretion of proteins (enzymes, hormones) is enhanced or suppessed.

The chemical structure of several of these receptors has been elucidated. In man this has allowed the analysis of mutations that impair hormone action and cause hormone-resistance syndromes.

1.2 Endocrine disorders

Endocrine disorders occurring in the dog and the cat can be divided into the following six broad categories, most of which can be further sub-divided:

Deficient hormone production. Endocrine glands may be injured or destroyed by autoimmune disorders or by neoplasia and theoretically also by infection or hemorrhage, and the resulting hypofunction is said to be primary. Hypofunction can also be due to inadequate stimulation of the gland and is then said to be secondary. These principles as well as the ones to follow are

illustrated by drawings depicting a generalized hypothalamus-pituitary system in relation to a peripheral endocrine gland (Fig. 1–5).

Excessive hormone production. The most frequent causes of hormone excess syndromes are hypersecretion of hormone by a tumor of the endocrine gland (primary hyperfunction) or hypersecretion due to hyperstimulation, of which there may be several causes (secondary hyper-function) (Fig. 1–6). Excessive hormone production may also be traced to cells that are not normally the primary source of the hormone (ectopic hormone production). When hormones are used to treat nonendocrine diseases or when hormone replacement for an endocrine deficiency is excessive, the resulting syndrome of hormone excess is said to be iatrogenic (Fig. 1–5).

Defective hormone synthesis. Genetic defects can cause abnormalities in hormone synthesis. Sometimes this does not lead to hormone deficiency but to manifestations of a compensatory adaptation, such as goiter developing because of defective thyroid hormone synthesis (Fig. 1–7).

Resistance to hormone action. Hormone resistance is defined as a defect in the capacity of normal target tissues to respond to the hormone. Usually it is an inherited disorder involving one or more molecular abnormalities, including defects in receptors and in post-receptor mechanisms. Hormone resistance may also be caused by the

6

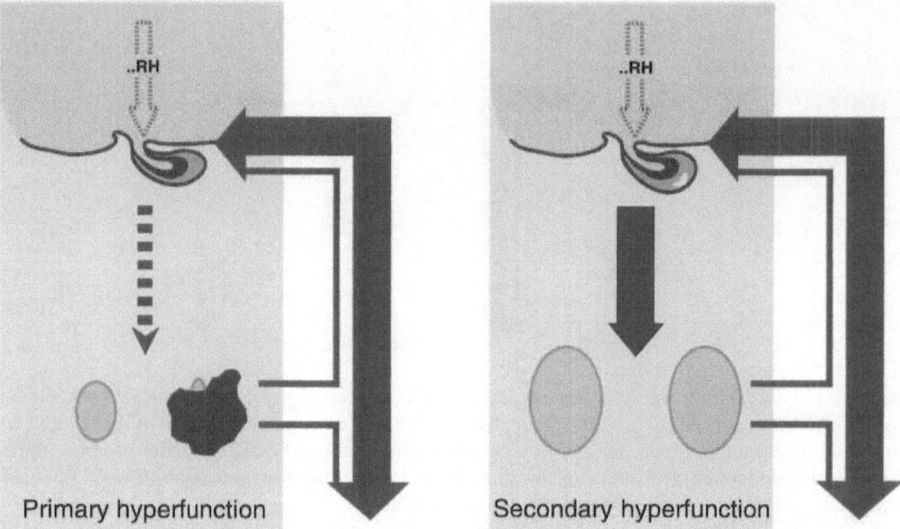

Fig. 1-6. Schematic illustration of two different forms of hormone excess: (1) tumor in peripheral gland (left), and (2) hormonally active lesion in the hypophysis (right). For explanation see also legend to Fig. 1–5.

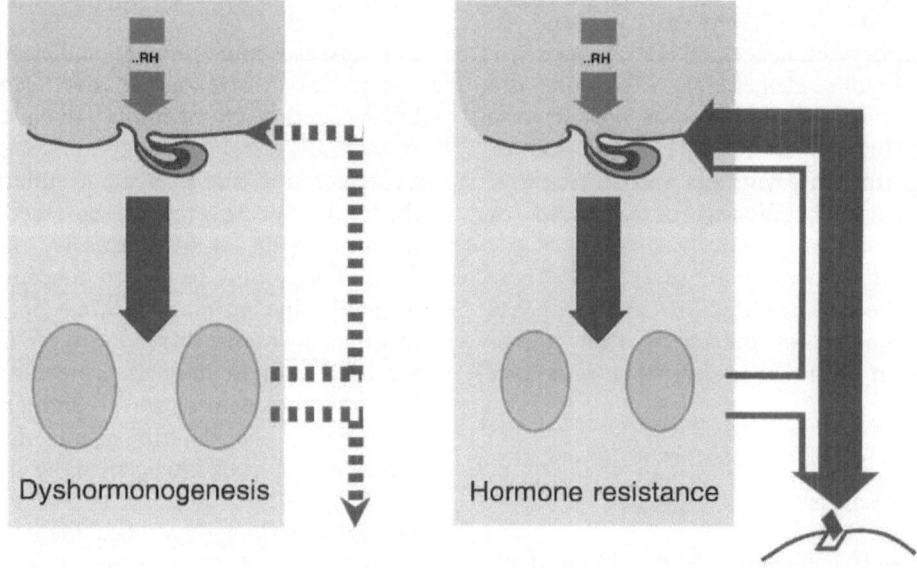

Fig. 1-7. Illustration of altered feedback control in situations of (1) defective hormone synthesis in the peripheral gland (left), and (2) resistance to hormone action due to a receptor defect (right). For explanation see also legend to Fig. 1–5.

development of antibodies to the hormone or to the hormone receptor. A common feature of hormone resistance is the presence of an elevated level of the hormone in the circulation of an individual with normal or deficient hormone action. The increased hormone levels are caused by the same defect, which is also present in (post)receptor functions involved in regulatory feedback control (Fig. 1–7).

Abnormalities in hormone transport. Feedback control of hormone production is mediated by the level of free hormone. Thus changes in the concentrations of transport or carrier proteins in the plasma usually only cause corresponding changes in the concentration of hormone in plasma but not in hormone production.

Finally, endocrine glands may be affected by *abnormalities not impairing function.* These include tumors, cysts, and infiltrative diseases not leading to significant impairment of hormone secretion.

1.3 Clinical assessment

History and physical examination. The diagnostic process is hampered by the inaccessibility for physical examination of all of the endocrine glands except the thyroid glands and the testes. However, deranged hormone secretion has consequences for the function of other organ systems, usually leading to multiple abnormalities which often have a characteristic pattern. The diagnosis of an endocrine disease thus often begins with the recognition of a pattern of characteristics in the medical history and in the findings by physical examination.[3]

Many syndromes of hormonal excess or deficiency lead to manifestations that are readily apparent at the time of the initial presentation of the patient for examination. Especially now that the definitive diagnosis can often be secured by laboratory data, veterinary clinicians have learned to recognize the patterns of physical characteristics of endocrine syndromes. Nevertheless, in some cases the changes are very subtle and it is necessary to rely completely on laboratory testing. This is especially true when endocrine disease is being considered in the differential diagnosis of common problems such as weakness, lethargy, and weight loss or gain.

Laboratory testing. The development of techniques for the measurement of hormones in biological fluids has made it possible to assess endocrine function in quantitative terms by the following approaches:

- *Plasma levels.* The total concentration of steroid and thyroid hormones in plasma ranges between 1 nM and 1 µM, while that of peptide hormones is generally between 1 pM and 0.1 nM. The application of radioimmunoassay, radioreceptorassay, chromatographic, and more recently molecular biological techniques has transformed endocrinology from a largely descriptive discipline to a more quantitative one. Yet there are only a few situations in which a single measurement of the concentration of a hormone in plasma may provide a

reliable assessment of hormone production. There are several reasons for caution in assessing isolated measurements of hormone concentration in plasma:

a) Several hormones are secreted in a pulsatile manner (Fig. 1–8) and/or their con-

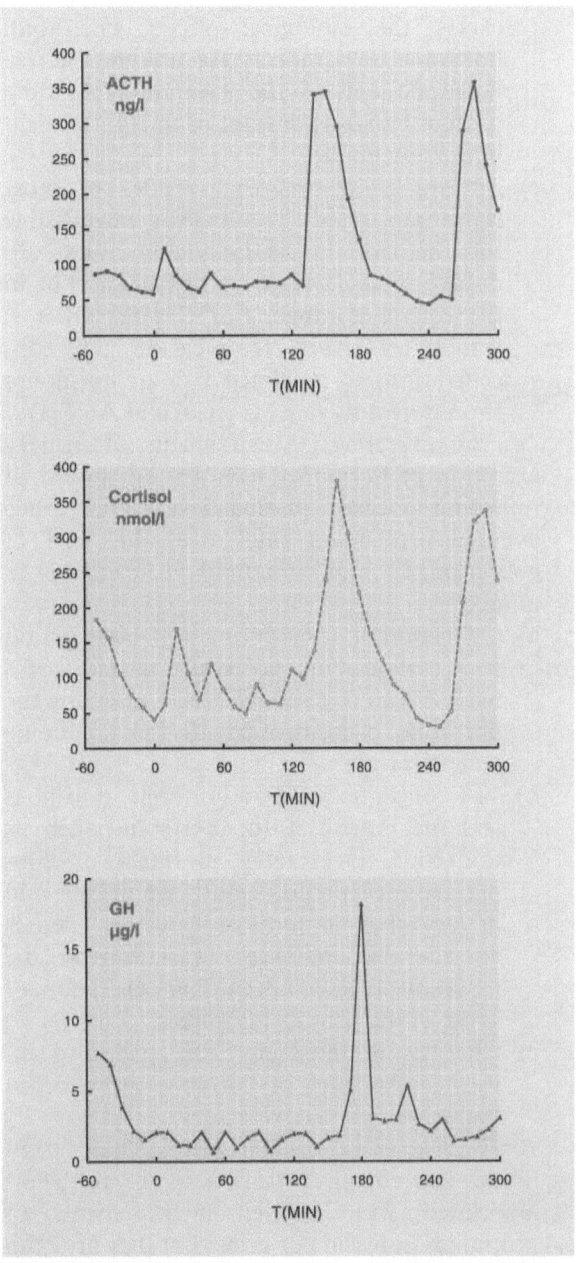

Fig. 1-8. Results of measurements of cortisol, ACTH and growth hormone (GH) in frequently collected blood samples of a healthy adult dog. At time 0′ a meal was given. The figure clearly illustrates the pulsatile character of hormone secretion.

centrations may vary in a diurnal rhythmicity, as well as with the sexual cycle, pregnancy, and season.

b) Steroid and thyroid hormones are transported in plasma largely bound to proteins. The small percentage (< 1–10 per cent of the total) of unbound hormone exerts the biological effect. The total hormone level reflects the amount of free hormone only if the amount of binding protein remains constant or fluctuates within narrow limits.

c) The range of reference values of most hormones is fairly broad. Thus it is possible for the level in an individual animal to double or to decrease by half but still be in the reference range. For this reason it is sometimes useful to measure the concentrations of a related pair of hormones simultaneously (e.g., cortisol and ACTH).

– *Urinary excretion.* Measurements of urinary excretion of hormones have the advantage of reflecting average plasma levels and hence average production rates over the time of collection. Certain limitations must be kept in mind:

a) Collection of urine during a 24-hour period is a cumbersome procedure in most animals. It can be circumvented by relating the hormone concentration to the creatinine concentration.

b) The concentration of a hormone in urine is less meaningful if the hormone, such as thyroxine, is excreted in intact or conjugated form predominantly via the bile and in very small amounts in the urine. There is considerable individual variation in the metabolism, and hence urinary excretion, of some of the peptide hormones.

c) Changes in renal function may also influence the rates of hormone excretion in the urine.

– *Production and secretion rates.* These techniques can circumvent many of the problems associated with isolated measurements of hormones in plasma or urine, but they are both difficult to perform and require administration of radionuclides and are therefore not generally available.

– *Dynamic endocrine tests.* Dynamic testing provides additional information. It involves either the stimulation or the suppression of endogenous hormone production. Stimulation tests are utilized most often when hypofunction of an endocrine organ is suspected. In the most commonly employed stimulation tests a trophic hormone is administered to test the capacity of a target gland to increase hormone production. The trophic hormone can be a hypothalamic releasing hormone such as corticotropin releasing hormone (CRH), in which case the target gland is the pituitary and the measured response is the increment in the plasma level of ACTH, or a pituitary hormone such as ACTH, with the adrenal cortex as the target gland being assessed by the measurement of the increment in the plasma level of cortisol. Suppression tests are utilized when endocrine hyperfunction is suspected. They are designed to determine whether negative feedback control is intact. A hormone or other regulatory substance is administered and the inhibition of endogenous hormone secretion is assessed. Dynamic tests continue to be of importance in the diagnosis of certain disorders but in circumstances in which hormone pairs can be measured accurately they are required only occasionally.

– *Hormone receptors and antibodies.* The measurement of hormone receptors in biopsy material from target tissues may become increasingly useful in companion animal endocrinology, especially in the diagnosis of hormone resistance. Also, measurements of antibodies to hormones may be essential to the characterization of certain endocrine abnormalities as autoimmune phenomena. In addition in some cases these antibodies may interfere with diagnostic procedures such as radioimmunoassays.

Diagnostic imaging. The inaccessibility of most of the endocrine glands for direct physical examination has been overcome during the past decade with the introduction of diagnostic imaging techniques such as ultrasonography and computed tomography. The former technique is relatively inexpensive but requires extensive operator experience, whereas the latter is easier to perform but requires expensive equipment.

1.4 Treatment

Endocrine deficiencies are usually treated by administering the hormone that is deficient. In some cases this is not possible or expedient and another compound must be given as, for example, vitamin D or one of its analogues instead of PTH in the treatment of hypoparathyroidism.

Tumors causing hormone excess are removed when possible and hyperplastic glands may be removed or may be destroyed by chemotherapy. In recent years neurotransmitter-modulating drugs and long-acting analogues of natural hypophysiotropic peptides have been used effectively for the medical management of pituitary hyperfunction in man. Unfortunately, these drugs have not thus far proven to be very effective in the treatment of pituitary diseases in the dog and the cat.

2. Hypothalamus-pituitary system

2.1 Introduction

The hypothalamus and pituitary form a complex functional unit that transcends the traditional boundary between neurology and endocrinology. Many key elements of this system are neither purely endocrine nor purely neural. It consists of three major systems:

1. A neuroendocrine system connected to an endocrine system by a portal circulation. The neuroendocrine system consists of clusters of peptide- and monoamine-secreting cells in the anterior and middle portions of the ventral hypothalamus. Their products are transported along nerve fibers to terminals in the outer layer of the median eminence (Fig. 2-1). Here they are released into the capillaries of the hypothalamic-hypophyseal portal system and transported to regulate the secretion of the hormones of the anterior lobe (AL) of the pituitary (Fig. 2-2; Table 2-1).

2. A neurosecretory pathway that starts in the anterior hypothalamus, traverses the ventral hypothalamus, and terminates in the neurohypophysis or posterior lobe (PL) on fenestrated blood vessels (Fig. 2-2).

3. A pars intermedia (PI) directly innervated by predominantly aminergic nerve fibers from the hypothalamus. This direct neural control is largely a tonic inhibitory influence.

During embryogenesis the adenohypophysis develops from Rathke's pouch, which arises from

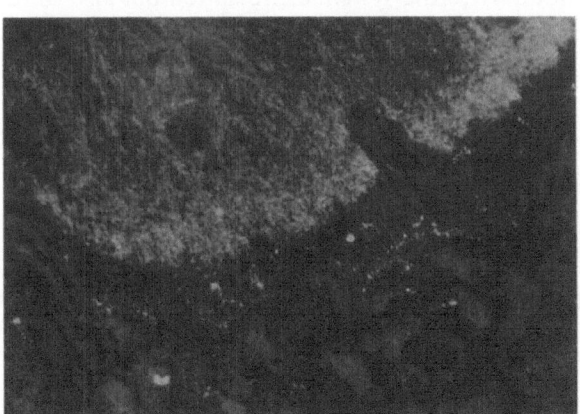

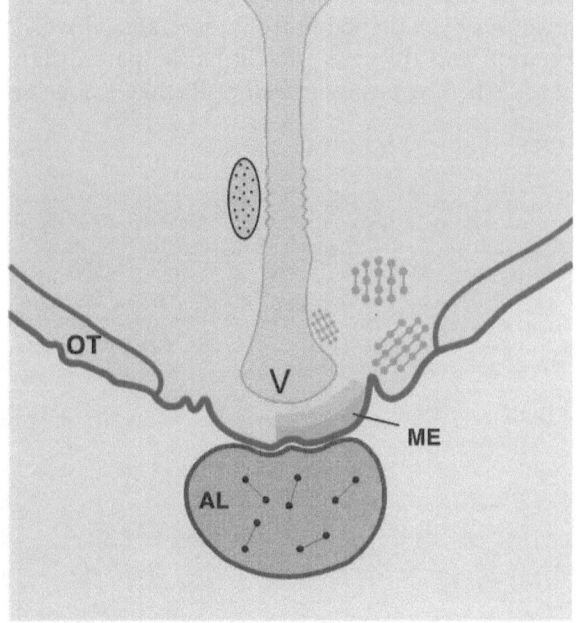

Fig. 2-1. Left: Nerve fiber terminals containing corticotropin-releasing hormone (CRH) in the outer layer of the median eminence of a dog, visualized by indirect immunofluorescence. Note the presence of CRH-immunoreactive fibers outside the terminal zone in close proximity to the capillary system. Right: Schematic representation of the distribution of cell bodies and nerve fibers detected by immunostaining for CRH in a transverse section through the canine hypothalamus in the caudal part of the median eminence (ME). Cell bodies are indicated as black dots at the left and fibers are at the right. OT = optic tract; V= third ventricle; AL = pituitary anterior lobe.[33]

11

A. Rijnberk (ed.), Clinical Endocrinology of Dogs and Cats, 11–34.
© *1996 Kluwer Academic Publishers.*

Table 2-1. Terminology for the parts of the hypophysis (glandula pituitaria) according to the Nomina Anatomica Veterinaria (N.A.V.) and the variants in Nomina Histologica Veterinaria (N.H.V.) and Nomina Anatomica (=for man).[35]

N.A.V.	N.H.V.	N.A.
Adenohypophysis (Lobus anterior)		
Pars infundibularis adenohypophysis	Pars proximalis adenohypophysis	Pars tuberalis
Pars intermedia adenohypophysis		Pars intermedia
Pars distalis adenohypophysis		Pars distalis
Neurohypophysis (Lobus posterior)		
Pars proximalis neurohypophysis (Infundibulum)		Infundibulum
Pars distalis neurohypophysis		Lobus nervosus

For practical reasons in this book the terminology is confined to the denotation of three functional units: Anterior lobe (= Pars infundibularis and Pars distalis of the adenohypophysis), Pars intermedia and Posterior lobe (see also Fig. 2-2).

the roof of the primitive mouth in contact with the base of the brain. Rathke's pouch subsequently separates by constriction from the oral cavity. The anterior wall thickens and forms the pars distalis of the AL. The posterior wall of Rathke's pouch is closely apposed to the neural tissue of the PL to form the pars intermedia, remaining separated from the AL by the hypophyseal cleft or cavity, which was the lumen of Rathke's pouch. In the dog and the cat the adenohypophysis also extends as a cuff or collar around the proximal neurohypophysis and even envelops part of the median eminence (Fig. 2–3).

The uniquely organized capillary plexus of the median eminence is in close proximity to nerve terminals of the hypophysiotropic neurons. The blood-brain barrier is incomplete in the area of the median eminence, which permits protein and peptide hormones as well as other charged particles to move to the intercapillary spaces and the nerve terminals contained therein. These terminals respond to humoral and neuronal stimuli by secreting releasing and inhibiting factors into the portal system. The portal capillaries coalesce into a series of vessels that descend through the pituitary stalk and form a second capillary plexus that surrounds the AL cells (Fig. 2–2).

Inferior hypophyseal arteries supply the PL. From the primary plexus of the PL blood flows not only to the systemic circulation but also to the AL and the hypothalamus. There is also some degree of circulatory flow within the pituitary, i.e., from the AL to the PL, from there to the infundibulum, and then back to the AL. The

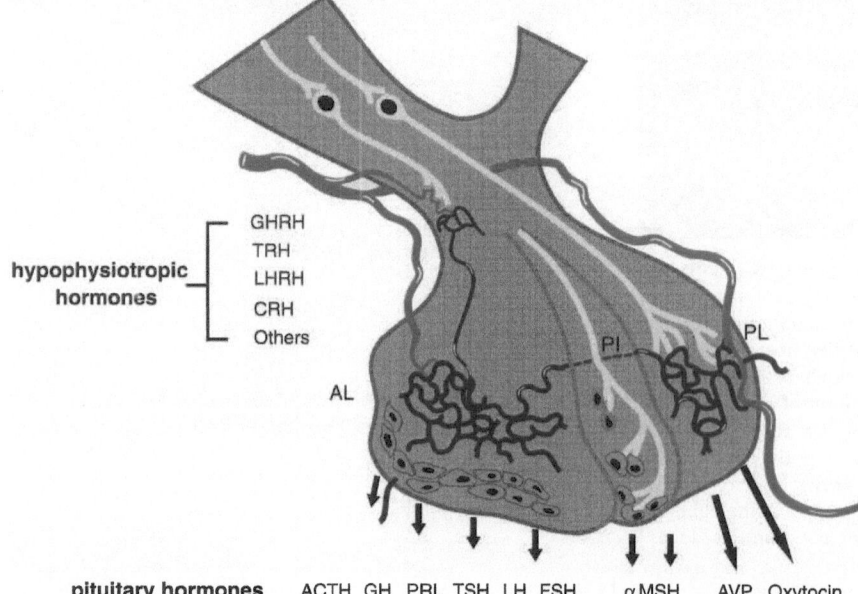

hypophysiotropic hormones
- GHRH
- TRH
- LHRH
- CRH
- Others

AL   PI   PL

pituitary hormones   ACTH GH PRL TSH LH FSH   αMSH   AVP Oxytocin

Fig. 2-2. Schematic representation of the relationship between the hypothalamus and the pituitary. The hypothalamus exerts control over the anterior lobe (AL) through releasing and inhibiting factors that reach the AL cells via capillaries of the pituitary portal system. The posterior lobe (PL) of the pituitary is a downward projection of the hypothalamus. The pars intermedia (PI) is under direct neurotransmitter control.

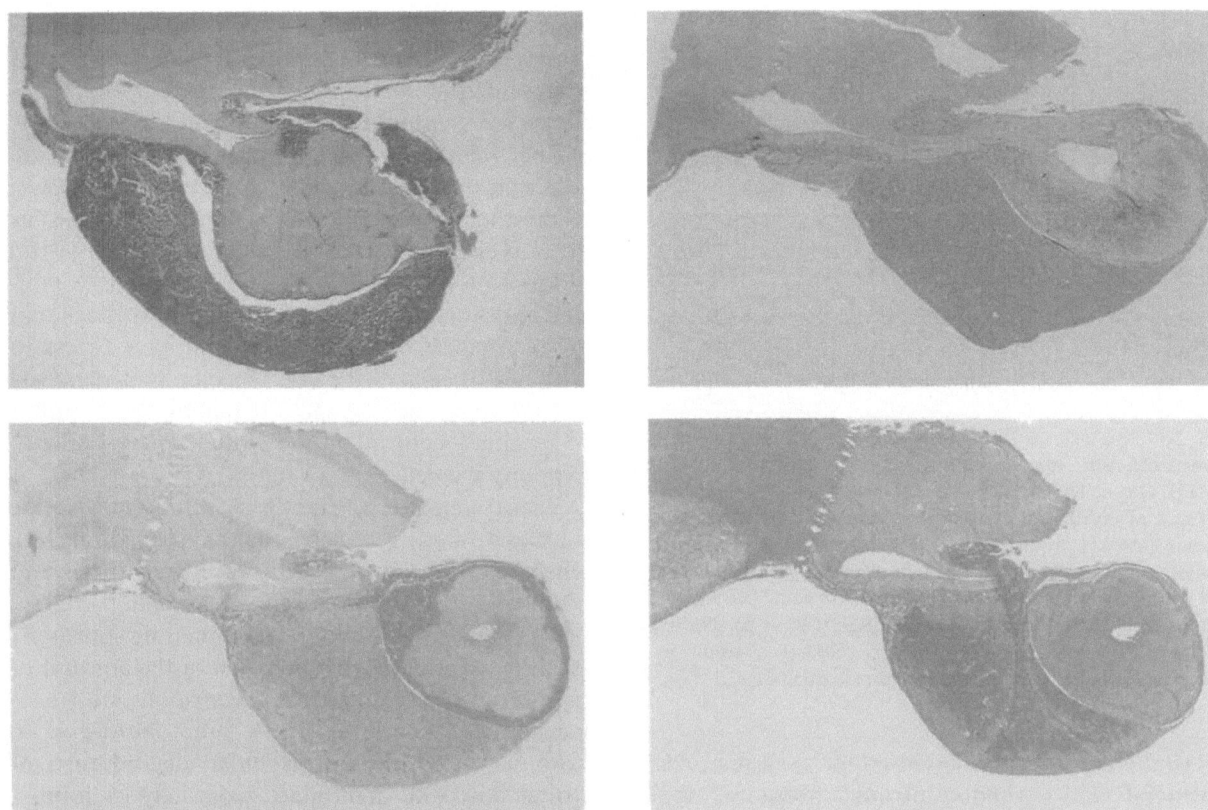

Fig. 2-3. Upper left: Sagittal section of a dog pituitary. The AL is separated from the PI and PL by the hypophyseal cavity and surrounds it up to the pituitary stalk and median eminence. The PI is a narrow zone around the periphery of the PL. H & E stain. (Courtesy of Dr. B.E. Belshaw.) Upper right: PAS-Alcian Blue-orange G stain of a sagittal section of a cat pituitary. The third ventricle runs deep into the PL (blue), which is surrounded by a thin rim of PI. Bottom: Sections of a cat pituitary stained with an antibody against α-MSH (left) and ACTH (right). The latter picture clearly illustrates that in the cat also the AL extends upwards around the pituitary stalk. (Courtesy Prof. Dr. H.J.Th. Goos and Mrs. A. Slob)

vascularization of the PI is closely linked to that of the PL. However, in spite of the rich blood supply of the PL, the PI is a poorly vascularized structure. Blood-borne factors play a relatively less significant role in control of PI function.

2.2 Anterior lobe

The peptide hormones secreted by the AL can be divided into three categories[1]: (1) the somato-mammotropic hormones growth hormone (GH) and prolactin (PRL), (2) the glycoprotein hormones thyrotropin (TSH), follicle-stimulating hormone (FSH), and luteinizing hormone (LH), and (3) the corticomelanotropins, which include α-melanotropin (α-MSH), adrenocorticotropin (ACTH), β-endorphin (β-END), and β-lipotropin

(β-LPH). The latter group of hormones is derived from the precursor proopiomelanocortin, which is synthesized not only in the corticotropic cells of the AL but also in cells of the pars intermedia (Fig. 2–4). They will be discussed in more detail in Chapter 4.

The cells of the AL are classified according to their specific secretory products: somatotrophs (secreting GH), lactotrophs (secreting PRL), thyrotrophs (secreting TSH), corticotrophs (secreting corticotropin and related peptides), and gonadotrophs (secreting LH and FSH). The somatotrophs account for 50% or more of the AL cells. The other types of AL cells each represent about 5–15% of the gland.

For the regulation of the basal plasma concentration each of the six major AL hormone systems (ACTH, LH and FSH, TSH, GH, and

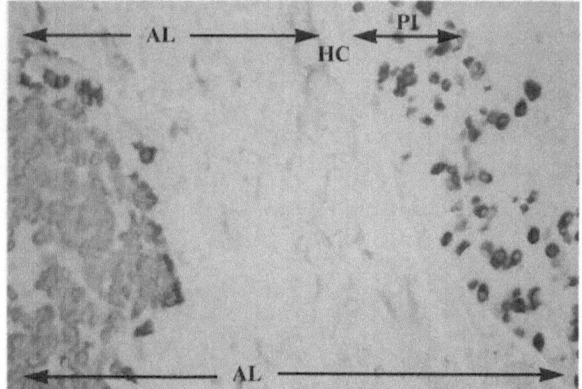

Fig. 2-4. Pituitary of a dog with pituitary-dependent hyperadrenocorticism, immunostained with an antibody against ACTH. On the left there is immunopositivity in a hyperplastic cell nest of corticotropic cells in the anterior lobe (AL). The excessive ACTH production by this microadenoma has caused loss of immunoreactivity in the nonneoplastic part of the AL, due to negative feedback. In the pars intermedia (PI), on the other side of the hypophyseal cavity (HC), there is persistence of immunoreactivity in corticotropic cells as a result of insensitivity to negative feedback by glucocorticoids.

PRL) there is a feedback (closed loop) system. AL hormone and hypophysiotropic hormone secretions are suppressed by the products of target endocrine glands such as the thyroids, adrenals, and gonads (see also Chapter 1). Apart from this long-loop feedback, some hormones such as PRL regulate their own secretion directly by acting on the hypothalamus (short-loop feedback). Upon this powerful feedback control with primary blood-borne signals, other signals are superimposed. These may originate within the central nervous system (open loop) and can be mediated

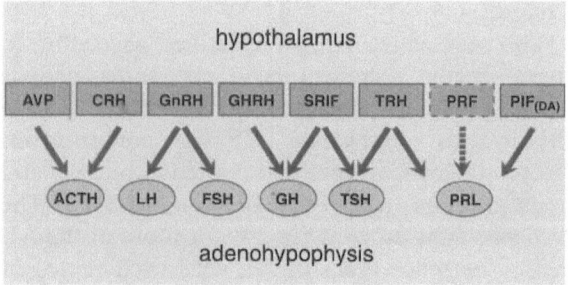

Fig. 2-5. Hypophysiotropic regulation of the secretion of hormones in the adenohypophysis. Solid lines denote hormones whose structures have been determined. Dashed lines indicate a factor whose identity is still uncertain.

by neurotransmitters and hypophysiotropic hormones (Fig. 2–5). Thus influences are exerted that represent the environment (temperature, light-dark), stress (pain, fear), and intrinsic rhythmicity.

The releasing and inhibiting hormones are stored in nerve terminals in the median eminence, where their concentrations are 10 to 100 times as great as elsewhere in the hypothalamus. The portal blood flow to the pituitary is not compartmentalized and thus the hypophysiotropic hormones that are secreted into the portal system have access to all types of cells in the AL. Specificity is achieved not by anatomic segregation but by the presence of specific receptors on individual types of adenohypophyseal cells.

These regulatory factors influence peptide synthesis and/or release in adenohypophyseal cells, where each of the steps in hormone synthesis and ultimate secretion represent a potential control point in the regulation of circulating hormone levels (see Fig. 1–3). Modulation of the amount of mRNA, the efficiency of transcription and translation, the processing from preprohormone to hormone, and the intracellular degradation of stored hormone determine, separately or jointly, the amount of hormone available for release.

The hypophysiotropic hormones whose structures have been elucidated are, with one exception, peptides with sequence lengths ranging from 3 to 44 amino acids (Fig. 2–6). With increasing length, species variation in amino acid sequences may occur. The structures of TRH, GnRH, and SRIF (3, 10 and 14 amino acids, respectively) are identical in all mammals studied and although some species specificity might be expected in the structures of GHRH and CRH (44 and 41 amino acids), the structure of CRH has been found to be identical in man, the dog, and the rat.

The only nonpeptide hypophysiotropic hormone is dopamine. In addition to its major role as a neurotransmitter, it is the most important inhibitor of prolactin secretion. The existence of a separate prolactin-releasing factor (PRF) has been a matter of debate for a long time. Recently it was found that the posterior pituitary contains such a PRF, which suggests a relation with the suckling reflex.[2]

Somatotropin and lactotropin. Somatotropin or growth hormone (GH) and lactotropin or

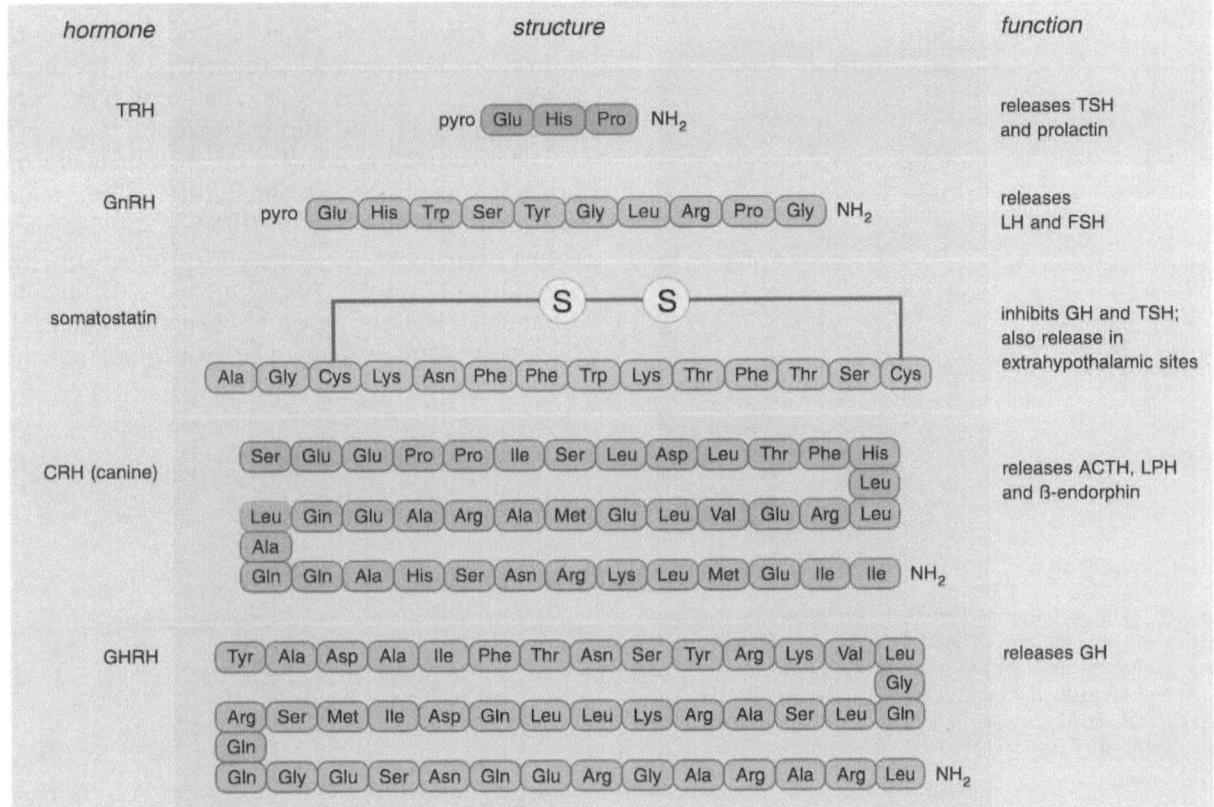

hormone	structure	function

Fig. 2-6. Structure and function of hypothalamic hypophysiotropic hormones. The structure of canine CRH was recently found to be identical to the structure of human, rat and equine CRH.[36]

prolactin (PRL) have similarities in amino acid composition and share some biological activities and thus they are classified together as somato-lactotropic hormones. They are rather large single-chain polypeptides containing about 200 amino acids and having two (GH) or three (PRL) intrachain disulfide bridges. Their molecular weights are approximately 22 and 23 kDa respectively. For both hormones there is a good deal of variability in the amino acid sequences in different species. The amino acid sequence of canine GH has recently been elucidated.[2a,2b] The amino acid sequences of canine PRL and feline GH and PRL are not yet known.

GH release is characterized by rhythmic pulses and intervening troughs (Fig. 1–8). The GH pulses predominantly reflect the pulsatile delivery of GHRH from the hypothalamus, whereas GH levels between pulses are primarily under soma-tostatin (= somatotropin-release inhibiting factor = SRIF) control. The effects of GH can be divided into two main categories: rapid or metabolic actions and slow or hypertrophic actions. The acute catabolic responses are due to direct inter-action of GH with the target cell and result in enhanced lipolysis and restricted glucose transport across the cell membrane due to insulin resistance. The slow anabolic effects are mediated via a growth factor that is synthesized in the liver and is known as insulin-like growth factor (IGF-I). In its chemical structure IGF-I (as well as IGF-II) has approximately 50% sequence similarity with insulin, suggesting it has evolved from a common ancestral molecule. Contrary to insulin, the IGFs are bound to carrier proteins in plasma. As a result they have a prolonged half-life, which is consistent with their long-term growth-promoting action. Insulin and IGF seem to complement each other, insulin being the acute and IGF the long-term regulator of anabolic processes.

Circulating IGF-I is an important determinant in the regulation of body size. In dog breeds of

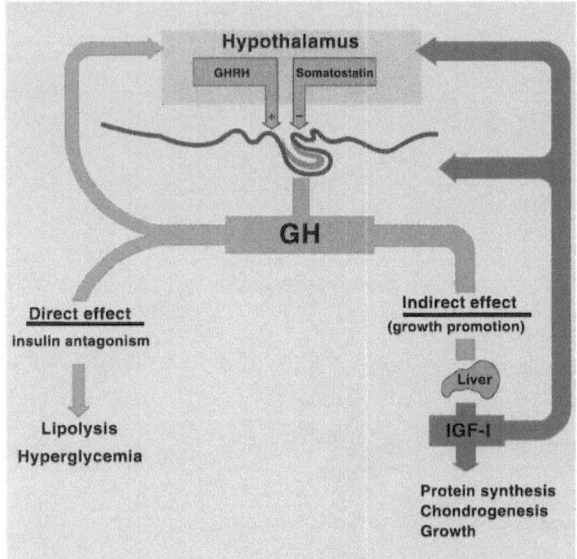

Fig. 2-7. The secretion of GH is under inhibitory (somatostatin) and stimulatory (GHRH) hypothalamic control and is also modulated by a long-loop feedback control by IGF-I, a peptide formed in the liver under the influence of GH. The direct catabolic (diabetogenic) actions of GH are shown on the left side of the figure and the indirect anabolic actions on the right.

widely-differing body sizes, similar GH concentrations are usually found in plasma, but the total IGF-I levels are .quite different and positively correlated with body size.[3] In addition IGFs exert an inhibitory effect on GH release, most probably by stimulating the release of somatostatin and by a direct inhibitory influence at pituitary level (Fig. 2–7).

As a closing remark on the actions of GH it should be mentioned that the separation of the two opposing biological actions is not as strict as suggested above. There is increasing evidence that GH exerts its growth-promoting effect not only via IGF-I produced in the liver but also by a direct effect on cells in the growth plate. Here it stimulates cell differentiation directly and clonal expansion indirectly through the local production of IGF-I. This fits in with the recent observation that not circulating IGF-I but rather GH is the major determinant of body size. It appears that young dogs of large breeds go through a period of GH excess, i.e., gigantism (Fig. 2–8).[4]

Like GH, PRL is also secreted in a pulsatile manner, with fluctuations during different stages of the reproductive cycle. In dogs PRL concentrations in plasma tend to increase in the luteal phase of the sexual cycle and very high concentrations are found during lactation.

The predominant effect of the hypothalamus on prolactin secretion is inhibitory. The main prolactin-inhibiting factor (PIF) is the biogenic amine dopamine, a secretory product of the tuberohypophyseal dopaminergic pathways. Although TRH and serotonin can stimulate PRL release, they are probably neither the only nor the

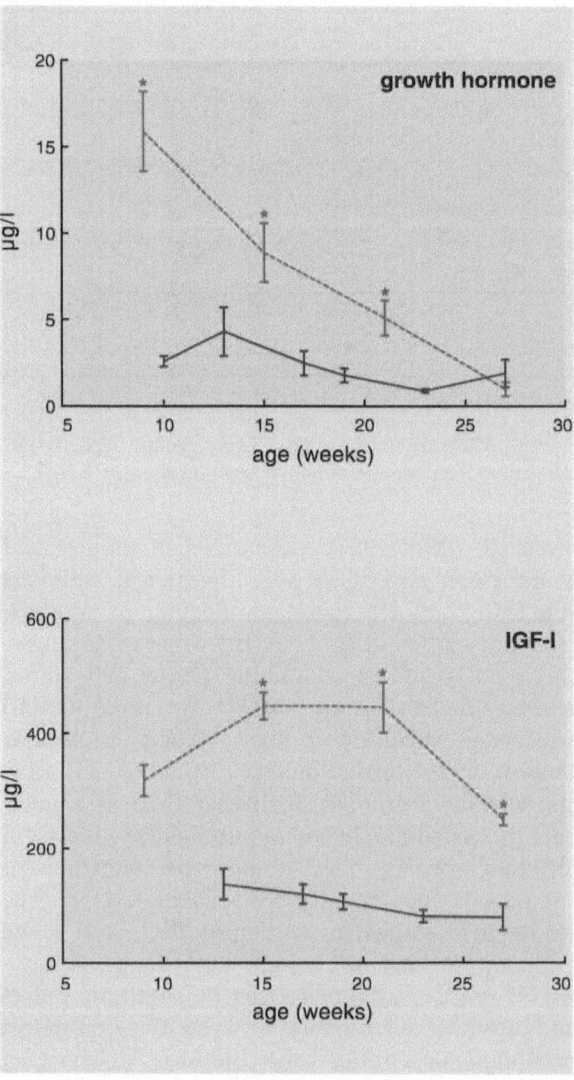

Fig. 2-8. Plasma concentrations (mean ± SEM) of growth hormone (upper panel) and IGF-I (lower panel) during growth in 6 Miniature Poodles (green lines) and 5 Great Danes (red lines). (Courtesy of Dr. R.C. Nap.[4])

major physiological prolactin-releasing factors (PRF). There is accumulating evidence that apart from the hypothalamic-AL axis there is a PL-AL axis which is primarily activated by neuronal impulses, e.g., those generated by suckling.[2] When this occurs, dopamine release is suppressed and the release of an unidentified PRF is augmented.

The most familiar role of PRL in mammals is stimulation of mammary gland growth and lactation. PRL increases mitosis of mammary gland epithelial cells during development and also during pregnancy and lactation. It also affects gonadal function.

2.2.1 Congenital growth hormone deficiency

Inadequate GH secretion early in life causes retardation of growth. There have been occasional reports of dwarfism in dogs and cats, but GH-deficiency dwarfism seems to occur primarily as a genetically transmitted condition (autosomal recessive inheritance) in German shepherd dogs[5] and Carelian bear dogs. The condition is due to pressure atrophy of the AL by cysts of Rathke's pouch.[6]

Clinical manifestations. The animals are usually presented at the age of 3–5 months because of poor growth and an abnormally soft and woolly hair coat (Fig. 2–9). The latter is due to retention of lanugo or secondary hairs and lack of primary or guard hairs. This stagnant development of skin and coat finally results in alopecia and a thin and grayish-brown pigmented skin (Fig. 2–9).

Initially the dogs are lively and alert. They have a characteristic pointed muzzle and a facial expression resembling that of a fox (Fig. 2–10). They remain small but do not have a disproportionate body contour and in most cases there is no remarkable delay in dentition. In the first year or two of life the functions of the other adenohypophyseal cells are usually not seriously disturbed, so that the function of the thyroids and gonads remains normal or near normal (Fig. 2–10), and the growth plates close before one year of age.

However, with time and most probably with progression of cyst formation in the pituitary, the animals become less active. Inappetence may also develop, finally resulting in a thin, dull, and hairless dog with a somewhat sad appearance. This situation is usually reached at the age of two to three years and is commonly associated with severe secondary hypothyroidism and impaired renal function. The latter may have both a renal and a prerenal component, i.e., maldevelopment of glomeruli due to lack of GH and low filtration pressure due to lack of glucocorticoids and thyroxine.

Differential diagnosis. Congenital hypothyroidism may be the most important differential diagnosis, although the appearance of these animals is quite different from that seen in hypothyroidism (see 3.2). The possibility should also be considered that the apparently dwarfed animal is the result of an unexpected and unwanted mating with a small-

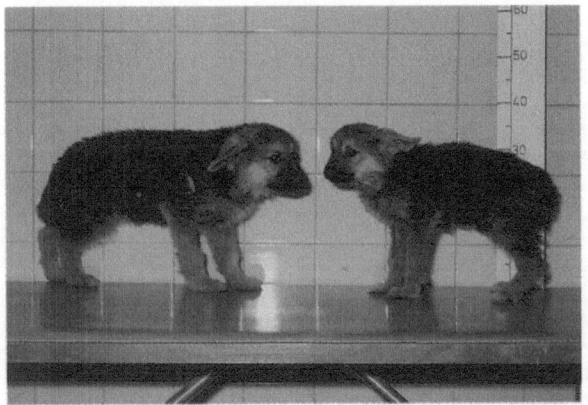 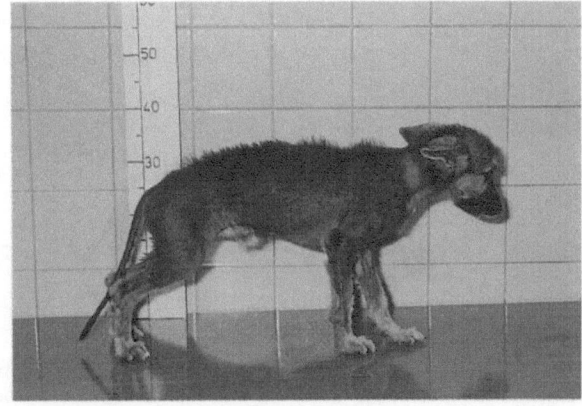

Fig. 2-9. Left: Two three-month-old German Shepherd dogs with pituitary dwarfism. The woolly appearance of the coat is due to the complete lack of development of primary guard hairs. Right: A German Shepherd dwarf at one year of age. There is almost complete truncal alopecia. The scale is in centimeters.

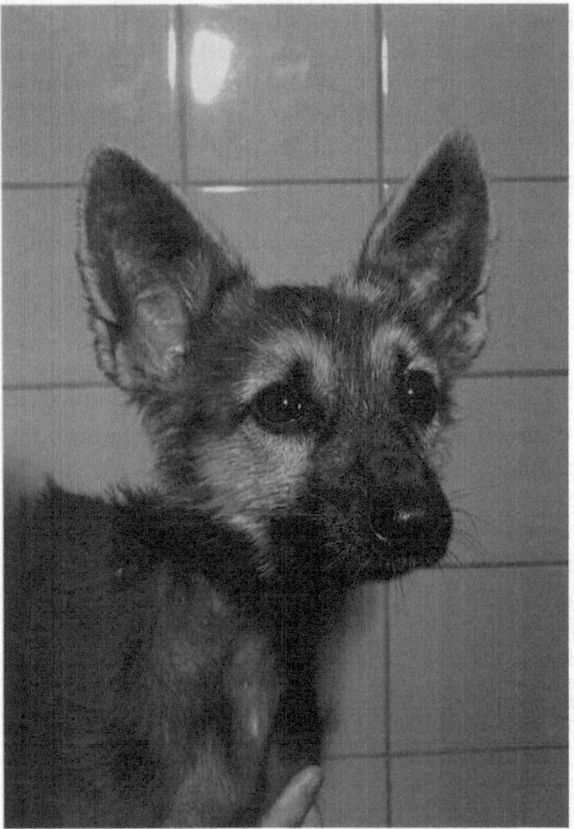
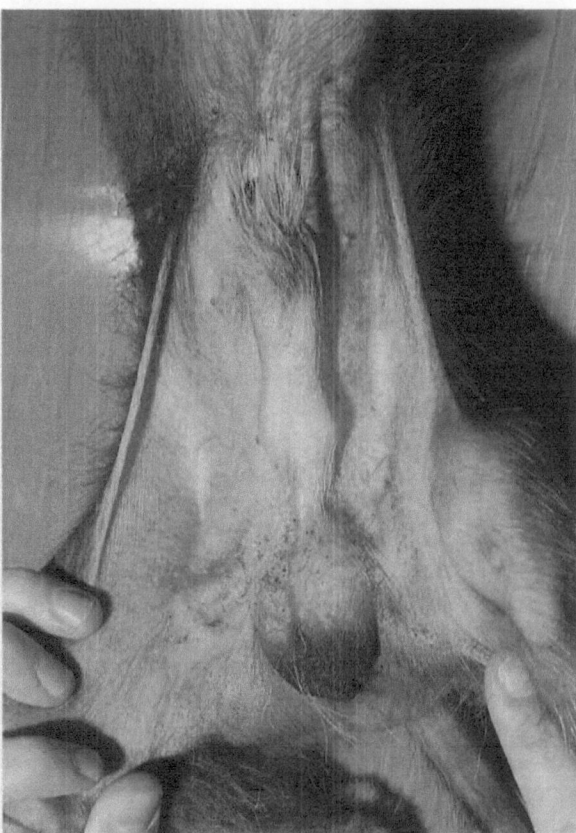

Fig. 2-10. Left: A German Shepherd dwarf at one year of age. The alert, fox-like face is characteristic of these animals. Right: The testicles were well-developed and semen contained motile sperm.

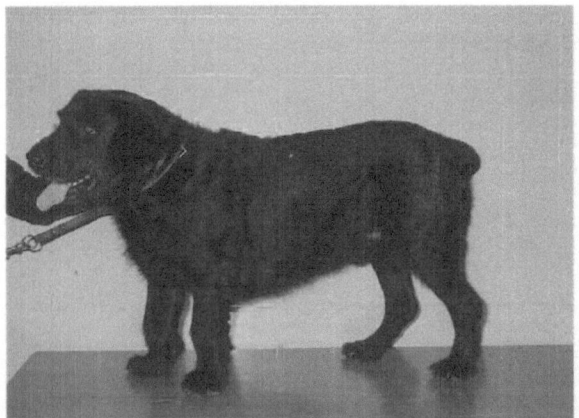
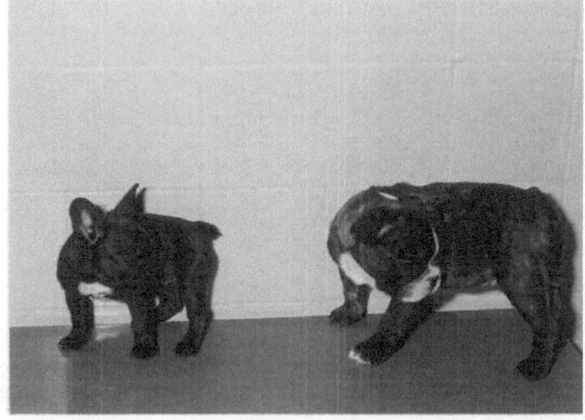

Fig. 2-11. Left: A one-year-old male dog, purchased as a Bouvier des Flandres and referred for examination because of its small stature. The achondroplastic forelegs and the tracing of its history indicated that it was the result of a mismating and not a purebred. Right: Two 12-week-old male French Bulldog littermates, the one on the left referred for examination because of its retarded growth. This could be explained by its small size at birth and its often losing in the competition for suckling. With supplemental feeding it became a healthy adult French Bulldog, although of small size.

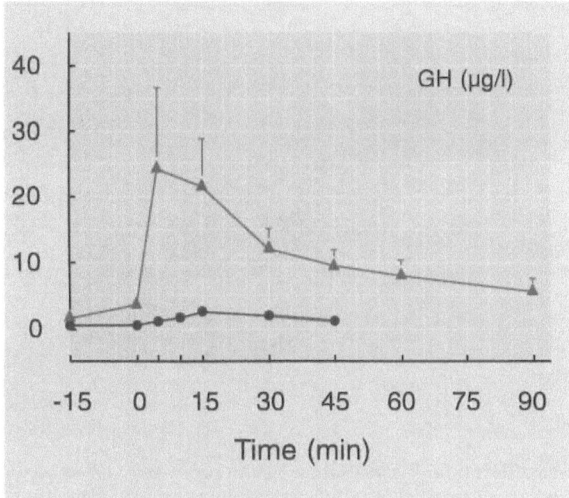

Fig. 2-12. The effect of intravenous administration of 1 μg GHRH per kg body weight on plasma GH concentrations in healthy dogs (mean ± S.E.M., red line) and in the Poodle shown in Fig. 2–13 (blue line).

sized dog, or is simply a small individual within the normal biological variation (Fig. 2–11). Retardation of growth can also be the result of undernutrition or of congenital abnormalities of vital organs such as the heart, liver, and kidneys. Corticosteroid administration at an early age also quite rapidly retards growth (see 4.3.3).

Diagnosis. Although the clinical diagnosis may be very obvious, definitive diagnosis requires meas-

urement of GH in plasma, employing a homologous radioimmunoassay. Since basal GH values may also be low in healthy animals, a stimulation test should be performed (Figs. 2–12, 2–16; Chapter 13). The amino acid sequence of IGF-I is less species specific than that of growth hormone and therefore it can be measured in a heterologous assay. In German shepherd dwarfs the IGF-I concentrations in plasma are usually low, even when age and size are taken into account,[3,7] but these measurements do not provide such a definitive diagnosis as do measurements of GH before and after stimulation.

In order to assess the presence of secondary hypothyroidism a TSH-stimulation test should be performed (Chapter 13).

Treatment. Canine GH is not available for therapeutic use and hence there have been attempts to treat affected dogs with porcine, bovine, or human GH in thrice weekly subcutaneous doses of 0.1–0.3 IU per kg body weight. Some regrowth of hair has been reported, but the overall results have been poor. For the use of human GH this has been explained by the development of antibodies against the heterologous GH.[8] Thyroid hormone replacement should be started (see 3.3.1) as soon as there is evidence of secondary hypothyroidism.

Prognosis. By the age of 3 to 5 years the animal has usually become a bald, thin, and dull dog.

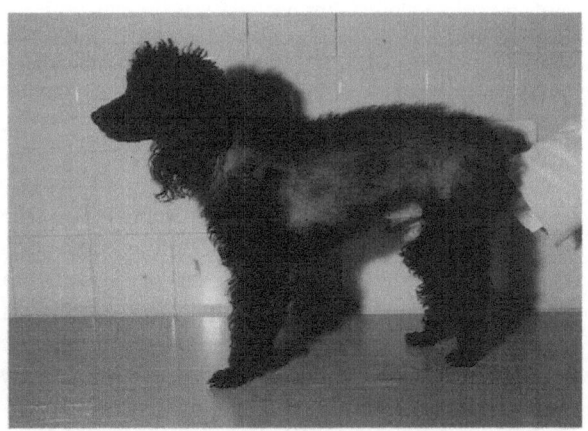 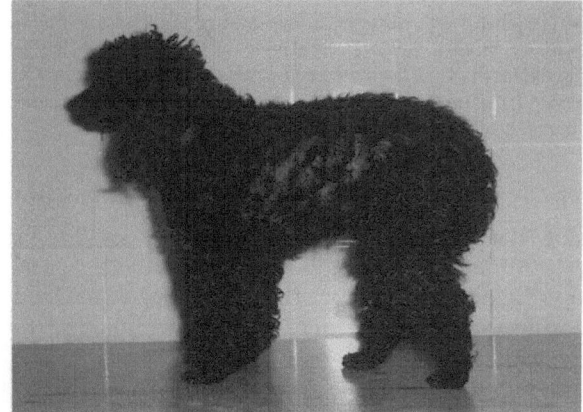

Fig. 2-13. Left: A six-year-old male Poodle with truncal alopecia. The absence of other physical or laboratory signs of a known endocrine disease led to the suspicion of disturbed GH secretion. Basal GH levels in plasma were low (< 0.3 and 0.8 μg/l) and increased very little following stimulation (0.8 and 2.5 μg/l). Right: The same dog after destruction of the adrenal cortices with o,p'-DDD. The dexamethasone screening test had not indicated hyperadrenocorticism but repeated measurements of urinary corticoid excretion had suggested mild hyperadrenocorticism (see Chapters 4, 13).

20

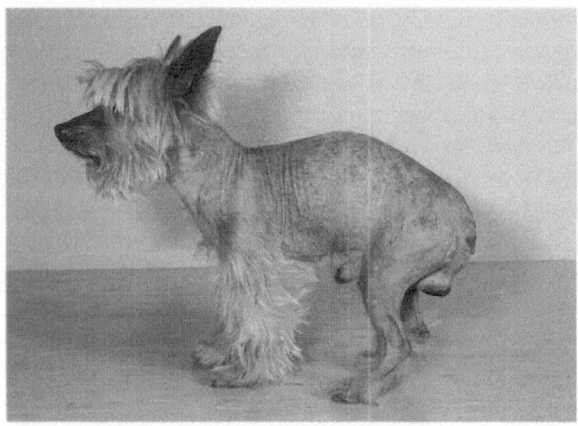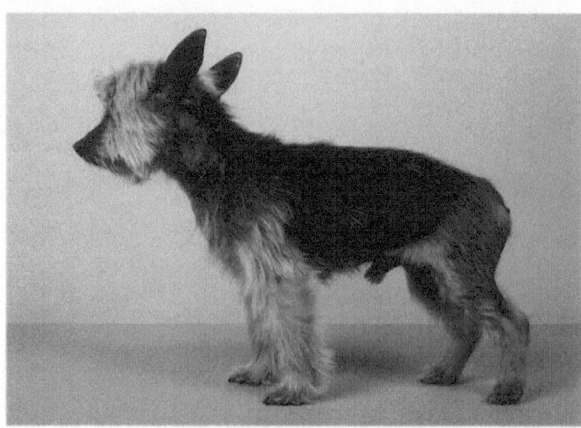

Fig. 2-14. Left: An 8-year-old Yorkshire Terrier with alopecia of two years duration. Plasma GH concentrations were low and did not respond to stimulation with GHRH. The results of both the dexamethasone secreening test and the urinary corticoid/creatinine ratios were around the upper limit of the reference range. Destruction of the adrenal cortices with o,p'-DDD resulted in new hair growth (right).

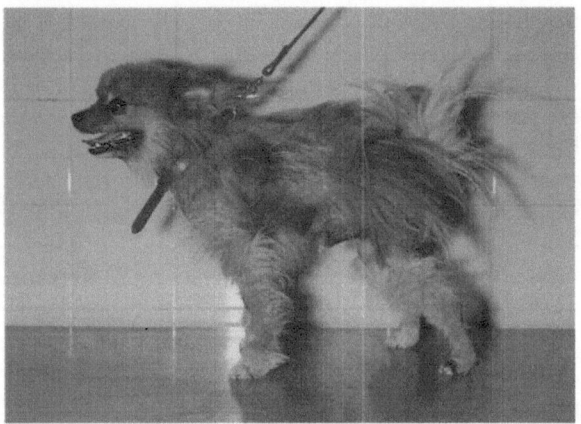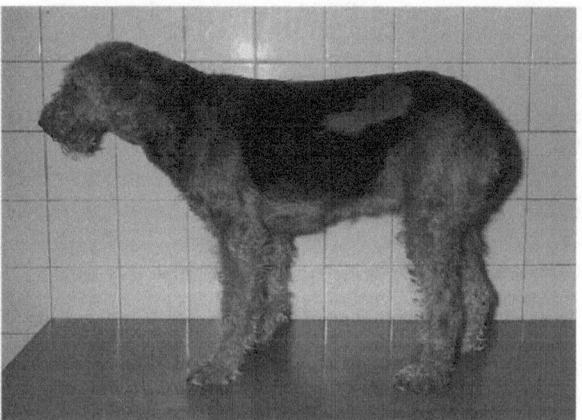

Fig. 2-15. Left: An eight-year-old male Pomeranian in which progressively increasing alopecia for one year was the only problem. Although this type of alopecia has been presumed to be due to GH deficiency, low levels of GH that do not respond to stimulation have also been found in Pomeranians without alopecia. Right: A two-year-old female Airedale Terrier with the type of alopecia on the flanks that has been ascribed to GH deficiency. There was a slow but complete regrowth of hair during the following 6 months without any treatment. This is a condition of unknown cause and it is referred to as "seasonal flank alopecia", although the seasonal character of the alopecia is not always evident.[34]

These changes seem to be the result of progressive loss of pituitary functions and usually cannot be prevented by treatment of the secondary hypothyroidism. In addition, the continuing expansion of the pituitary cyst may impair the function of adjacent brain tissue and thus contribute to the animal's misery. At this stage the owners usually request that the animal be euthanized, if they have not done so long before this.

2.2.2 Acquired disturbances of growth hormone release (many unresolved questions)

In recent years there have been reports on the occurrence of an isolated growth hormone deficiency in mature dogs. It has been proposed that such a deficiency may explain some forms of alopecia that do not seem to be caused by classic diseases known to be associated with skin atrophy and hair loss (hypothyroidism and hyperadrenocorticism). Injections with heterologous GH have been reported to be beneficial in these cases of alopecia, which mainly involve the trunk and the caudal surfaces of the thighs but not the legs (Figs. 2–13, 2–14). This form of alopecia has been reported to occur in male Pomeranians, poodles, chow chows, and Airedale terriers at any age but usually beginning at 1–2 years of age. (Fig. 2–15). These observations and the results of treatment with heterologous GH, although poor to moderate, have led to names such as "adult-onset growth hormone deficiency" and "growth-hormone responsive dermatosis".

The entity does not seem to be well-defined, for in about one-third of the cases a normal GH response to stimulation has been found. Yet in some cases in which there was a normal response to stimulation, treatment with GH was reported to be effective. In others, seemingly unrelated measures such as castration or administration of testosterone were followed by the appearance of a new

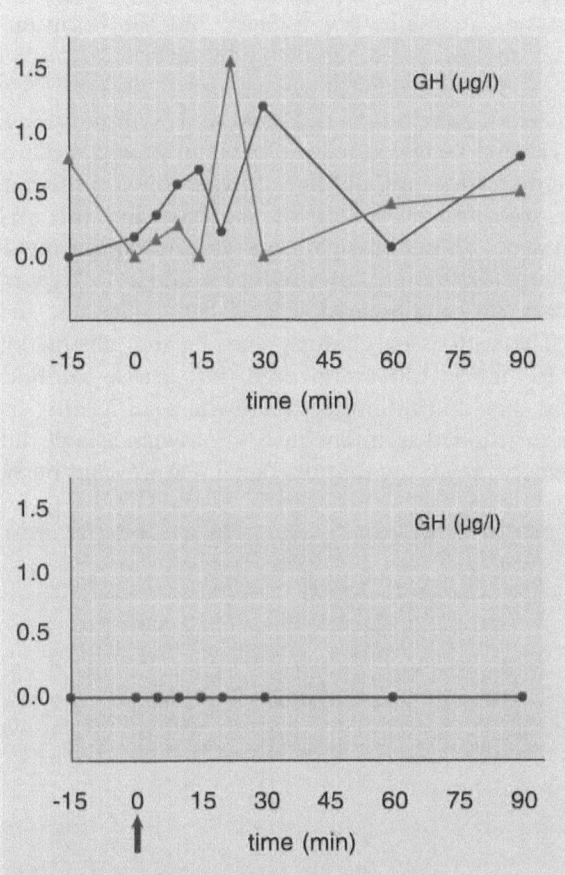

Fig. 2-16. The influence of GHRH (1 µg/kg i.v.) administration on plasma GH concentrations in two middle-aged Poodles with alopecia and disturbed GH release (upper panel) and two young German Shepherds with congenital GH deficiency of pituitary origin.[7] Note that in the Poodles there was still some basal GH secretion.

hair coat.[9] Furthermore, in a study in Pomeranians, both with and without alopecia, the mean circulating GH concentrations did not increase significantly in either group after stimulation.[10]

Thus the proposed relation between some forms of this adult-onset alopecia and decreased growth hormone secretion is not on very solid ground. It is even unlikely that a true growth hormone deficiency exists, for when IGF-I concentrations in plasma have been measured, they have invariably been within the reference ranges. Also, in contrast to dogs with congenital GH deficiency, these dogs usually have measurable GH concentrations in plasma (Fig. 2–16).

The fact remains that in some mature dogs with or without alopecia there is no response or only a weak response of plasma GH to stimulation with either GHRH (1 µg/kg), or the α-adrenergic agonist clonidine (10 µg/kg), or its structural analog xylazine (100 µg/kg). This lack of response is most likely an isolated disturbance, for there is no evidence of involvement of other pituitary hormones.

The cause of this disturbed GH secretion is unknown. Of the possible explanations, i.e., (1) a primary pituitary lesion, (2) decreased suprapituitary stimulation by GHRH, or (3) increased suprapituitary inhibitory control, the latter seems the most likely in some of the cases. It includes the possibility that an increased inhibitory control of GH secretion by somatostatin overrides the stimulatory influence of GHRH. The most likely candidate for inducing this change in the balanced control of GH release are glucocorticoids, hormones well known to suppress the GH response to various stimuli in the dog.[11] Indeed, there is evidence suggesting that in at least some of the dogs with alopecia and nonresponsive GH levels, there is a very mild form of hyperadrenocorticism (see Figs. 2–13, 2–14; also Section 4.3).[7] In others this does not seem to be the case and their alopecia remains unexplained at present.

For treatment the reader is referred to Section 2.2.1, but it is once more emphasized that the use of heterologous GH may give rise to formation of antibodies (Fig. 2–17), which may make treatment ineffective and lead to anaphylactic reactions.[8]

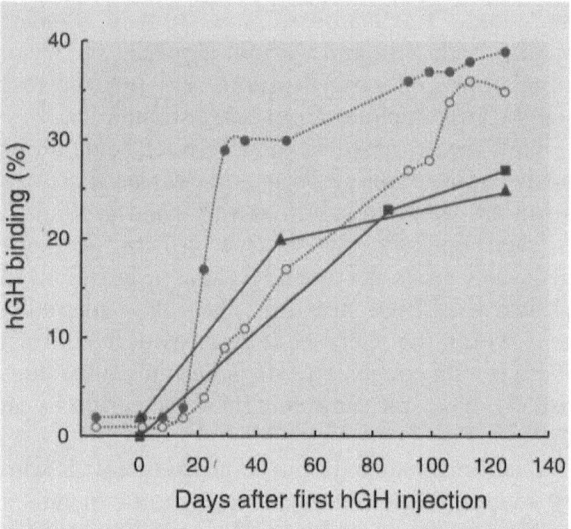

Fig. 2-17. Illustration of antibody formation following administration of heterologous growth hormone by depicting the binding of biosynthetic human growth hormone (hGH) to plasma proteins in two German Shepherd pups with congenital growth hormone deficiency (red lines) and in two Poodles with supposedly acquired GH deficiency (blue lines) that finally proved to be mild hyperadrenocorticism.[8] Very recently it has been reported that, although there is no 100% homology at genomic level, the translated GH molecules of pigs and dogs are identical.[2a,2b] Thus adverse reactions are not to be expected with the use of highly purified or biosynthetic porcine GH, if available.

2.2.3 Growth hormone excess

GH hypersecretion in the adult results in acromegaly, an insidious disease associated with bony and soft tissue overgrowth. The condition is known to occur in middle-aged female dogs and middle-aged and elderly, predominantly male, cats.

Pathogenesis. The pathogenesis of the GH excess is completely different in the two species. In female dogs either endogenous progesterone (metestrus) or exogenous progestagens (used in estrus prevention) may give rise to GH hypersecretion that results in acromegaly and glucose intolerance.[12] This progestin-induced GH excess originates from foci of hyperplastic ductular epithelium in the mammary gland (Fig. 2–18).[13] This mammary GH is biochemically identical to pituitary GH.[2b]

In the cat acromegaly is caused by primary pituitary tumors that secrete excessive amounts of GH.[14] Also in cats progestagens induce GH expression in mammary tissue[2b], but the hormone does not seem to reach the systemic circulation.[15]

Clinical manifestations. Signs and symptoms of GH hypersecretion tend to develop slowly and are characterized initially in both the dog and the cat by soft tissue swelling of the face and the abdomen. These changes are readily appreciated when, fortunately, photographs taken 1 2 years apart can be compared (Fig. 2–19).

The soft-tissue changes may be the reason for presentation but more often they are so gradual that they do not impress the owners sufficiently to be mentioned spontaneously. Yet when asked, the owners may reply that the facial features and body

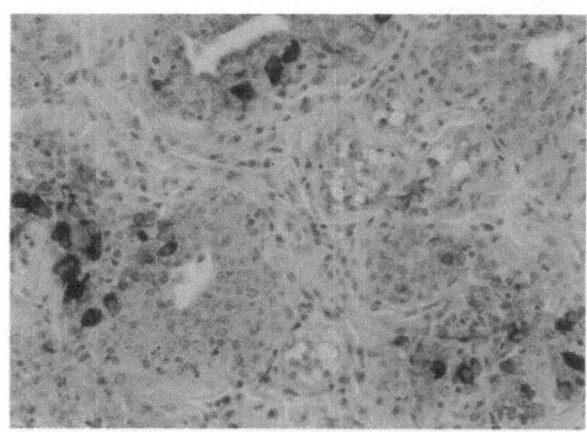

Fig. 2-18. Left: Effect of mammary resection on plasma GH levels in a dog with progestin-induced acromegaly. Time zero is the moment of the first surgical incision. The dotted line indicates the upper limit of the reference range for basal plasma levels of GH. Right: Histologic section of the mammary gland of a progestin-treated dog, indirectly immunostained with monkey anti-canine GH. The immunopositive staining is located in cells of hyperplastic ductular epithelium.[13]

23

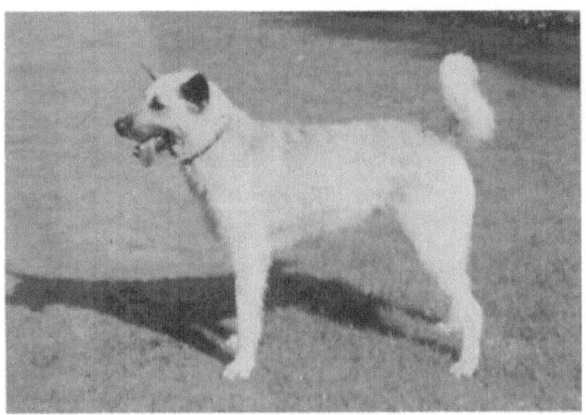 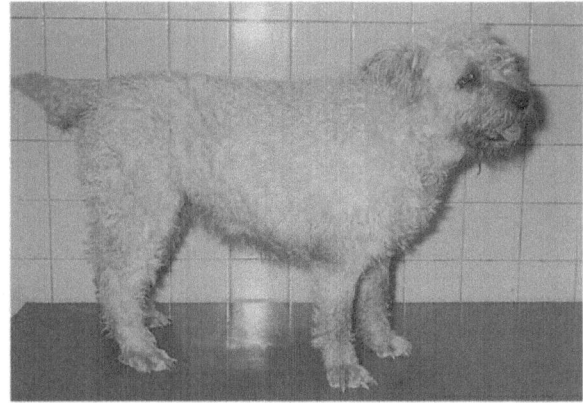

Fig. 2-19. Left: A female mongrel Belgian Shepherd at the age of 3 years, photographed in the owner's garden. Right: The same dog when presented two years later for examination because of decreased endurance, intolerance to warmth (frequent panting, preference for cool places), exaggerated growth of the coat, increase in abdominal size, and inspiratory stridor. The high GH concentrations in plasma (≥ 45 µg/l) had been induced by thrice yearly injections of medroxyprogesterone acetate for prevention of estrus.

dimensions have indeed increased. As the owner of a female golden retriever answered: "She almost looks like a male now".

In some dogs severe hypertrophy of soft tissues of the mouth, tongue, and pharynx causes snoring and even inspiratory dyspnea. Those dogs in which the condition has developed during the luteal phase of the estrous cycle are usually presented with polyuria (and sometimes polyphagia) as the leading symptom. The polyuria is usually without glucosuria, but manifest diabetes mellitus can develop after repeated exposure to GH excess during metestrus.

In cats the reason for suspicion of GH excess is almost exclusively insulin-resistant diabetes mellitus. Cats with acromegaly which have been

described thus far have had diabetes mellitus that could only be controlled with doses of insulin in excess of 30 U/day. Affected cats may also have dyspnea due to congestive heart failure.[14]

Physical examination reveals variable degrees of soft tissue and bony changes, including a heavy head and thick folds of skin, especially in the neck, and prognathism and wide interdental spaces (Fig. 2–20). In cats the head may also become somewhat massive and may have rather pronounced features, probably due in part to overgrowth of the bony structures bounding the paranasal sinuses (Fig. 2–21).

Prolonged GH excess also leads to generalized visceromegaly involving the tongue, salivary glands, and abdominal organs. The latter causes

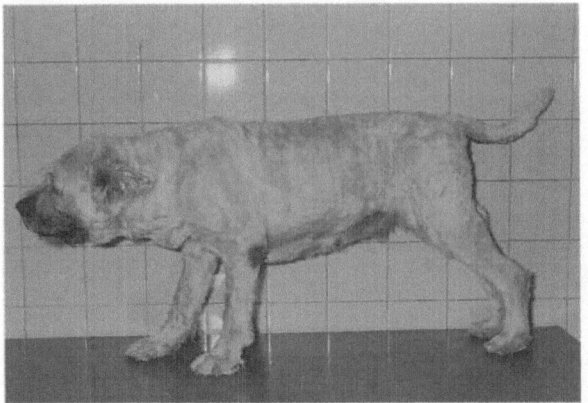 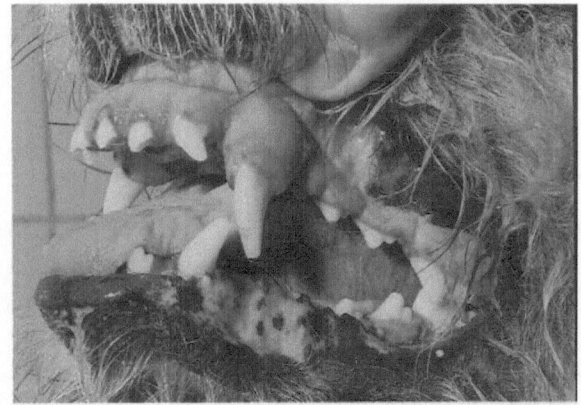

Fig. 2-20. The dog shown in Fig. 2–19, after its coat had been clipped. Left: The head, trunk, and limbs have a coarse and heavy appearance and the skin on the neck is thrown into folds. Right: Prognathism, wide spacing of the teeth, and a relatively large tongue.

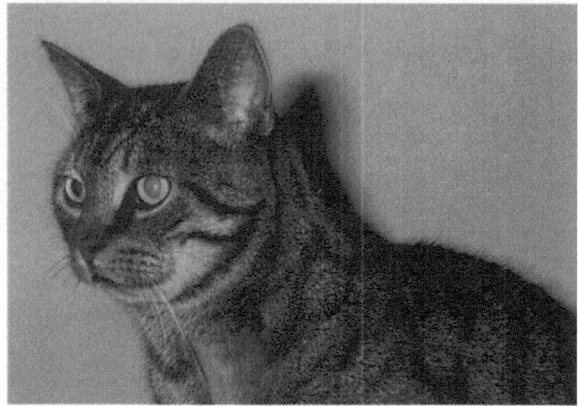 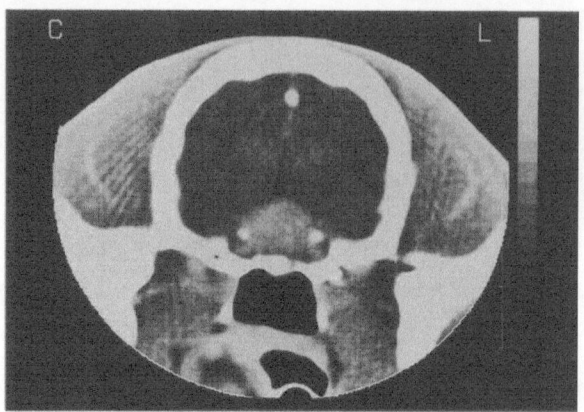

Fig. 2-21. Left: A 10-year-old castrated male cat with diabetes mellitus and acromegaly. It is a sturdy cat with possibly somewhat coarse facial features, although according to the owner its appearance had not changed. Right: Contrast-enhanced CT image through the pituitary fossa in this cat revealed a large pituitary tumor.

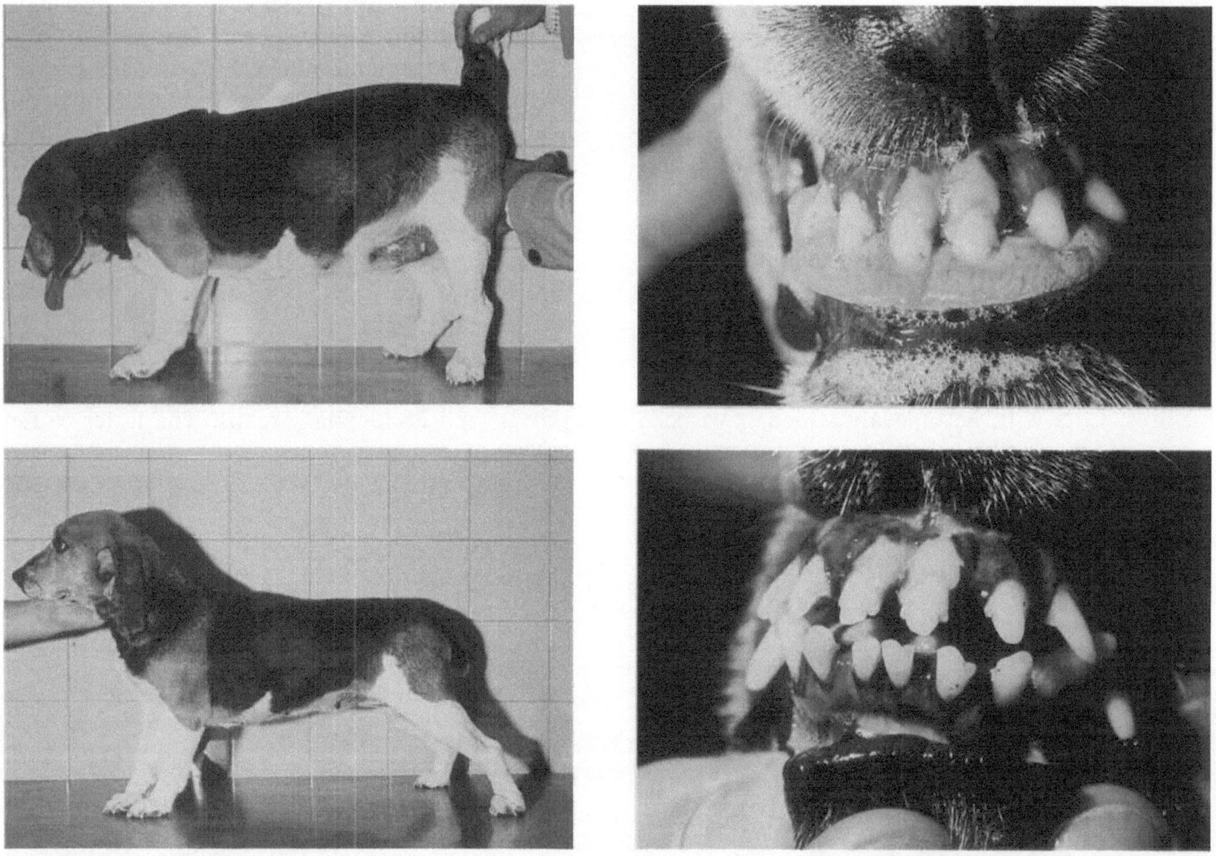

Fig. 2-22. Top: An 8-year-old female Beagle dog with severe acromegaly and diabetes mellitus that had developed during the concurrent metestrus. Note the body size and large tongue. Bottom: The same dog, three months after ovariohysterectomy. The soft-tissue overgrowth has been reversed but not the bony changes such as prognathism and widened interdental spaces.[12]

abdominal enlargement (Fig. 2–22).

Routine laboratory investigations will often reveal hyperglycemia, especially in cats. In dogs plasma levels of alkaline phosphatase may also be increased. This may be due in part to the glucocorticoid activity which is intrinsic to progestagens.[16]

Radiographic examination of dogs will not enlarge upon the physically observed signs of overgrowth of bone and soft tissue. In cats the disease may be complicated by degenerative arthritis with periarticular periosteal reaction, which may require radiographic examination.[14]

Differential diagnosis. In pronounced cases the clinical features, including the specific medical history in both dogs and cats, are not easily confused with those of other diseases. However, in some dogs the metabolic changes lead to polyuria, polyphagia, and hyperglycemia which, together with the increase in abdominal size, may mimic the signs of hyperadrenocorticism. The redundant folds of skin on the head may suggest the possibility of hypothyroidism.

Diagnosis. The diagnosis of GH excess can generally be established by measuring basal GH concentrations in plasma. Feline GH can also be measured in a homologous radioimmunoassay developed for the dog. The basal values in this condition often exceed the upper limit of the reference range (6 μg/l) and so a single measurement might be diagnostic. However, if the disease is mild or is just beginning, basal GH concentrations may be only slightly elevated. Conversely, a high value may be the result of a secretory pulse in a normal subject. There are also disease conditions associated with anorexia and malaise in which GH secretion may be increased. Especially in dogs, three to five repeated measurements at 10-minute intervals may be helpful, since plasma GH concentration does not fluctuate in acromegalic dogs as it does in healthy dogs. Nonresponsiveness of normal or elevated GH levels to stimulation (Chapter 13) may also support the diagnosis in dogs.

The measurement of IGF-I may also contribute to the diagnosis. As mentioned above, the IGF-I concentration in plasma is GH dependent. Being bound to a transport protein, it is much less subject to fluctuation than is GH. IGF concentrations are commonly higher in acromegalic dogs than in healthy control dogs of similar body size, but there may be more overlap than for GH.

In cats the excessive GH is secreted by a pituitary tumor. Thus when GH hypersecretion has been demonstrated in a cat, the pituitary should be visualized by computed tomography, if possible. Documentation of the size and expansion of the pituitary tumor is of value for the prognosis and also for monitoring the response to treatment.

Treatment. Canine acromegaly can be treated easily and effectively by withdrawal of exogenous progestagens and/or ovariohysterectomy. The animal may then change dramatically (Fig. 2–22), due to the reversal of the soft tissue changes. The size of the abdomen decreases, as does the thickening of soft tissues in the oropharyngeal region and hence the associated snoring. The bony changes appear to be irreversible but do not seem to cause problems to the animal. In cases in which the GH excess did not lead to complete exhaustion of the pancreatic β cells, the elimination of the progesterone source by the ovariohysterectomy may prevent persistent diabetes mellitus (Fig. 2–23).

Serious problems can arise in dogs in which the progestagen causing the acromegaly has been

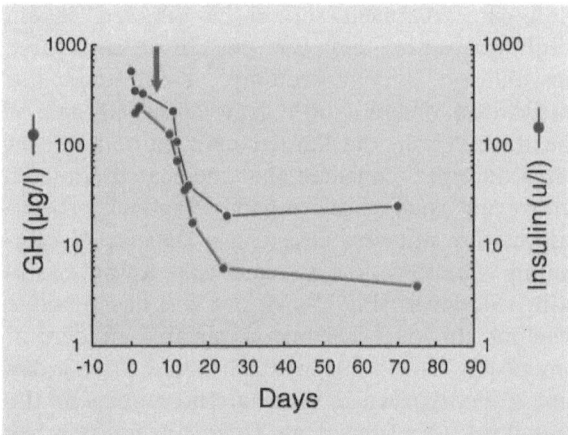

Fig. 2-23. Plasma GH and insulin concentrations (log scales!) in the dog shown in Fig. 2–22, immediately before and after ovariohysterectomy (arrow). The dog was in the luteal phase of the sexual cycle and had developed persistent hyperglycemia. Following elimination of the insulin resistance, i.e., the progestin-induced GH excess, both the hyperinsulinemia and the hyperglycemia disappeared.

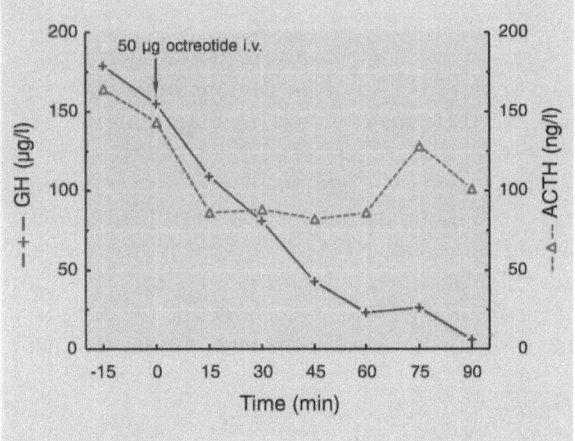

Fig. 2-24. GH and ACTH concentrations in plasma of a 10-year-old castrated male cat (Fig. 2–21) with diabetes mellitus and acromegaly, before and after intravenous administration of 50 μg of the somatostatin analogue, octreotide.

administered only recently. Its action may persist for several months and there is no alternative but to wait for the cessation of its effect. An alternative would be especially helpful in these cases, but thus far only the use of a synthetic antiprogestagen (RU 486) has proved to be effective.[17] There is as yet no experience with long-term administration of this drug and as it is a glucocorticoid antagonist as well, it should be used with caution. In the end one may even decide for total mammectomy (Fig. 2–18).

In cats treatment should be directed at the pituitary tumor and for this there are three possibilities: hypophysectomy, irradiation, and medication. There is little experience with any of the three. From the limited number of reported cases one may conclude that medical treatments with drugs such as the dopamine agonist bromocriptine are not very effective in the cat. A long-acting somatostatin analogue[a] can lower circulating GH levels (Fig. 2–24), but it is questionable whether this will become applicable in clinical practice as it has to be injected several times a day and is very expensive. There are no reports on the long-term use of this drug. Cobalt irradiation has resulted in temporary improvement in one cat.[14] Hypophysectomy may become the treatment of choice for the smaller pituitary tumors.

[a] Sandostatine® (Octreotide), Sandoz AG, Basel, Switzerland

Prognosis. In dogs with progestagen-induced GH excess the prognosis is good following elimination of the progestagen source. Diabetes mellitus resulting from the GH excess is sometimes reversible following reversal of the GH excess. Persistence of the GH excess is accompanied by insulin resistance, which can be quite severe (see also Section 5.2.1).

In cats the short-term prognosis is relatively good, but although the insulin-resistant diabetes mellitus can generally be managed satisfactorily, this requires large daily doses of insulin, at considerable expense. Complications such as congestive heart failure or an expanding pituitary tumor usually result in death or euthanasia within 1–2 years.

2.2.4 Prolactin and pseudopregnancy in the dog

Pseudopregnancy is a syndrome which more or less accompanies the extended luteal phase of all nonpregnant ovarian cycles in the bitch. If the nature of the syndrome is mild it is generally referred to as a physiological or covert pseudopregnancy. In contrast, in overt or clinical pseudopregnancy, mammary development and/or behavioral changes are barely distinguishable from the changes of late pregnancy or lactation. Some breeds such as the Afghan hound and the Basset hound appear to be especially predisposed to development of overt pseudopregnancy.

Pathogenesis. The secretion of progesterone during the luteal phase and during pregnancy is in bitches (not queens) quite similar (see Chapter 7). It is, therefore, not amazing that in some dogs conditions develop which very closely mimic pregnancy. During the second half of pregnancy plasma PRL concentrations increase. In most nonpregnant bitches the prolactin concentrations vary only slightly during the follicular and luteal phases (around 7 μg/l). However, in dogs which develop overt pseudopregnancy in the second half of the luteal phase, elevated PRL levels of around 35 μg/l are found. This may be a consequence of a rapid decrease in progesterone secretion. A rapid decline in progesterone secretion, as for example occurs following ovariectomy during the luteal phase, appears to be an important precipitating factor for pseudopregnancy.

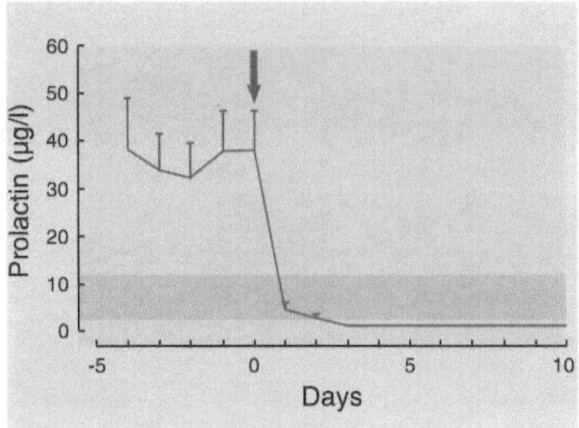

Fig. 2-25. Mean (± SEM) PRL concentrations in plasma of 6 bitches with pseudopregnancy before and during 10 days of metergoline administration (twice daily 0.1 mg/kg). The arrow marks the start of treatment. The horizontal bar indicates reference ranges in anoestus bitches. (Courtesy of Drs. K.J.W. van Cleef, E.H.H. Grevelt and A.C. Schaefers-Okkens.)

Clinical manifestations. About 4–8 weeks after estrus some bitches with pseudopregnancy may exhibit behavior which can be interpreted as nest building and caring for offspring; it may include reluctance to leave the home, aggression, and the mothering of objects. Others may become restless, somewhat anorectic and may exhibit frequent licking of their abdomen. The mammary glands can develop to such an extent that the body contour closely resembles that of late pregnancy or lactation. The mammary secretion varies from only a few drops of a clear or brownish fluid to considerable amounts of true milk.

Prognosis and treatment. In most dogs the signs of pseudopregnancy will cease spontaneously after a couple of weeks. In some cases, however, the changes are so severe and long lasting that the owners cannot cope with them and ask for treatment.

Prolactin levels can be suppressed and pseudopregnancy terminated by administration of:
1. The dopamine-agonist bromocriptine[b] at a dose rate of 10 µg/kg twice daily for 10–14 days. Vomiting which frequently occurs can be avoided by reducing the dose by half for the first four days and by administering the drug after meals.

[b] Lactafal®, Eurovet B.V., The Netherlands (Bromocriptine, Sandoz A.G., Switzerland).

2. The serotonin antagonist metergoline[c] at a dose rate of 0.1 mg/kg twice daily for 8 days. This drug lowers PRL release (Fig. 2–25) without the risk of vomiting, but hyperexcitation, some increase in aggression, and frequent whining may occur.

2.2.5 Pituitary tumors

The manifestations of pituitary tumors may be both endocrine and nonendocrine. The endocrine aspects comprising hormone excess are discussed in the previous sections and in Section 4.3.1. The nonendocrine manifestations result from pressure by the tumor on adjacent structures in the brain. In addition, such patients may have anterior pituitary failure. As is the case with expanding cysts in the pituitary in young dogs (see 2.2.1), large pituitary masses can cause partial or complete anterior pituitary hormone deficiency. In principle, deficiency of all six major hormones (LH, FSH, GH, TSH, ACTH, and PRL) can occur. The pituitary enlargement may also have consequences for PL function (see 2.3.1).

Endocrine manifestations. In the adult, GH deficiency is not easily recognized as a pathological syndrome, although longstanding GH deficiency is said to cause atrophy of skin and adnexa, leading to alopecia (see 2.2.2). TSH deficiency occurs relatively late in the course of hypopituitarism and is discussed in Section 3.3.2. Secondary adrenocortical failure may occur late in the development of large pituitary tumors. The resulting cortisol deficiency (see also 4.2.2) may contribute to the gradual deterioration of the animal and a relatively trivial illness or anesthesia may precipitate vascular collapse. Gonadotropin deficiency in female dogs may remain unnoticed because of the naturally long interestrous intervals. In the rare case of a tumor producing excess PRL, anestrus may be associated with galactorrhoea. In male dogs the continuing decrease in gonadotropin secretion results in testicular atrophy (Fig. 2–26). The testes are very small and soft and the unchanged epididymis is more easily delineated than it normally is. Posterior pituitary failure is

[c] Contralac®, Virbac (tablets of 0.5 and 2 mg metergoline).

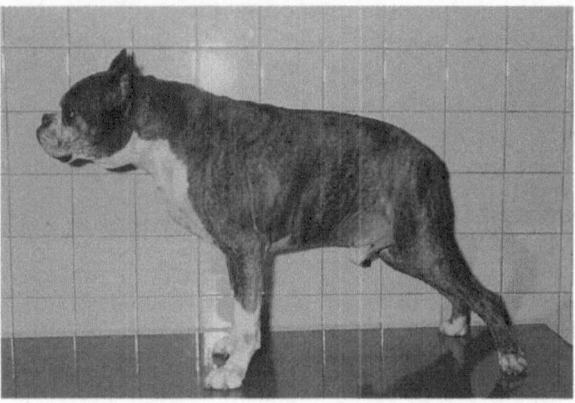 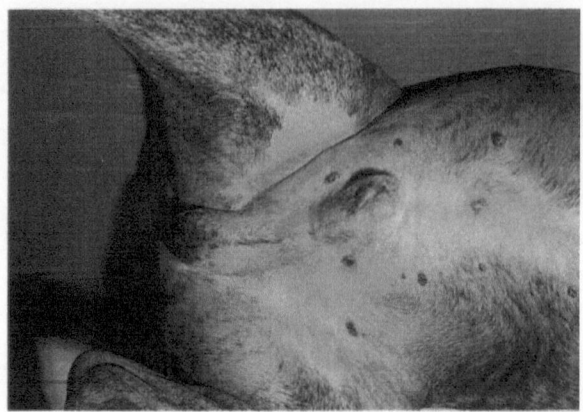

Fig. 2-26. A nine-year-old male Boxer dog with a large pituitary tumor and secondary hypothyroidism, only manifested by somnolence, slight alopecia in the groins and flanks, and a thin coat (left). There was marked atrophy of the testes (right). There were as yet no neurologic symptoms.

unusual in primary anterior pituitary disease, although it has been found in association with very large tumors (see also 2.3).

Mass effects. Continued suprasellar expansion of the tumor exerts pressure on the diaphragma sellae mater, the hypothalamus and, if the expansion is sufficiently rostral, the optic chiasm. This can be expected to cause headache and visual field defects in the dog and cat, as in man, but because of the lack of an autoanamnesis, the veterinarian must rely on rather vague and nonspecific symptoms. These include lethargy, a tendency to seek seclusion, and a decrease in appetite.[18,19] The suspicion of a mass effect from a pituitary tumor may be supported by the owner's description of the animal's tendency to lower its head to avoid being patted. Progressive enlargement of the mass may give rise to severe neurological abnormalities such as pacing, head pressing, and circling. Seizures usually do not occur. In the dog and cat pituitary tumors seldom appear to cause pressure on the optic chiasm to such an extent that visual disturbances are noticed by the owner.

Physical examination can reveal a variety of signs, including dullness, one or more of the above neurological signs, weight loss due to increasing anorexia, and occasionally mydriasis with or without anisocoria. Ophthalmoscopic examination rarely reveals papilledema.

Differential diagnosis. In part due to the nonspecific character of the signs and symptoms, the differential diagnoses range from other neurologic diseases such as parasellar lesions and increased intracranial pressure to metabolic disorders such as hypothyroidism and hepatic encephalopathy.

Diagnosis. Evidence of low basal functions of peripheral endocrine glands, i.e., a low plasma concentration of thyroxine and a low urinary corticoid excretion, may support the suspicion of anterior pituitary failure. However, the diagnosis of partial or total hypopituitarism should preferably be made by demonstrating the deficiencies of pituitary hormones. This can be accomplished by stimulation tests with hypophysiotropic hormones such as GHRH, GnRH, CRH, and TRH. Measurements of the respective pituitary hormones – GH, LH, ACTH, and PRL – permits assessment of pituitary reserve capacity. Although these tests can in principle be performed in an outpatient setting, it is cumbersome to do so when the tests are performed separately. Hence a combined anterior pituitary test has been developed, in which the four hypophysiotropic hormones are injected within 20 s and blood samples are collected for measurements of all 4 pituitary hormones in each sample (Chapter 13).

Contrast-enhanced computed tomography provides imaging of the pituitary (Fig. 2–27 with high spatial and contrast resolution, allowing the identification of pituitary enlargement and its relationship to surrounding structures. Magnetic resonance imaging has even greater potential than computed tomography.

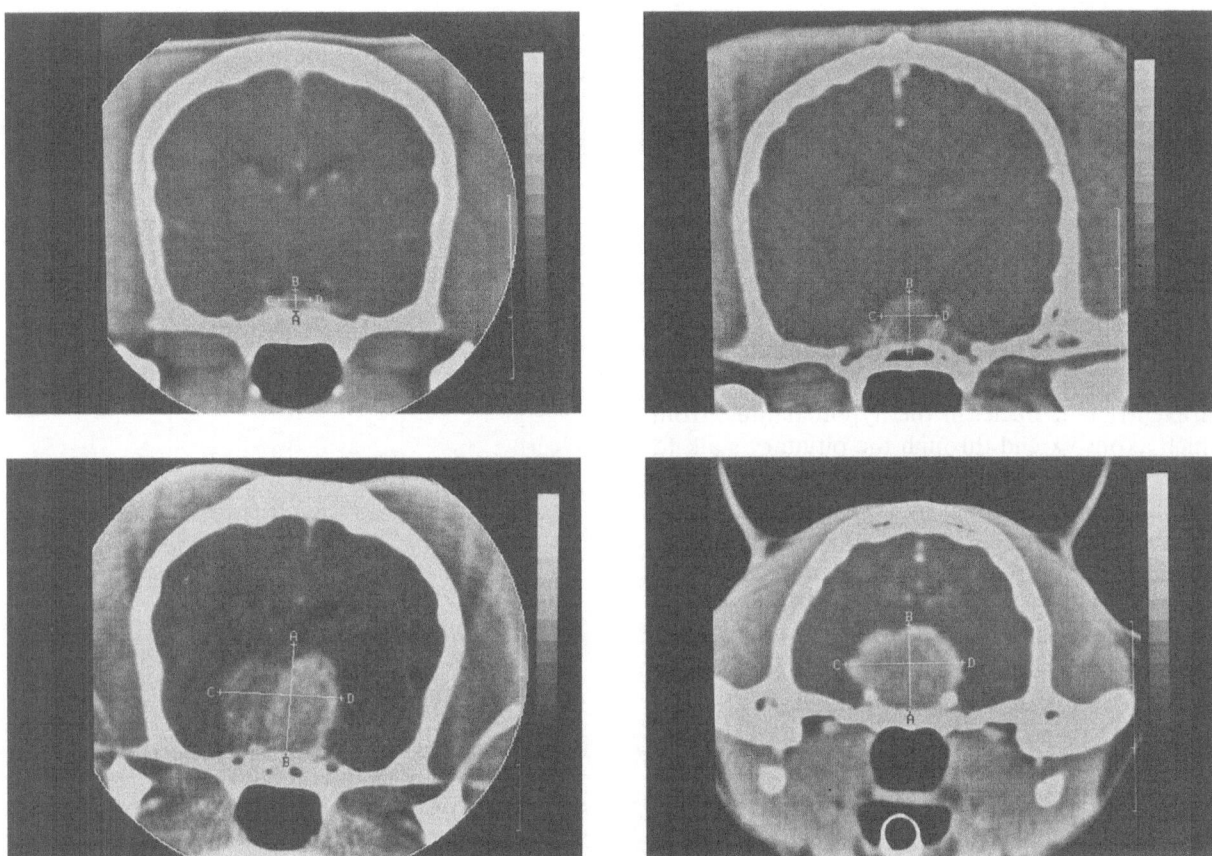

Fig. 2-27. Transverse CT images of the skulls of three dogs and one cat. Left top: A healthy Beagle dog. Contrast enhancement enabled the visualization of a normal-sized pituitary, the margins of which are indicated by A-B (3.6 mm) and C-D (5.0 mm). Right top: A 12-year-old female mongrel Greyhound with pituitary-dependent hyperadrenocorticism. Contrast enhancement revealed a definitely enlarged pituitary (A-B = 8.6 mm and C-D = 9.2 mm). Left bottom: A 10-year-old female Australian Terrier with dexamethasone-resistent pituitary-dependent hyperadrenocorticism without noticeable neurologic symptoms. Contrast enhancement revealed a very large pituitary (A-B = 16.6 mm; C-D = 17.7 mm). Right bottom: A 14-year-old castrated male domestic shorthair cat presented with mild signs and symptoms of pituitary-dependent hyperadrenocorticism and central blindness. A very large pituitary was revealed by contrast enhancement (A-B = 13.6 mm; C-D = 17.9 mm).

Treatment. Anterior pituitary failure can be treated by substituting for the deficient hormone production by the target glands. Since gonadal hormones are not essential, treatment amounts to oral administration of thyroxine (10 µg/kg twice daily) and cortisone (0.25–0.5 mg/kg twice daily). The owners usually report that this treatment brings about some improvement in alertness and also in appetite if the animal had been anorectic. Especially when by virtue of its size the tumor has already had neurological effects, the improvement, if any, will be only temporary.

In principle there are three treatment options: medical therapy, hypophysectomy, and radiation therapy (see also discussion on the treatment of GH excess in the cat in the previous section). Attempts to reduce the size of the tumor with neuropharmacological drugs such as the dopamine agonist bromocriptine and the serotonin antagonist cyproheptadine have been unsuccessful thus far. Although hypophysectomy is used successfully in the treatment of pituitary-dependent hyperadrenocorticism (see 4.3.1), the technique employed does not yet allow the complete removal of very large pituitary tumors. A temporary relief may be obtained by a subtotal removal of the tumor. In some cases the animal can resume a normal life for many months.

30

Pituitary irradiation with megavoltage radiation has been succesful in decreasing the size of the pituitary mass. Adverse effects include hearing impairment and central vestibular disease.[20]

2.3 Posterior lobe

As illustrated in Fig. 2–2, the posterior lobe or neurohypophysis is an extension of the ventral hypothalamus. The two neurohypophyseal hormones are synthesized in both the supraoptic and paraventricular nuclei in the hypothalamus, from which axons extend through the pituitary stalk to the posterior pituitary. The hormones vasopressin and oxytocin are formed by separate neurons and migrate down the axons as part of precursor proteins. They are stored in secretory granules within the nerve terminals in the neurohypophysis and are released by exocytosis into the bloodstream in response to appropriate stimuli. As in most mammals, in dogs and cats arginine-vasopressin (AVP) or antidiuretic hormone (ADH) (in pigs: lysine-vasopressin) plays a vital role in water conservation. Oxytocin stimulates uterine contractions and milk ejection. This section will concentrate on vasopressin.

The nonapeptide AVP is synthesized as part of a large precursor molecule that is composed of a signal peptide, the hormone, a carrier protein termed neurophysin and a glycopeptide. The major determinant of the release of vasopressin is plasma osmolality. In addition, significant changes in circulating blood volume may influence the setting of the osmoregulation. Specialized neurons called osmoreceptors are concentrated in the anterolateral hypothalamus, which is near but separate from the supraoptic nuclei. This area is supplied with blood by small perforating branches of the anterior cerebral arteries.

The major role of vasopressin is to regulate body fluid homeostasis by affecting water reabsorption. The antidiuretic effect is achieved by promoting the reabsorption of solute-free water in the distal and collecting tubules of the kidney. The cellular mechanism of AVP activity in the renal tubule involves binding to specific contraluminal V_2-receptor sites, an adenylate cyclase reponse, and phosphorylation of membrane proteins that lead to transient insertion of water channels in the

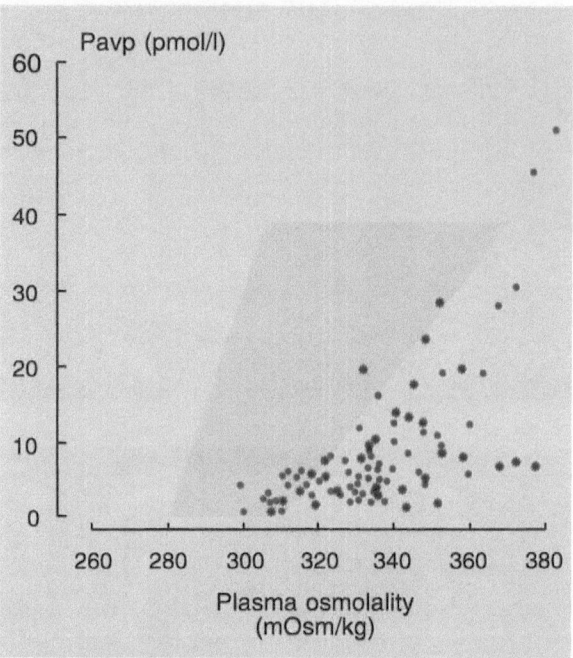

Fig. 2-28. Relation of plasma vasopressin (Pavp) to plasma osmolality in 9 dogs with pituitary-dependent hyperadrenocorticism (red dots) and 6 dogs with hyperadrenocorticism due to an adrencortical tumor (blue asterixes) during hypertonic saline infusion. The green area represents the range in healthy dogs.

luminal membrane of the cell. In the presence of these channels water molecules can move passively along an osmotic gradient, i.e., from the distal and collecting tubules to the hypertonic renal medulla.

Cations, drugs, and hormones can influence the action of AVP, thereby causing polyuria. Calcium inhibits the adenylate cyclase response to vasopressin. Glucocorticoids also interfere with the action of AVP, although in dogs loss of reactivity of the osmoreceptor system also seems to contribute to the corticosteroid-induced polyuria[21] (Fig. 2–28). Even physiological increases in cortisol inhibit basal vasopressin release in dogs.[22]

2.3.1 Vasopressin deficiency; central diabetes insipidus

Diabetes insipidus refers to the passage of large quantities of dilute urine and is actually synonymous with polyuria. In central diabetes insipidus the polyuria results from a lack of sufficient AVP to concentrate urine. The disease is characterized by three primary findings: (1) dilute urine despite

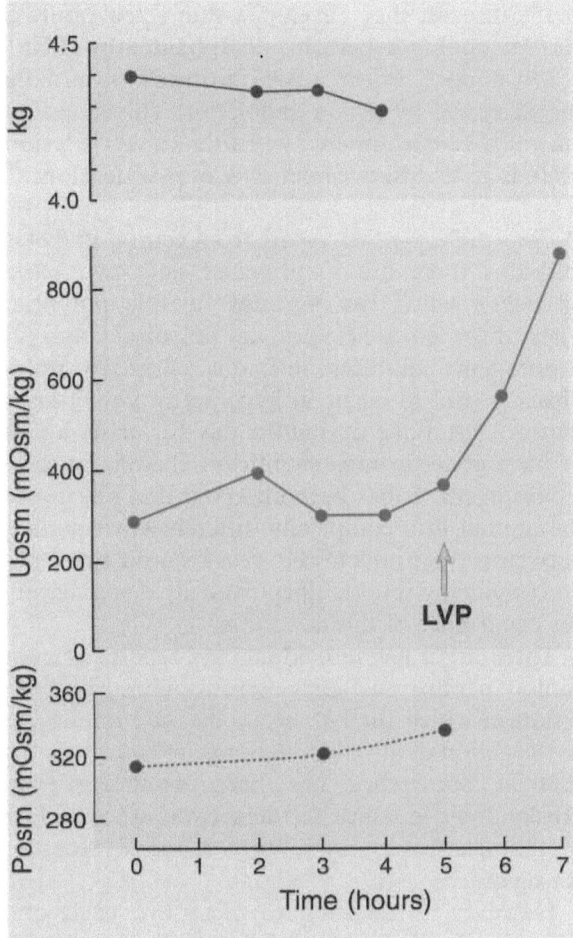

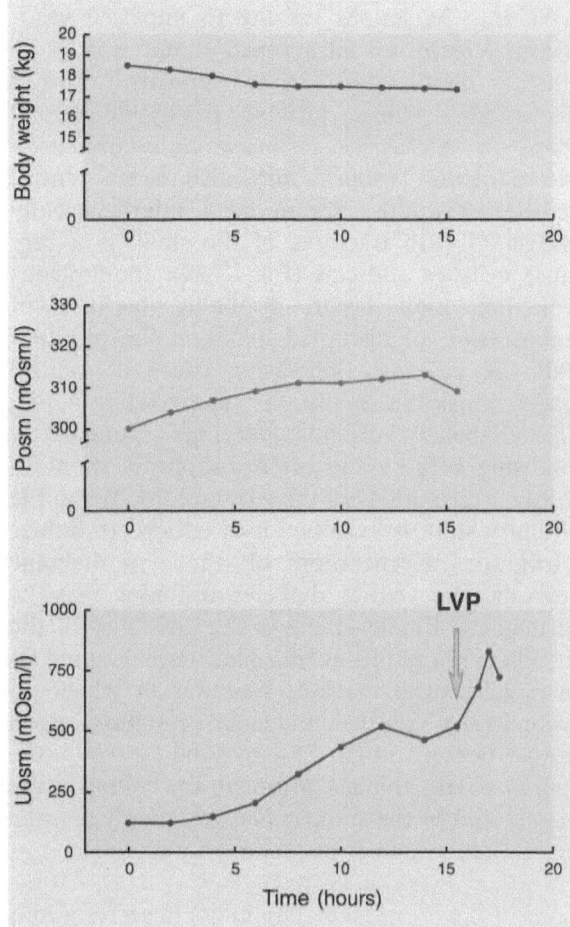

Fig. 2-29. The effect of water deprivation on body weight, plasma osmolality (Posm) and urine osmolality (Uosm) in a 4-year-old castrated male cat with a history of head trauma. The arrow represents an injection of aquous vasopressin (lysine-vasopressin, LVP). In this case the dehydration-induced rise in Posm did not lead to an increase in Uosm. This in combination with the sharp rise in Uosm following vasopressin administration justified the diagnosis of complete central diabetes insipidus.

Fig. 2-30. In a 5-month-old mongrel dog presented for polyuria, water deprivation led to a slow, subnormal rise in urine osmolality (Uosm). At maximal Uosm, i.e., when a "plateau" was reached, vasopressin (lysine-vasopressin, LVP) administration caused a 60% increase in urine osmolality. These observations are compatible with partial central diabetes insipidus.

strong osmotic stimuli for AVP secretion, (2) absence of renal disease, (3) a rise in urine osmolality following the administration of vasopressin.

Pathogenesis. Insufficient AVP release may be caused by defects at several functional sites in the chain of events which regulates discharge of the hormone into the blood. As a result, different forms of central diabetes insipidus can be distinguished. In dogs and cats only two forms have been recognized: complete and partial central

diabetes insipidus. In the first type there is very little rise in urine osmolality with increasing plasma osmolality. These animals are essentially devoid of releasable AVP (Fig. 2–29). In the second type AVP is released with increasing plasma osmolality but is subnormal in amount (Fig. 2–30). In some cases this moderate AVP release only starts at rather high plasma osmolality values and therefore it may be said that not only is the secretory capacity limited but that there is also a high setting of the osmoreceptor.

Among the lesions leading to impaired vaso-pressin release, an intracranial tumor is a likely cause in middle-aged and old animals.[23] This is most often a primary pituitary (or hypothalamic) neoplasm. Metastatic lesions and inflammatory and parasitic lesions[24] may also cause central diabetes insipidus. Severe head injury, usually associated with fractures of the skull, is a rare cause in dogs and cats (Fig. 2–29); spontaneous remission may occur, probably because of regeneration of disrupted axons in the pituitary stalk. A currently increasing cause of central diabetes insipidus is pituitary surgery (see 4.3.1). The diabetes insipidus develops immediately following surgery and often disappears spontan-eously after periods of days to months. When the pituitary stalk is sectioned high enough to induce retrograde degeneration of the hypothalamic neurons, the central diabetes insipidus may be permanent. Finally, there is the possiblity of the so-called idiopathic form. This term is used in cases of central diabetes insipidus in which no lesion in the hypothalamic and/or pituitary region can be demonstrated. This may be especially the case in young animals, although the course of the disease and/or the autopsy may eventually reveal a lesion that could not be identified initially.[25]

Clinical manifestations. The major manifestations are polyuria, polydipsia, and a near-continuous demand for water. These symptoms may be sudden in onset and the maximum urine flow reached in one or two days. In severe cases water intake and urine volume may be immense, requir-ing micturition almost every hour throughout day and night. However, in the incomplete forms the urine volume may be only moderately increased. In the severe cases the enormous water intake may interfer with food intake and result in weight loss. It will be clear that animals in which a large neo-plasm is the underlying cause may have additional neurologic signs (see 2.2.5).

The urine concentration will be below that of plasma (s.g. < 1.010 and Uosm < 290 mosmol/kg) but in the mild cases higher osmolalities (up to 600 mosmol/kg) may be found. Blood examination usually does not reveal abnormalities except for a slight hypernatremia due to commonly inadequate replenishment of the excreted water. When water is withheld from animals with the complete form

of the disease, they develop within a few hours a life-threatening hypertonic encephalopathy (PNa^+ > 170 mmol/l; Posm > 375 mosmol/kg), initially characterized by ataxia and sopor. This situation may also be encountered when the causitive lesion extends to the thirst center and adipsia develops.[26]

Differential diagnosis. Apart from central diabetes insipidus there are in principal only two basic disorders which can account for the polyuria. These disorders are (1) primary polydipsia, and (2) nephrogenic diabetes insipidus. Primary poly-dipsia is said to occur in hyperactive young dogs that are left alone during the day for many hours or have gone through significant changes in their environment. It has been observed that placing of the animal in a completely different environment may stop the problem. However, so far there are no convincing reports unequivocally documenting the occurrence of this condition.

There are a few individual case reports of con-genital nephrogenic diabetes insipidus, the con-dition in which the kidney tubules are insensitive to the action of antidiuretic hormone. Recently the familial occurrence has been documented in Husky dogs, in which the defect was ascribed to a mutation affecting the affinity of the V_2 receptor for ligand.[27]

However, in addition to these two basic and infrequently encountered differential diagnoses, a wide variety of conditions cause polyuria. In the young animal this may be congenital kidney disease, whereas at all ages acquired kidney disease may lead to polyuria. Especially in the middle-aged and elderly animals (endocrine) conditions such as diabetes mellitus, hyperadreno-corticism, hyperthyroidism, pyometra, progestin-induced (luteal phase) growth-hormone excess, hyperparathyrodism, hypercalcemia of malig-nancy, and the syndrome of inappropriate vasopressin secretion (see 2.3.2) have to be con-sidered. Then there are conditions such as hepato-encephalopathy and heart failure that may be associated with polyuria, although in these diseases polyuria is seldom a presenting symptom. This range of possiblities may make it a difficult task to come to a diagnosis in an animal with polyuria. In Chapter 15 an algorithm is presented that may be helpful.

Diagnosis. The water deprivation test combined with vasopressin adminstration, as examplified in Figs. 2–29 and 2–30 and described in detail in Chapter 13, is most commonly used for differentiating the causes of polyuria. The test is difficult to perform correctly, unpleasant for the animal, relies heavily on the emptying of the bladder, and is indirect because changes in urinary concentration are used as an index of vasopressin release. Furthermore, the stimulus to vasopressin release is a combination of hypertonicity and hypovolemia, especially towards the end of the period of dehydration.

A more direct way to differentiate between the three basic causes of polyuria rests on the measurement of plasma vasopressin during osmotic stimulation by hypertonic saline infusion (Figs. 2–28, 2–31; Chapter 13). As in man[28] this approach can improve the diagnostic accuracy. The advantage is not in the severe forms of central diabetes insipidus, as in these conditions the standard indirect test will give a correct diagnosis. In all other categories of polyuria, i.e., in animals that concentrate their urine to various degrees during dehydration, the indirect test may be less reliable. Dogs in which the polyuria had initially been attributed to renal disease or to primary polydipsia proved to have partial central diabetes insipidus in the direct test. However, with regard to primary polydipsia some reservation in the interpretation is needed, as it was recently demonstrated for humans that this chronic overhydration downregulates the release of AVP in response to hypertonicity.[29]

The use of this direct approach has been limited but it is worth considering in the few unresolved cases that remain after exclusion of the many other causes of polyuria (see algorithm in Chapter 15). It is often a question of whether the animal must endure for,may years a life hampered by thirst, a large bladder, and unwanted behavior.

Treatment. As for almost all peptides, orally administered vasopressin is ineffective. Aquous (lysine-)vasopressin[d] may be administered subcutaneously in doses of 2–5 U, and will act for only about 3 h, and therefore the effect may be hardly noticeable by the owner. Its main use may

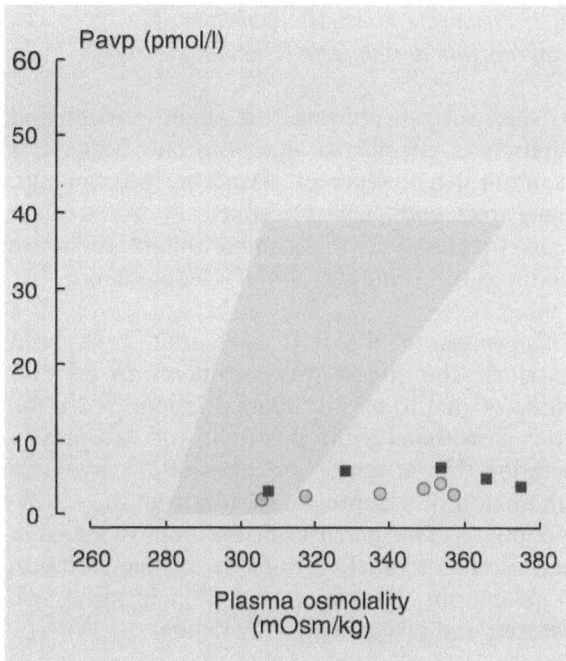

Fig. 2-31. Relation of plasma vasopressin with plasma osmolality (Pavp) during hypertonic saline infusion in two dogs with central diabetes insipidus caused by pituitary tumor.[23] See also legend to Fig. 2–28.

be in the rare case of hypertonic encephalopathy.

The vasopressin analogue desmopressin, DDAVP (1-deamino, 9-D-arginine vasopressin)[e], provides antidiuretic activity for about 8 h. One drop (= 1.5–4 µg DDAVP) placed twice daily in the conjunctival sac sufficiently controls the polyuria in most dogs with central diabetes insipidus. With the administration of three drops a day the urine production usually returns to normal.

Prognosis. In the absence of a neoplastic lesion the long-term prospects are good. With appropriate treatment the animals become asymptomatic. Especially untreated animals with the complete form are always at risk of developing life-threatening dehydration when left without water for longer than a few hours. Animals with diabetes insipidus due to a pituitary tumor may lead acceptable lives for many months until the lesion has reached such size that mass effects develop (see 2.2.5).

[d] Vasopressin-Sandoz® (lypressin), Sandoz A.G., Basel, Switzerland

[e] Minrin®, Ferring AB, Malmö, Sweden (0.1 mg DDAVP/ml); also available as injection preparation, spray and tablet (= less effective).

2.3.2 *Vasopressin excess; syndrome of inappropriate antidiuresis (SIAD)*

In this rare syndrome the high vasopressin secretion is considered inappropriate because it occurs in the presence of plasma hypoosmolality. Apart from endogenous vasopressin excess, there is also the possiblity that similar abnormalities are produced by administration of vasopressin.

Pathogenesis. In the few cases that have been described, the disease was considered to be idiopathic or due to an intracranial lesion.[30,31] In the latter case there is the possibility of vasopressin secretion by a tumor or nonspecific irritative stimulation of vasopressin release from the neurohypophysis. The long list of conditions reported in man as causes of SIAD include ectopic secretion by neoplasms, eutopic secretion in intrathoracic diseases, and drugs such a vincristine.

Clinical manifestations. The hypotonicity leads to generalized cellular edema. Unlike extracranial tissues that can expand freely, the distending brain is compressed against the unyielding cranium. The resulting hypotonic encephalopathy causes weakness and lethargy, which may proceed to convulsions, coma and death as hypotonicity worsens.

Besides these neurologic manifestations, the dogs described so far also had polyuria, which seems to be somehwat paradoxical in these situations of vasopressin excess. It may be explained by the experimental observation that chronic exposure of the kidney to increased amounts of vasopressin eventually leads to impaired responsiveness to the hormone.

Differential diagnosis. When the diagnosis of SIAD is considered, other conditions that may be associated with hyponatremia have to be excluded: e.g., primary adrenocortical insufficiency, heart failure, and hypothyroidism.

Diagnosis. The combination of hypotonicity and detectable amounts of circulating vasopressin is diagnostic for SIAD. Additional measurements during hypertonic saline infusion allow the

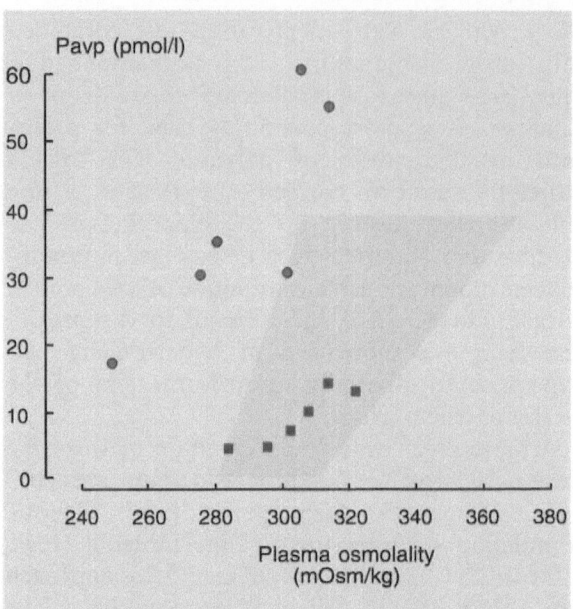

Fig. 2-32. Relation of plasma vasopressin (Pavp) to plasma osmolality during hypertonic saline infusion in two dogs with the syndrome of inappropriate antidiuresis (SIAD). In one of the dogs there was already a strong increase in vasopressin values at a very low threshold (blue dots). In the other dog there was an inappropriate elevation of the unstimulated basal vasopressin levels, and the level only started rising when plasma osmolality reached the normal range (red squares); this is regarded as a constant nonsuppressible "leakage" of vasopressin from the neurohypophysis, with otherwise normal osmoreceptor function.[30] See also legend to Fig. 2–28.

distinction of different forms of inappropriate vasopressin release (Fig. 2–32).

Treatment. In the cases in which the underlying cause of the SIAD cannot be corrected, water intake should be restricted to prevent severe hyponatremia. The vasopressin antagonists developed so far have not proven to be sufficiently effective for clinical application.[32]

Prognosis. In the idiopathic form of the disease, water restriction will allow the animals to live an almost normal life for several years. Their behavior will indicate continuing thirst but the neurological signs will only reappear when accidentally too much water is given. If the disease is caused by a tumor, the degree of malignancy and/or the rate of expansion will determine the prognosis.

3. Thyroids

3.1 Introduction

In the dog and cat the thyroid glands are separate lobes lying beside the trachea from about the third to the eigthth tracheal ring. They are covered ventrally by the sternohyoid and sternothyroid muscles. Normal thyroid glands are not palpable.

Embryologically the thyroids originate from a midline evagination of the pharyngeal epithelium. Also lateral primitive cells migrate medially to fuse with the median-derived tissues, and these primarily contribute the parafollicular or C cells. Thus the so-called thyroglossal duct is formed. During its descent remnants of tissue may persist along the course of this tract. Rarely, these remnants are the sole functioning thyroid tissue. In such cases, its secretion may not be sufficient to maintain a normal metabolic (euthyroid) state (see 3.2.1).

The basic functional unit of the thyroid is the follicle, a hollow sphere of cells, about 30–300 μm in diameter. The wall of the follicle is a single layer of thyroid epithelial cells. These follicular cells are cuboical when quiescent (Fig. 3–1) and columnar when active. The lumen is filled with a protein-aceous colloid that contains a large glycoprotein called thyroglobulin, within the sequence of which the thyroid hormones are synthesized and stored. The C cells are largely located in the interfollicular spaces and secrete calcitonin (Fig. 3–1).

Hormone synthesis and secretion. The main secretory hormonal product of the thyroid gland is L-thyroxine or $3,5,3',5'$-L-tetraiodothyronine (T_4). The other thyroid hormone, $3,5,3'$-L-triiodo-thyronine (T_3), is secreted in much smaller quantities (about 20% of that of T_4). Most of the circulating T_3 is produced in peripheral tissues by outer ring deiodination of T_4. Inner ring deiodination results in the metabolically inactive $3,3',5'$triiodothyronine (reverse T_3, rT_3) (Fig. 3–2).

Iodide, the main building block of the thyroid hormones, is actively transported ("trapped") from the extracellular fluid into the thyroid follicular cells, resulting in thyroid/plasma-concentration ratios of around 25. Tissues other than the thyroid, such as gastric mucosa, salivary glands and choroid plexus, also have an active

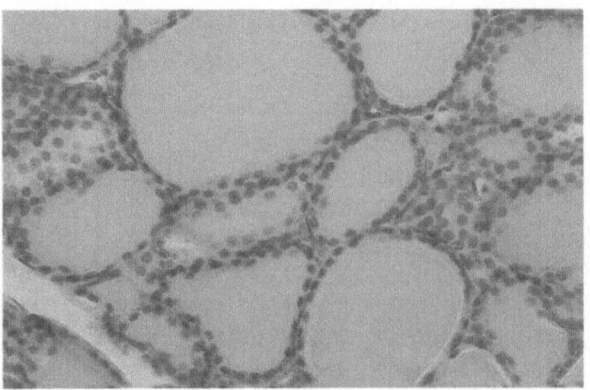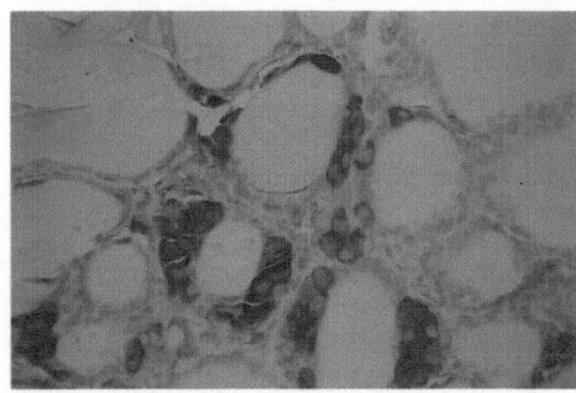

Fig. 3-1. Left: Microscopic picture of the thyroid gland of a healthy adult dog, illustrating the variable sizes of the thyroid follicles. Right: Immunoperoxidase stain for the calcitonin-secreting C cells or parafollicular cells in a healthy adult dog.

A. Rijnberk (ed.), Clinical Endocrinology of Dogs and Cats, 35–59.

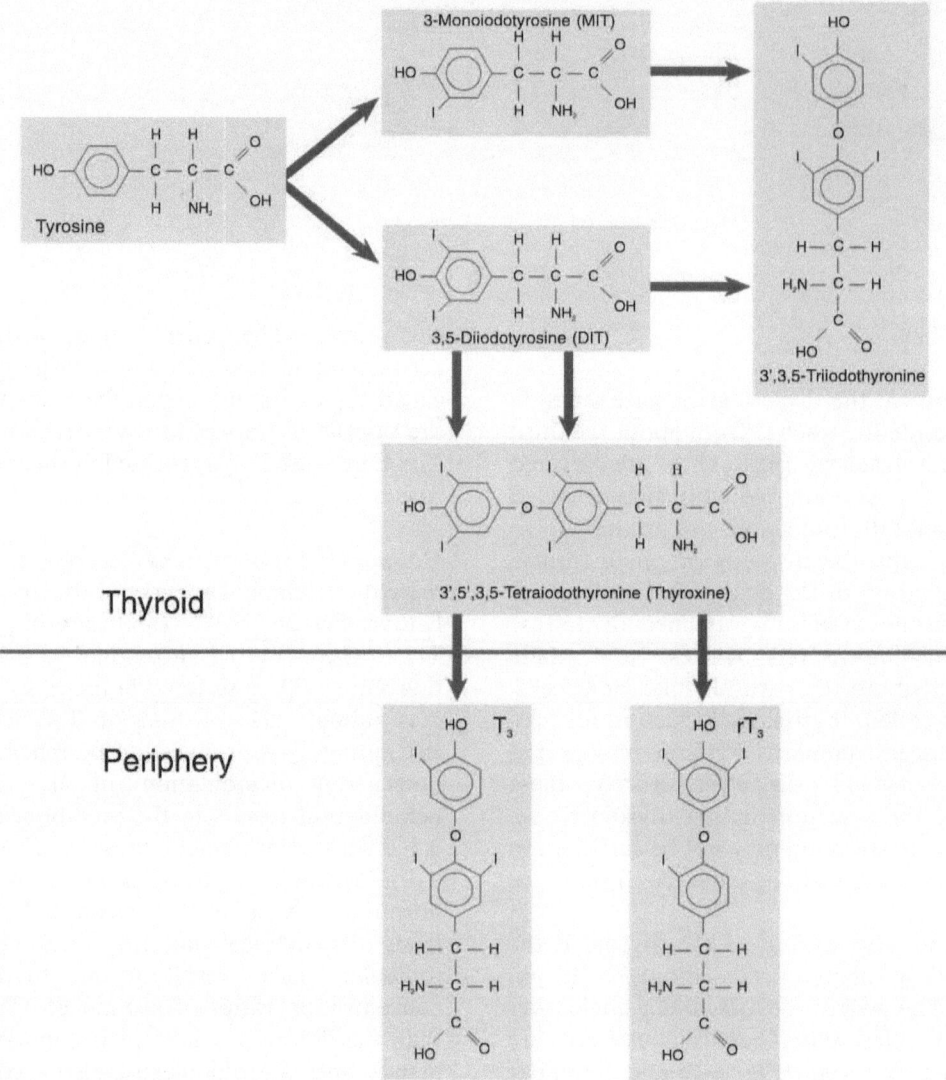

Fig. 3-2. Structures of the amino acid tyrosine, intrathyroidally formed iodotyrosines (MIT and DIT) and iodothyronines (T_4 and T_3), and two products of peripheral deiodination of T_4, i.e., T_3 and reverse T_3 (3′,5′,3-triiodothyronine).

transport mechanism for iodide. In contrast to the thyroids, these tissues do not have the capacity for organic binding of iodide.

All of these iodide-concentrating tissues are also capable of concentrating other structurally related monovalent anions such as thiocyanate (SCN^-), perchlorate (ClO_4^-) and pertechnetate (TcO_4^-). However, unlike iodide, these ions are also not organically bound in the thyroid and hence their duration within the thyroid is short. This property together with its short physical half-life, makes the radioactive isotope of pertechnetate ($^{99m}TcO_4^-$) a valuable radionuclide for imaging the thyroid by scintillation scanning.

Once within the thyroid cell, inorganic iodide is rapidly oxidized by thyroid peroxidase in the presence of H_2O_2 into a reactive intermediate that is then incorporated into tyrosine residues of acceptor proteins, mainly thyroglobulin. These iodotyrosines (MIT and DIT) in thyroglobulin can combine to form iodothyronines (Fig. 3–2). Both organic binding of iodide and coupling of iodotyrosines can be inhibited by thiourea compounds, which are used in the treatment of

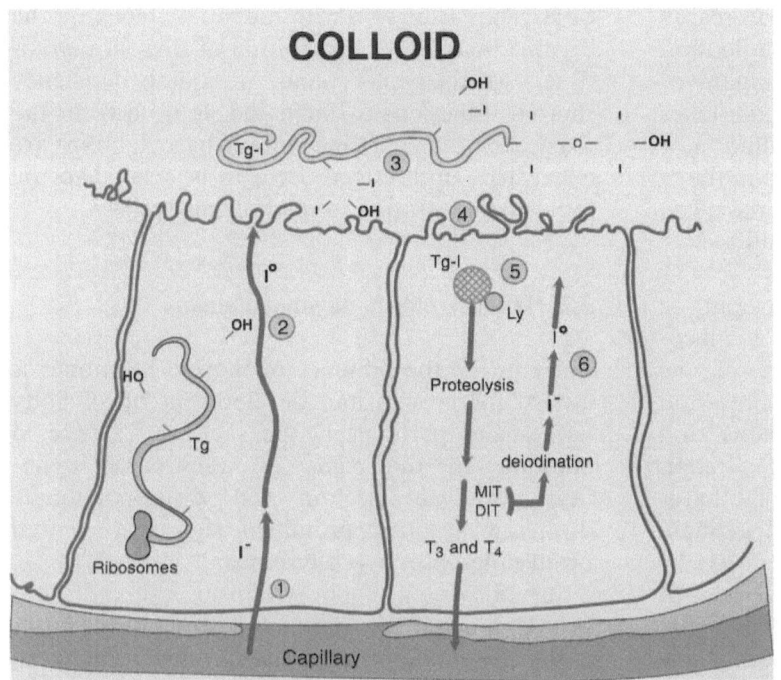

COLLOID

Fig. 3-3. Schematic representation of thyroid hormone biosynthesis (left) and secretion (right): (1) Active transport of iodide from the blood into the thyroid cell, (2) oxidation of the iodide by peroxidase and transfer of this oxidized iodide to tyrosyl residues of thyroglobulin (Tg), (3) coupling of two DIT molecules or MIT + DIT to form respectively T_4 and T_3 (see also Fig. 3–2), (4) endocytosis or pinocytosis of colloid droplets, (5) fusion of colloid droplets with lysosomes (Ly) and subsequent hydrolysis of Tg with release of T_3 and T_4, (6) deiodination of free iodotyrosines and intrathyroidal reutilization of iodide.

hyperthyroidism (see 3.4.1). The thyroglobulin is iodinated at the apical (follicular) border of the cell and is then brought into the colloid by exocytosis (Fig. 3–3).

For secretion, thyroglobulin is resorbed into the thyroid cell via pinocytosis of colloid droplets (Fig. 3–3). Each colloid droplet is enclosed in a membrane derived from the apical border. This is combined with a lysosome and as the phagolysosome moves toward the basal aspect of the cell the droplet becomes smaller and more dense with progression of the hydrolysis of the thyroglobluin by the lysosomal proteases (Fig. 3–3).

Hormone transport and metabolism. Plasma T_4 and T_3 are largely bound to protein. Less than 0.05% of T_4 and less than 0.5% of T_3 circulate "free", in the unbound state. It is this free hormone concentration that is maintained constant by the feedback regulatory system and that appears to parallel the rate of cellular uptake of these hormones. Thus it is the free hormone concentration that determines the thyroid status irrespective of the total plasma concentration. The levels of circulating binding proteins (the high affinity binding globulin, TBG and a low affinity albumin and pre-albumin) may be changed by a variety of

diseases and pharmacologic agents, e.g., salicylates and phenytoin. Especially alterations in the TBG concentration may have considerable effect on total plasma hormone concentration as it usually measured, although the concentration of free hormone may remain unchanged.

Deiodination of the iodothyronines is the most significant metabolic transformation of the thyroid hormones. About 80% of the secreted T_4 is deiodinated to form T_3 and rT_3, predominantly in liver and kidney and catalyzed by Type-I deiodinase.[1] T_3 has approximately three to four times the metabolic potency of the parent hormone, which means that almost all of the metabolic action of T_4 can be ascribed to the action of T_3. The notion that the thyroid itself contributes little to the T_3 pool does not apply to states of hyperfunction. In these situations the T_3/T_4 ratio of the secretory product increases.

As mentioned above, rT_3 has little if any metabolic activity and therefore the relative rates of outer- and inner-ring monodeiodination of T_4 determine the quantity of metabolically active hormone available. Factors that impair T_3 formation, such as fasting and several nonthyroidal diseases, almost invariably increase plasma rT_3 concentrations. Selective impairment of deio-

38

dination of the outer ring causes both decreased conversion of T_4 to T_3 and decreased degradation of rT_3 to $3,3'$-T_2. An important determinant of whether 5-deiodination or 5'-deiodination takes place is the conjugation with sulfate. Sulfation of T_4 and T_3 appears to be a facilitating step in the 5-deiodination process by the Type I deiodinase, i.e., the formation of rT_3-sulfate and $3,3'T2$-sulfate.

Regulation of thyroid function. Thyrotropin or thyroid-stimulating hormone (TSH), a glucoprotein secreted by the anterior lobe of the pituitary, promotes thyroid hypertrophy and hyperplasia, and stimulates the synthesis and secretion of thyroid hormones. This TSH secretion by the pituitary is inhibited primarily by T_3, that is produced locally from T_4 by Type II deiodinase (catalyzes deiodination exclusively at the 5'-position) and also by T_3 derived from the pool of free T_3 (Fig. 3–4).[1] The setting of this T_4/T_3-TSH feedback loop is modulated by a hypothalamic tripeptide, TSH-releasing hormone (TRH) (see Fig. 1–2), that stimulates TSH release, whereas somatostatin (see Fig. 2–5) and possibly other neuropeptides inhibit TSH release.

There is also an intrathyroidal regulation of thyroid function, which is especially important in situations of insufficient or excessive iodine supply. This autoregulation enables an immediate adaptation to acute iodide excess (e.g., disinfection of large areas of skin with iodine) by blocking the organic binding, i.e., inhibition of thyroid peroxidase. On the other hand, in iodine deficiency thyroid function is increased long before the thyroidal organic iodine stores (thyroglobulin) are exhausted. Both effects seem to be related to the iodide concentration in the follicular cell.

3.2 Hypothyroidism in young animals

Early in life the presence of thyroid hormones is crucial for growth and development of all body tissues and particularly the skeleton.[2] Hence in addition to the signs of adult-onset hypothyroidism (see Section 3.3), disproportionate dwarfism may be a prominent sign of congenital or juvenile-onset hypothyroidism.

Juvenile-onset hypothyroidism can be congenital or acquired. Among the causes of the latter is the classic iodine deficiency, which occurred in times when owners took too literally the notion that dogs and cats are carnivores. A diet consisting of meat alone is deficient in many respects and certainly in iodine. The lack of the essential building block of the thyroid hormones results in TSH-induced thyroid hyperplasia. In mild deficiencies the increased capacity for hormone production compensates sufficiently and euthyroidism is maintained. However, in severe iodine

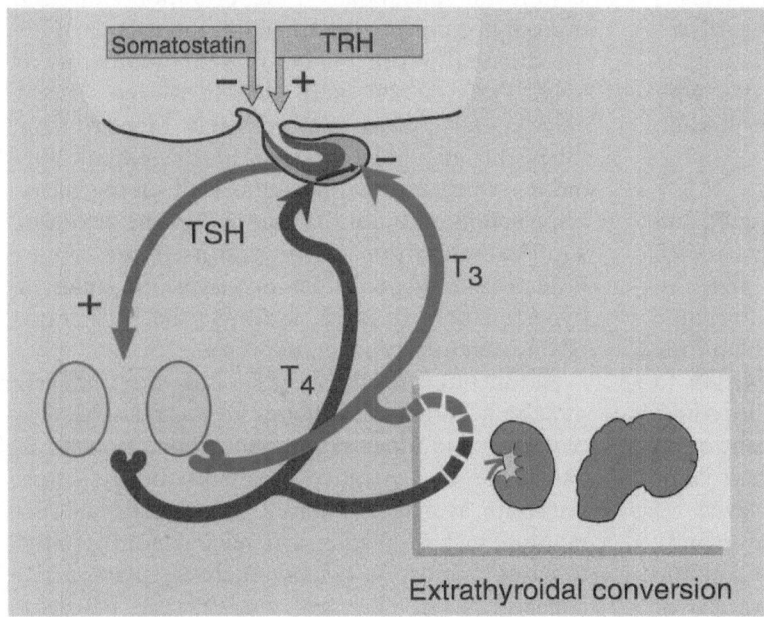

Fig. 3-4. Schematic illustration of the hypothalamus-pituitary-thyroid axis. Hypothalamic TRH reaches the thyrotropic cells in the anterior lobe of the pituitary by the local portal vessels and enhances TSH secretion. Thyroid hormones and particularly systemic and locally produced T_3, reduce the number TRH receptors on the thyrotropic cell, thus impairing its responsiveness to TRH.

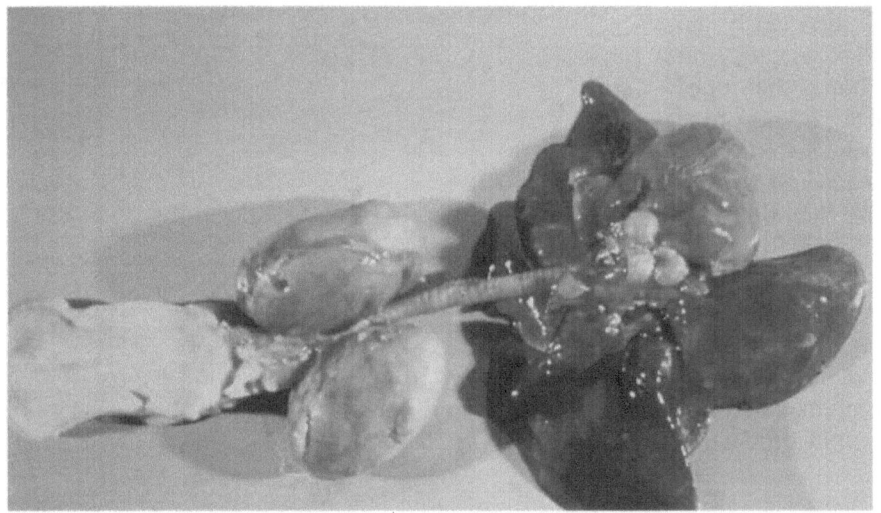

Fig. 3-5. Autopsy specimen from a 6-week-old Newfoundland puppy, whose mother had been fed only tripe. On the left is the large tongue in front of two enormous thyroid glands (goiters), that have become enlarged as the result of iodine deficiency. On the right are the heart and the lungs. At the base of the heart are three goitrous nodules arising from ectopic thyroid tissue.

deficiency there is insufficient production of thyroid hormone despite the compensatory thyroid hyperplasia. Animals with severe iodine deficiency are presented with the combination of large goiters (Fig. 3–5) and signs of hypothyroidism such as sluggishness and retarded growth. This entity is no longer seen in countries in which it is customary to feed manufactured diets, which are rather rich in iodine.

Another, although also very rare, cause of acquired juvenile-onset hypothyroidism is lymphocytic thyroiditis. This is the common cause of primary hypothyroidism in the adult dog. Rarely the process of autoimmune destruction of the thyroid glands occurs during adolescence and as a consequence the animal may be slightly retarded in growth, in addition to developing the signs of hypothyroidism of the adult.

In the dog and cat two forms of congenital hypothyroidism are known to occur, i.e., thyroid dysgenesis and defective thyroid hormone synthesis.

3.2.1 Thyroid dysgenesis

Ectopia of thyroid tissue is common in the dog. In most cases it is the result of the descent of primitive thyroid tissue together with the aortic sac during embryonic life. This explains the occurrence in about 50% of adult dogs of thyroid tissue embedded in the fat on the intrapericardial aorta. Aberrant thyroid tissue may also lie cranial to the thyroid glands as a remnant of the thyroglossal duct. Its existence may be an incidental finding later in life during scanning for other reasons (Fig. 3–6). It may also be associated with the absence of normal thyroid tissue and the function of the ectopic thyroid tissue may be insufficient to prevent hypothyroidism (Fig. 3–7). Complete athyreosis has also been found (Fig. 3–8). In man, it has been proposed that a partial failure of development of thyroid tissue in its normal location may be due to maternal antithyroid antibodies.

Clinical manifestations. The manifestations of hypothyroidism due to thyroid dysgenesis vary according to the duration and severity of the disease before therapy is instituted. In complete athyreosis symptoms are noticed during the second or third month of life, although some animals may not reach this age. Abnormalities in the newborn that may suggest the hypothyroidism include a large fontanelle (which should be closed at birth in dogs but not in cats), hypothermia, hypoactivity, suckling difficulties, and abdominal distension.

As the puppy or kitten grows older, the head becomes relatively large and broad, the facial features become puffy, and the tongue becomes broad and thick (Fig. 3–8). Growth in height is slow and the affected animal engages in little physical activity in comparison with littermates. Mental development appears to be retarded. The coat may be thin and without guard hairs.

Radiography of the spine and long bones reveals

delayed skeletal maturation and abnormally short vertebral bodies that even may give rise to spinal cord compression. In the long bones the appearance of ossification centers is delayed and physeal growth is retarded. In addition the epiphyseal dysgenesis may also be associated with scattered focal areas of ossification, giving the epiphyses a granular appearance (see also Chapter 10).

Diagnosis. Measurements of circulating thyroxine before and after stimulation with TSH (Chapter 13) will confirm the diagnosis of primary hypothyroidism. Thyroid scintiscanning may reveal the cause to be ventral midline ectopia or complete athyreosis.

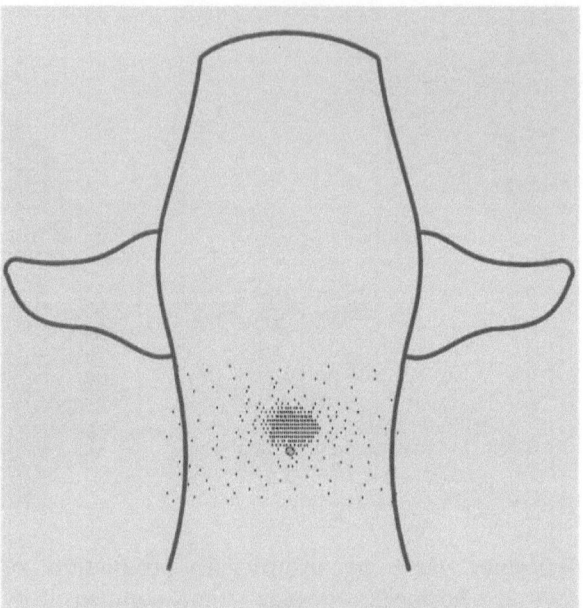

Fig. 3-7. Rectilinear ^{131}I-scintiscan of a four-year-old female German Pointer weighing 18 kg. The dog was presented because of longstanding bilateral symmetrical areas of alopecia on the flanks. The dog's growth had been retarded and it had disproportionately short legs. There were no signs of reduced mental or physical activity. The scan revealed only one small area of ^{131}I accumulation, in the midline, cranial to the normal site of the thyroid glands. Apparently this small remnant from the thyroglossal duct was insufficient to maintain euthyroidism. Substitution with thyroxine was followed by regrowth of hair.

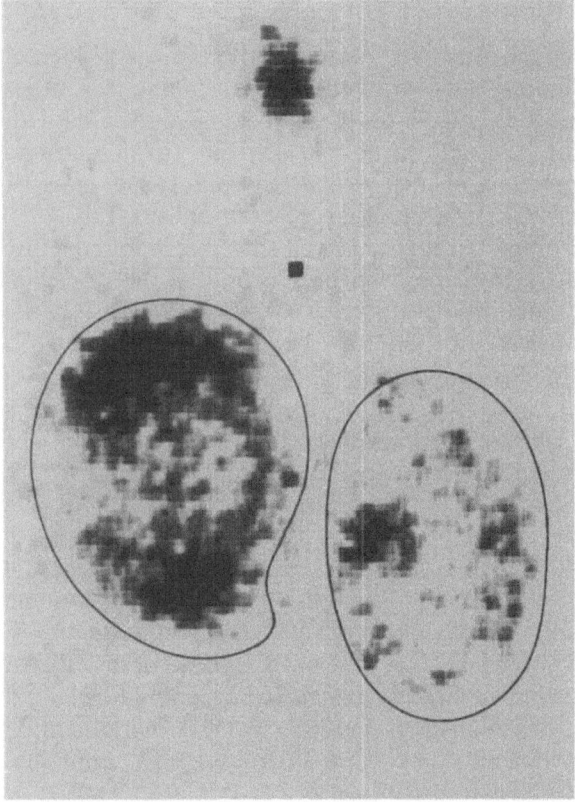

Fig. 3-6. Scintiscan of a dog with bilateral thyroid tumor (palpated outlines indicated by solid lines). The patchy distribution of the radioactivity is compatible with the heterogenous character of the tumors, i.e., areas without the capacity to trap radioiodine (anaplastic tumor, necrosis, and/or hemorrhage) intermingled with areas that accumulate radioiodine (predominantly follicular tumor tissue). Cranial to the reference mark (square dot) on the midline over the cricoid cartilage there is an accumulation of radioactivity in a thyroglossal duct remnant (at the level of the lingual bone).

Treatment. As soon as the condition is diagnosed, treatment should be started with thyroxine (10 μg thyroxine per kg body weight, twice daily). The animal will become much more lively and will develop a normal hair coat. When hypothyroidism is not detected early enough during skeletal maturation, the additional growth may be marginal because administration of thyroxine will also lead to closure of growth plates (Fig. 3–8). The mental sluggishness disappears, however, and usually there is little evidence of persistent mental retardation, a dreaded complication of late detection of congenital hypothyroidism in children.

3.2.2 Defective thyroid hormone synthesis

Congenital hypothyroidism may also occur because of an enzyme deficiency that prevents synthesis of thyroid hormones. Such congenital

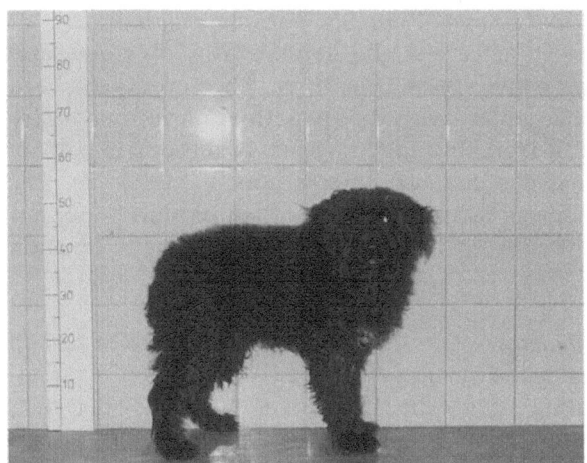

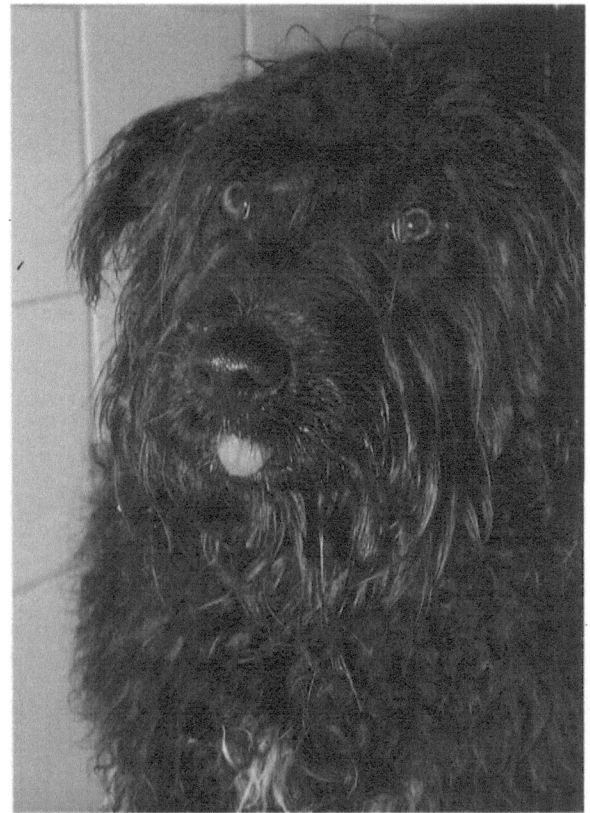

Fig. 3-8. Upper panels: A female Bouvier des Flandres presented at the age of one year for retarded growth and sluggishness. The dog was in good nutritional condition, but weighed only 13 kg. It had disproportinally short legs, a dull facial expression, and a large tongue. Radioiodine studies revealed complete athyreosis. Lower panels: The same dog after four months of oral substitution with thyroxine. Note the much more alert expression and the growth in height. Probably related to the rapidly ensuing sexual maturation (the dog came into estrus after 2 months of treatment), the growth plates closed and there was no further growth in height. The ages in months are indicated on the radiographs.

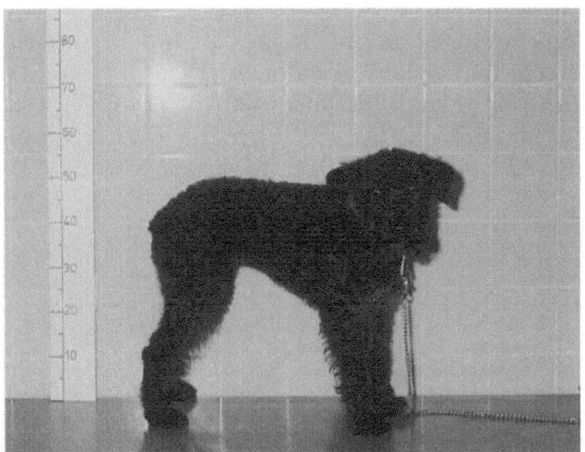

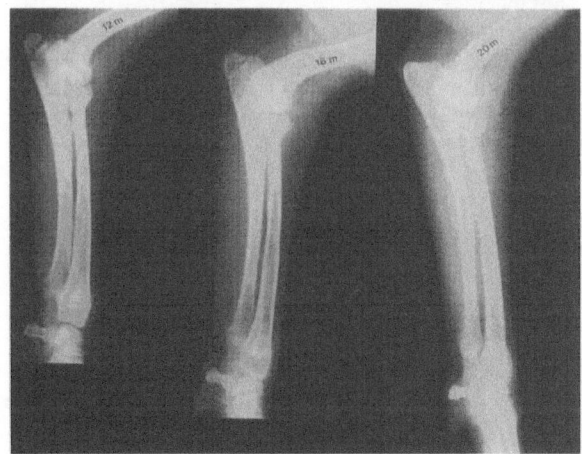

defects are rare and although in principle any step in thyroid hormone synthesis may be affected (see 3.1), thus far unresponsiveness to TSH[3] and defective peroxidase activity[4,5,5a] have been found in the dog and cat. Of these the latter seems to be the least rare form, and is especially seen in cats. Animals with this so-called organification defect concentrate iodide in the thyroid glands but have limited ability to use this iodide in thyroid hormone synthesis. The disorder appears to be heterogenous, for in some animals the defect is complete and no iodide peroxidase activity can be demonstrated, while in others it is partial. In the latter case the defect may be an abnormal localization of the enzyme within the thyroid cell.

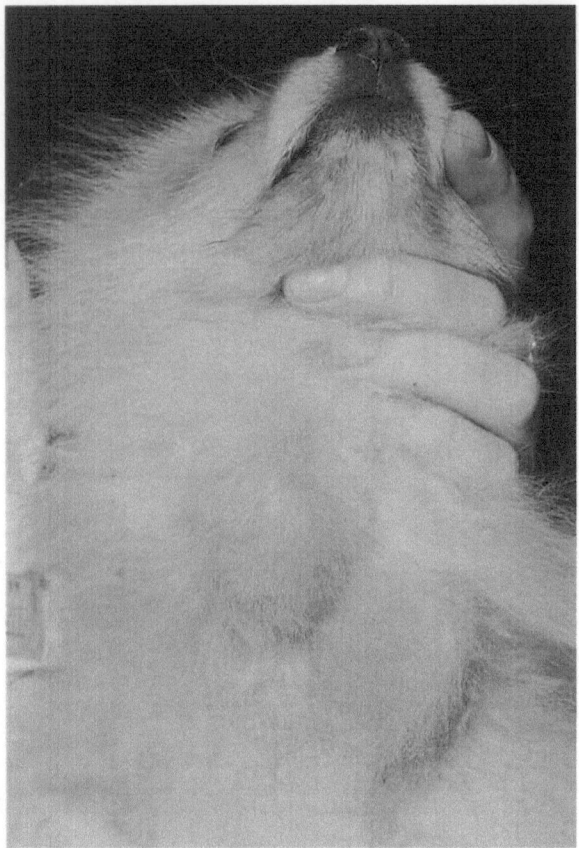

Fig. 3-9. Enlarged thyroid glands of an 11-month-old male Pomeranian. The goitrous glands were first noticed when the dog was 5 months old. There was a defect in organification of iodide by the thyroid glands. The animal was of about normal size but had a thin hair coat and retention of deciduous teeth after eruption of the permanent teeth.

Clinical manifestations. The clinical hallmark of most defects is the combination of goiter and hypothyroidism (Fig. 3–9). The severity of both the goiter and the hypothyroidism may vary considerably and it may also be difficult to palpate a goiter in a very young animal (Fig. 3–10). The clinical features of the hypothyroidism do not differ from those in thyroid dysgenesis (Section 3.2.1).

Diagnosis. The diagnosis of hypothyroidism can be made by measuring the concentration of circulating thyroxine. When a goiter is detected, stimulation with TSH is redundant, as the goiter is already evidence of increased endogenous TSH secretion.

The diagnostic challenge is the elucidation of the defect in thyroid hormone synthesis that is causing the increased TSH secretion. This requires in vivo studies with radioiodine. There is an elevated uptake of radioiodide by the thyroid but the iodide remains nonorganified, as is readily demonstrated by the precipitous discharge of the accumulated radioactivity from the thyroids when an ion that competes for uptake, such as perchlorate or thiocyanate, is given (Fig. 3–11).

Treatment. As in all forms of hypothyroidism except that caused by iodine deficiency, treatment consists of oral administration of thyroxine (see Section 3.2.1). This will lower the TSH secretion and as a result the goiter will shrink.

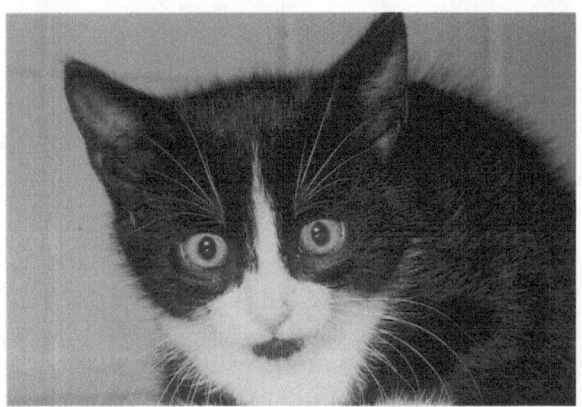
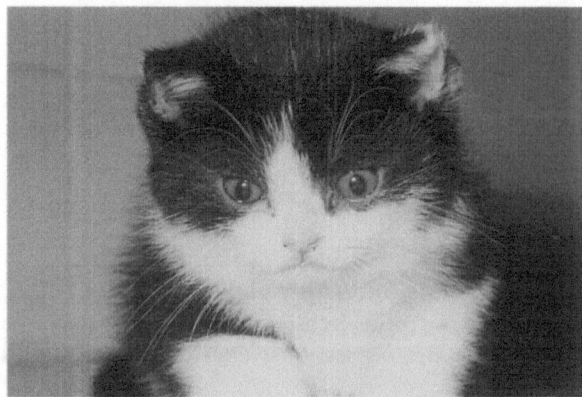

Fig. 3-10. Two 8-week-old littermate kittens. In comparison with its healthy littermate (left), the hypothyroid kitten (right) has a juvenile appearance manifested by a round head and small ears and also by blue irises, while those of the healthy kitten had changed to the yellow of adulthood. The thyroid glands could not be palpated. The hypothyroidism was caused by a complete absence of organification of the iodide taken up by the thyroid gland (Fig. 3–11).

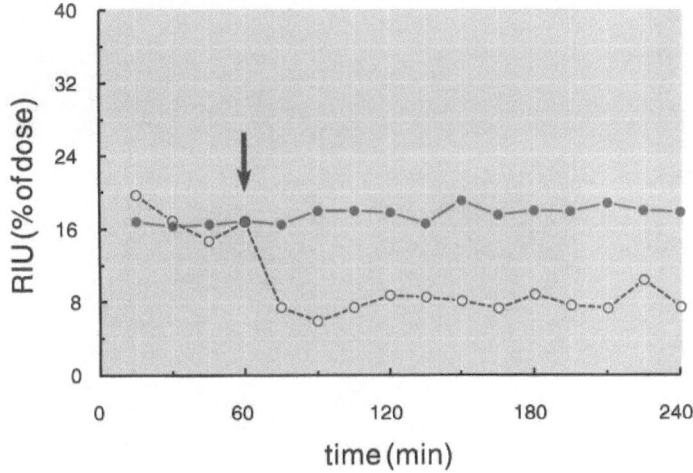

Fig. 3-11. Measurements of thyroidal radioiodide uptake (RIU) at 15-min intervals (solid red line) in a cat with defective organification. The iodide accumulated very rapidly in the thyroid glands and remained at a constant level of about 17% of the administered dose, due to release and re-uptake. The latter was demonstrated in a repeat test by intravenous administration of the competing ion perchlorate (arrow), which caused an abrupt discharge of radioactivity (interrupted blue line).

3.3 Hypothyroidism in adult animals

Hypothyroidism is the clinical syndrome resulting from deficient production of thyroid hormone. At adult age in approximately 95% of cases it is a primary thyroid disorder. Only in 5% or less of cases the disease is of (supra) pituitary origin.

3.3.1 Primary hypothyroidism

Pahogenesis. In the spontaneous form a progressive autoimmune process leads to lymphocytic infiltration and disappearance of thyroid tissue. Also the so-called idiopathic forms, in which there is thyroid atrophy without inflammatory infiltrate, are generally regarded as the end result of an autoimmune disorder. These immune-mediated destructions are slow processes. Clinical manifestations of hormone deficiency will become evident only after a considerable amount of tissue has been destroyed.

Although rare, there may coexist another hormone deficiency syndrome such as diabetes mellitus.[6] These multiple autoimmune endocrine deficiencies are known as polyglandular failure syndromes. The combination of hypothyroidism and hypoadrenocorticism is known as Schmidt's syndrome.[7]

In dogs with hypothyroidism and dogs with lymphocytic thyroiditis with or without overt hypothyroidism, circulating antibodies to thyroglobulin (Tg), a second colloidal antigen and to a thyroid microsomal antigen have been identified.

These autoantibodies and especially those against the microsomal fraction may initiate the complement cascade or antibody-dependent cell-mediated cytolysis resulting in further release of thyroid antigens.

Although they may not be of great pathogenetic importance, autoantibodies against Tg may have some virtue as markers of autoimmune thyroiditis. Circulating antibodies to Tg have been detected in over 50% of hypothyroid dogs. These Tg antibodies may also occasionally interfere with radioimmunoassays used to measure plasma concentrations of thyroid hormones, and especially T_3. The occasional occurrence of T_3 autoantibodies is due to antibodies recognizing a T_3-containing epitope of Tg that is different from the epitopes involved in eliciting the predominant population of canine Tg autoantibodies.[8,9] These rarely (< 1% of samples sent to diagnostic laboratories) occurring T_3 autoantibodies may cause falsely elevated or decreased (depending on the assay) values. T_4-autoantibodies are encountered much less frequently than T_3-autoantibodies; in routine diagnostic laboratories they are observed only once in several years.

Apart from spontaneous hypothyroidism there is the iatrogenic form. This is especially seen in cats as a result of the treatment of hyperthyroidism, a condition frequently occurring in this species. The hypothyroidism may be the result of radioiodine therapy or bilateral thyroidectomy.

Clinical manifestations. Generally thyroiditis remains unnoticed, although very rarely transient signs of hyperthyroidism (mainly characterized by polyuria) have been observed. Most probably this has to be ascribed to the release of thyroid hormone into the circulation during an acute phase of destructive thyroiditis. Eventually these animals will, like the great majority, present with signs referable to thyroid hormone deficiency.

Acquired primary deficiency of thyroid hormone is a condition of young and middle-aged dogs (1–6 years). Dogs of larger breeds are more frequently affected than smaller dogs. The incidence is equally distributed between male and females. So far there is only one convincing description on the occurrence of spontaneous primary hypothyroidism in a cat.[10]

The classical clinical picture of overt hypothyroidism involves simultaneous manifestations from nearly all organ systems. However, even in severe cases symptoms from a single organ system (e.g., locomotor system) may dominate in such a way as to distract from the causative disease.[11,12] Nevertheless, centrally in the syndrome usually there is the history of slowing of mental and physical activities. Most dogs with hypothyroidism have some degree of mental dullness, lethargy and disinterest in exercise (Fig. 3–12). These signs are gradual in onset, often subtle and may not be recognized by the owner until after treatment has been started. Changes of hair and skin are also common observable signs (Figs. 3–12 – 3–16).

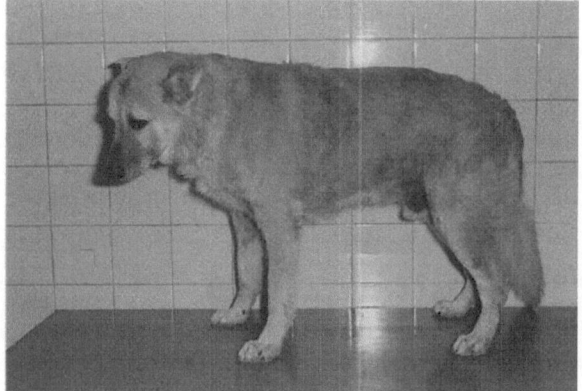

Fig. 3-12. A 4-year-old male mongrel Shepherd dog with primary hypothyroidism. The picture clearly shows the dog's lethargic appearance. In addition the dog had a thin coat with alopecia and some pigmentation in the flanks, groin and on the back of the nose.

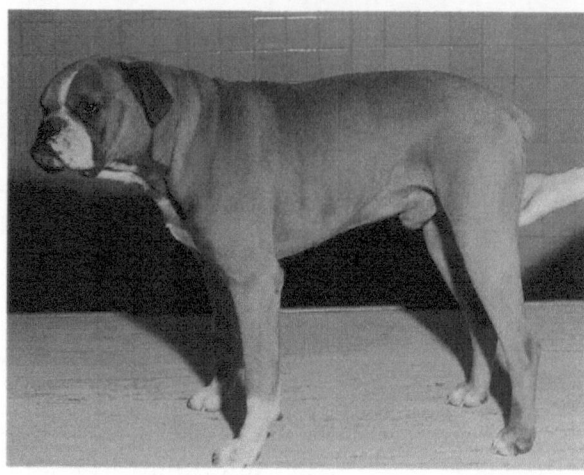

Fig. 3-13. A 4-year-old male Boxer dog with primary hypothyroidism. The skin was thick and inelastic. This being most noticeable in the thick skin folds in the shoulder area, on the lower parts of the forelegs, and above the eyes. The latter together with dropping of the upper eyelids (decreased sympathetic tone) had led to a somewhat tragic facial expression. The stiff gait had caused abnormal wear of the nails of the front feet.

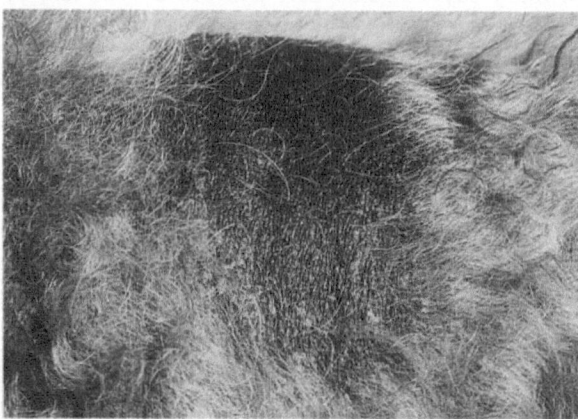

Fig. 3-14. Skin of a 6-year-old female Poodle with primary hypothyroidism, showing dark pigmentation and a somewhat rough surface comparable to emery paper.

Table 3–1 lists the signs and symptoms according to organ systems, of which some changes in the cardiovascular and nervous systems are illustrated in Figs. 3–17 and 3–18.

Differential diagnosis. As indicated above the presenting symptoms may vary widely and therefore the most common pitfall in the diagnosis of hypothyroidism is undoubtedly to overlook the possibility that the presented problem(s) could be

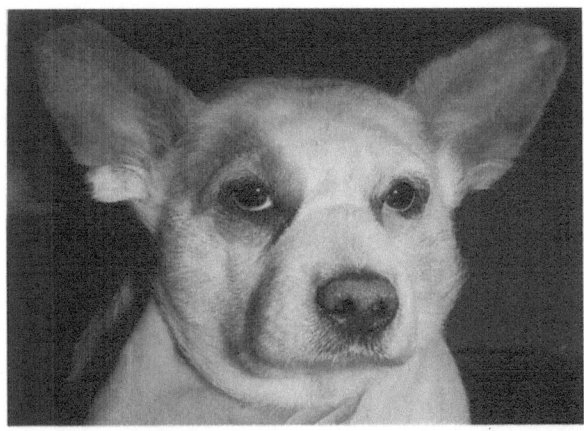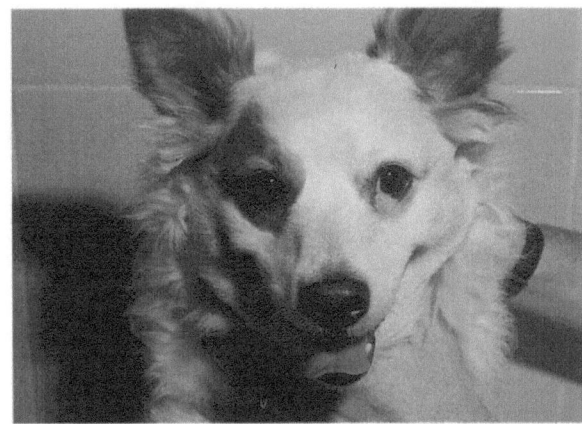

Fig. 3-15. A 6-year-old female mongrel dog with primary hypothyroidism. The puffy appearance due to mucopolysacharide accumulation (myxedema) gave the dog a tragic-/lethargic facial expression (left). A low sympaticotonus leading to blepharoptosis contributes to this appearance These changes were especially noticed in retrospect when the dog returned after four months of treatment (right).

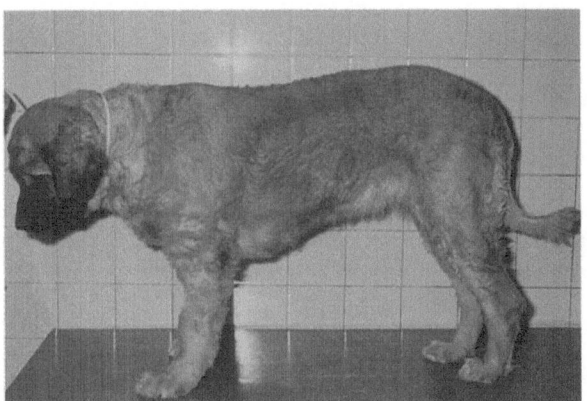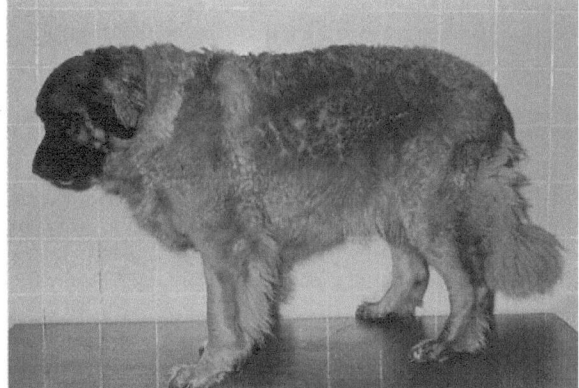

Fig. 3-16. A 2-year-old female Leonberger dog, in which the primary hypothyroidism had resulted in an almost complete loss of the hair coat. Only a sparse, coarse, and short coat had remained (left). Right: the same dog after 7 months of oral supplementation with thyroxine.

due to hypothyroidism. For example, it is not uncommon that dogs with hypothyroidism are presented in specialty areas such as cardio-pulmonology (lethargy misinterpreted as decrease in exercise tolerance) or orthopedics (locomotor disturbance). With regard to the most common problem, lethargy, the disease may be mistaken for metabolic (hepatoencephalophathy) or neurologic (encephalitis, hydrocephalus) cerebrocortical disease. As far as the atrophy of skin and adnexa is concerned, conditions such as estrogen excess (see 6.4), hyperadrenocorticism (see 4.3) and growth hormone deficiency (see 2.2) may also be considered.

Diagnosis. In man a low T_4 level in plasma combined with a high concentration of TSH establishes the diagnosis of primary hypothyroidism. Unfortunately this approach is impossible in the dog as a valid canine-specific assay for TSH is not available.* Therefore the diagnosis of hypothyrodism is still strongly based upon measurements of T_4 concentrations in plasma. As a measure of thyroid function T_4 has to be preferred over T_3, as T_4 is only produced from the thyroid gland. T_3 concentrations in plasma are largely derived from peripheral conversion (see 3.1) and

* See also addendum to section 13.3 (page 212).

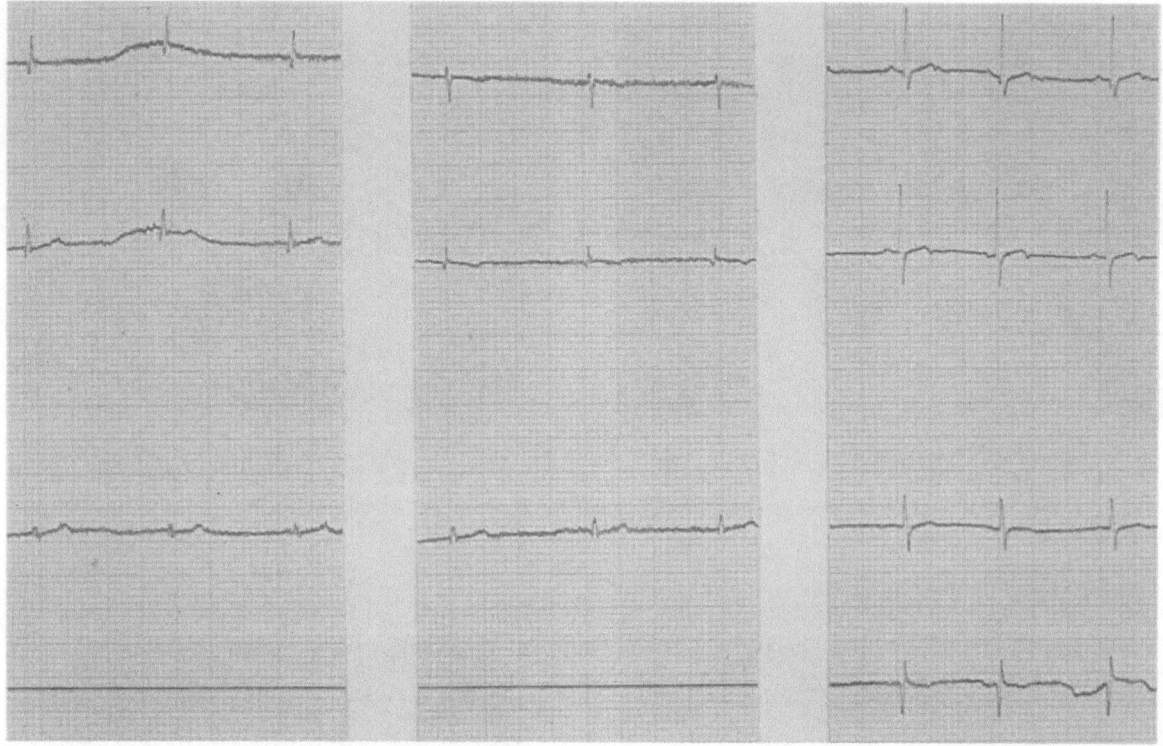

Fig. 3-17. ECG recording of a 4-year-old male Boxer dog with pronounced hypothyroidism (calibration: 1 cm = 1 mV; paper speed 25 mm/s). Left: Lead I, II and III. Middle: Lead aVR, aVL and aVF. Right: Precordial leads CV_6LU, CV_6LL, CV_6RL and V_{10}. There is low voltage of the deflections in all leads. It should be noted that in less pronounced (= less long-standing) cases the ECG changes may be less remarkable or even absent. (Courtesy A.A. Stokhof)

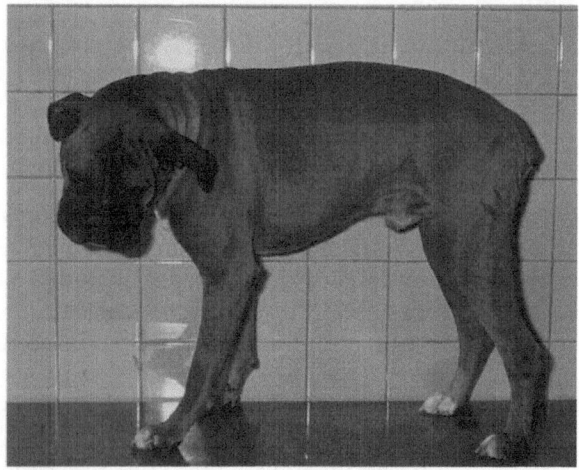

Fig. 3-18. A 3-year-old Boxer dog, in which the primary hypothyroidism was associated with vestibular signs, including head tilt and ataxia. In addition there was facial nerve palsy. Nerve lesions of hypothyroidism include peripheral nerve entrapment from myxedema in surrounding tissue.[11] This may give rise to problems when nerves pass narrow canals such as the facial canal (this dog) and the carpal canal.

may remain within normal limits in moderate hypothyroidism and may be low in many non-thyroidal diseases. In addition the T_3 measurements may be subject to artifactually high or low results due to T_3-autoantibodies (see above).

However, there are also many factors that can affect basal T_4 concentrations in euthyroid dogs, often leading to a false lowering and consequently a false positive diagnosis of hypothyroidism. Of these factors, concurrent illness and drugs (glucocorticoids, antiepileptics and analgesics) are the most relevant. Drugs such as glucocorticoids have multiple effects on peripheral T_4 and T_3 transfer, distribution and metabolism[13]. These effects include altered T_4 binding to plasma carrier proteins, resulting in altered free fraction levels of T_4. Probably due to the multiple character of these drug- and disease-induced effects, measurements of free T_4 concentrations (see also 3.1) in dogs have not provided improvement of the diagnostic accurary above that of measurements of total T_4.[14]

Table 3-1. Clinical manifestations of primary hypothyroidism in adult dogs.

System	Common	Less common/rare
Metabolism	Some weight gain. Unchanged or reduced appetite. Cold intolerance	Tendency to low body temperature
Skin and hair	Coarse and scanty coat. Non-pruritic truncal alopecia, starting over points of wear. Skin thickening due to mucopolysaccharide accumulation (myxedema)	Hyperpigmentation. Secondary pyoderma and/or seborrhea
Cardiovascular	Bradycardia and weak apex beat. Low voltage ECG (Fig. 3-17)	Poor peripheral circulation. Skin cold to the touch.
Reproductive/ Endocrine	Persistent anestrus. Loss of libido. Testicular atrophy	Gynaecomastia and galactorrhea. Polyglandular deficiency syndrome (Schmidt's syndrome)
Neuromuscular	Lethargy and somnolence. Stiff gait (elevated plasma creatinine kinase)	Head tilt, vestibular ataxia (Fig. 3-18), facial nerve paralysis, lameness (entrapment of median/facial nerve in carpal/facial tunnel/canal)
Gastrointestinal		Diarrhea
Hematologic	normochromic, normocytic hypoplastic anemia	

In addition it should be mentioned that drugs such as glucocorticoids may reduce TSH secretion and that the observed low concentrations of circulating thyroid hormone may even suggest a state of hypothyroidism, albeit mild and without the need of thyroid hormone supplementation.[15] However, when considering a completely independent parameter of thyroid function, it is questionable whether glucocorticoids induce a reduction in thyroid function (Fig. 3–19).

Thus the TSH-stimulation test continues to be the most conclusive test for the diagnosis of primary hypothyroidism. The test will distinguish depression of basal T_4 concentrations due to drugs and illness from advanced primary hypothyroidism, but not from secondary hypothyroidism and early stages of primary hypothyroidism (Chapter 13). Here scanning with $^{99m}TcO_4^-$ or even radioiodine-uptake studies may provide the final diagnosis.

Treatment. Although T_3 is the metabolically active thyroid hormone, it is not the supplement of choice. A primary advantage of providing the "prohormone" T_4 is that the body is given the opportunity to regulate the amount of T_3 generated by normal physiologic mechanisms. In fact appropriate T_4 therapy results in normal levels of both T_4 and T_3.

Both T_4-production rates and parenteral L-T_4 replacement doses required to maintain euthyroidism are around 5 µg per kg body weight per day.[16] However, when T_4 is administered orally the bioavailability is low and variable, due to incomplete and variable gastrointestinal absorption.[17] Oral supplementation with synthetic L-

48

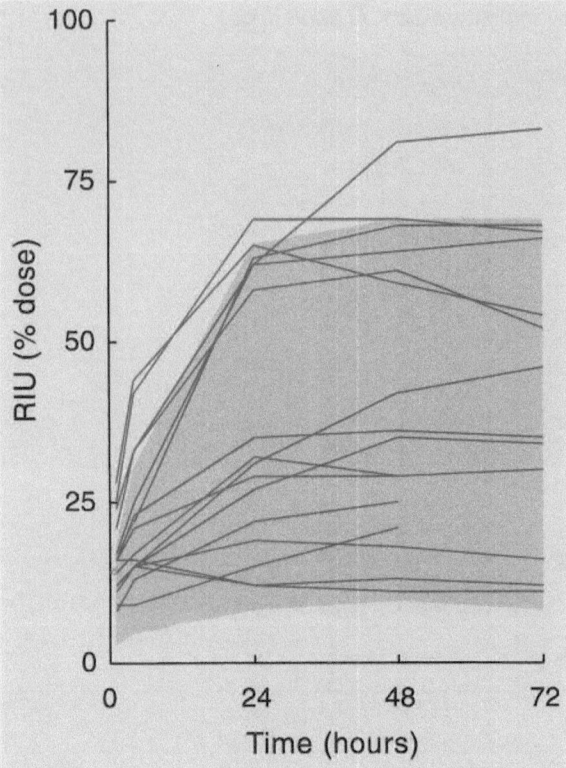

Fig. 3-19. Thyroidal radioiodine uptake in 16 dogs with hyperadrenocorticism[37] (lines) and in 48 healthy pet dogs (blue area) of similar body size.[38] The distribution of the uptake values in both groups was similar, indicating that long-term glucocorticoid excess does not induce a systematic reduction in thyroid function. Note: These measurements were performed in the 1960s, when it was not customary to feed manufactured diets, which are rich in iodine. This explains the rather wide range of uptake values.

thyroxine is started at a dose rate of 10 µg/kg twice daily. After two months a control examination is carried out. Blood is collected at 8-10 h after the last dose. Then the T_4 level in plasma should be between 20 and 40 nmol/l. If not, the dose should be adjusted. Because of the individual variation in intestinal absorption of T_4 further control examinations and adjustments may be needed.

Prognosis. Hypothyroidism is one of the most gratifying diseases to treat, because of the ease and completeness with which it responds to treatment. With appropriate treatment and follow-up examinations (every half year) all of the alterations associated with hypothyroidism are reversible, except for some of the neurologic chnges. The long-term prognosis is excellent.

3.3.2 Secondary hypothyroidism

In secondary or central hypothyroidism the thyroids are not primarily affected but deprived of stimulation by TSH. On histological examination there are no losses of follicles but rather characteristics of inactivity (Fig. 3–20). The condition is rare compared to primary thyroid failure. The spontaneous forms result from a tumor of the pituitary or adjacent regions. Central hypothyroidism may also result from surgical removal of pituitary tumors, whereby there is of course also the possibility that it was present initially.

Clinical manifestations. The clinical picture is similar to that of primary hypothyroidism, although generally less pronounced. There may be lethargy and some alopecia, but the tendency to thickening of the skin is less pronounced (Fig. 2–24). Often there is accompanying impairment in the secretion of other pituitary hormones such as growth hormone and gonadotrophins (Fig. 2–24).

Not uncommonly, the lesion causing low TSH secretion is a hormone-secreting tumor (e.g., ACTH). The symptoms and signs that arise from such a pituitary tumor may precede, accompany, and even obscure the manifestations of pituitary failure. In the example of an ACTH-secreting tumor the central hypothyroidism may only become manifest when the associated hyperadrenocorticism has been cured (see also 4.3.1).

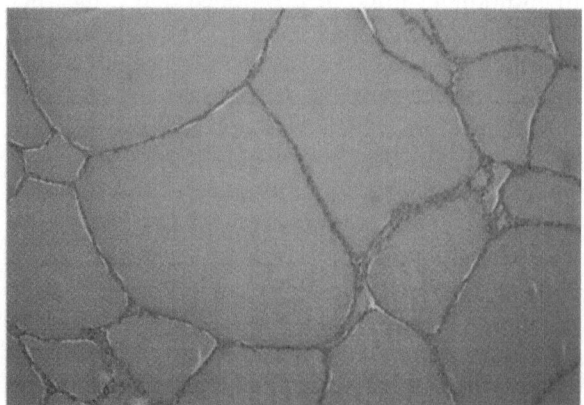

Fig. 3-20. H&E-stained histological section of a thyroid of a 9-year-old long-haired German Pointer with secondary hypothyroidism. Note the relatively large follicles as compared to the inactive (flat) follicular epithelium (see for comparison Fig. 3–1).

Diagnosis. The diagnosis of central hypothyroidism should be based upon the demonstration of low concentrations of T_4 in plasma that increase clearly in a TSH-stimulation test (Chapter 13). This is with the condition that in all likelihood the low T_4 concentration is not caused by illness or drugs.

Apart from thyroid function, diagnostic evaluation should include (1) the secretion of other pituitary hormones (see also 2.2.5 and Chapter 13), and (2) the pathology of the pituitary and adjacent areas (see 2.2.5).

Treatment. Treatment with L-thyroxine can be the same as in primary hypothyroidism (3.3.1). In addition, hypofunction of other endocrine glands resulting from pituitary hormone deficiencies should be corrected. In clinical practice this is usually confined to correcting only for a coexisting ACTH deficiency. It is even advisable to assess pituitary-adrenocortical function and to treat an eventual deficiency with cortisol supplementation (4.2.2) before T_4 therapy is begun. Otherwise there might be the risk of precipitation of a crisis due to glucocorticoid deficiency.

Prognosis. In the spontaneous forms the prospects are completely dependent upon the course of the causitive lesion in the hypothalamus-pituitary area. In the iatrogenic form, i.e., following total hypophysectomy, supplementation with thyroxine (and glucocorticoids!) enables the animal to live a healthy life for many years.

3.4 Hyperthyroidism and thyroid tumors

Neoplastic changes of thyroid epithelial cells may give rise to clinical problems in two ways. First, there is the possibility that the mass is noticed by the owner. This is the common confrontation with a thyroid tumor in the dog. Secondly, there is the possibility that the neoplasm has the capacity to produce thyroid hormone to such an extent that with increasing size an excess of thyroid hormone is produced (Fig. 3–21) and the animal is presented with signs of hyperthyroidism. This is almost invariably the case in cats and is only occasionally seen in dogs.

A disease entity comparable to Graves' disease

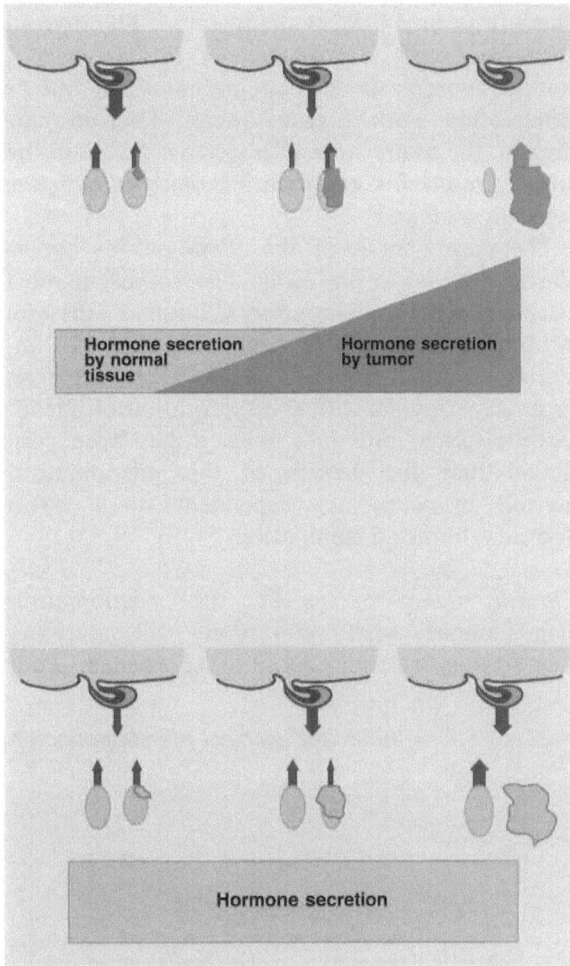

Fig. 3-21. Development of a functional thyroid tumor towards a state of hyperthyroidism (upper figure). As hypersecretion of thyroid hormone progresses, the TSH release successively declines and the remaining thyroid tissue becomes inactive. During development of nonfunctional destructive thyroid tumor (lower figure) thyroid hormone secretion is sustained via the feedback-controlled increased secretion from the contralateral lobe.

in man, i.e., a disease due to TSH-receptor antibodies that stimulate the thyroids, has not yet been observed in dogs or cats. As the clinical entities of thyroid neoplasia differ considerably between dogs and cats, they will be discussed separately in the next sections.

3.4.1 Hyperthyroidism in cats

Feline hyperthyroidism is a disease of middle-aged and old cats, with a mean age of 12 to 13 years.

There is no breed or sex predilection. The thyroid hormone excess is produced by thyroid adenomatous hyperplasia or adenoma, involving one or more often both thyroid lobes. Thyroid carcinoma, the main cause of hyperthyroidism in the dog, accounts for less than 2% of cases of feline hyperthyroidism.[18]

The pathogenesis of the adenomatous hyperplastic changes is not clear. The condition most resembles toxic nodular goiter (Plummer's disease) in humans. Searches for circulating thyroid-stimulating immunoglobulins have been negative. From experiments with transplantation of adenomatous tissue into nude mice it has been concluded that the growth of this adenomatous thyroid tissue is not dependent upon extrathyroidal humoral stimulations.[19]

Clinical manifestations. As the adenomatous glands remain small, very rarely will veterinary help be sought because of an observed mass. Thus acutally all signs and symptoms are due to effects of thyroid hormone excess on organ systems. The classic presentation of a hyperthyroid cat is that of a skinny, hyperactive, old cat with increased appetite and polyuria (Fig. 3–22). It may make a tense and anxious impression with an impaired tolerance for stress, such as restraint.[20] Many organ systems can be affected and the associated signs and symptoms are listed in Table 3–2.

In addition to this classic picture, in about 10% of cases the clinical picture may be quite different. In these cats weight loss remains an important feature, but there is lethargy and anorexia rather than hyperactivity and increased appetite. This form, called "apathetic hyperthyroidism", may represent an end-stage of the disease and may also be associated with cardiac disease (see also Table 3–2).

Differential diagnosis. There are at least two nonthyroid disorders that may simulate certain

Table 3-2. Clinical manifestations of hyperthyroidism in cats.

System	Common	Less common/rare
Metabolism	Weight loss despite increased appetite	Mild hyperthermia
Respiratory/ cardiovascular	Panting, tachycardia (gallop rhythm), "pounding" heart beat. Left ventricular hypertrophy (echography)	Dyspnea, cardiac murmur, cardiac arrhythmias, congestive heart failure
Neuromuscular	Restlessness (irritability)	Weakness, muscle waisting
Renal	Polyuria (low urine S.G.)	Mild elevations of plasma levels of urea and creatinine
Gastrointestinal	Increased faecal volume	Diarrhea, vomiting (after large meal)
Hair and skin	Umkempt hair coat	
Hematologic	Neutrophilic leukocytosis with eosinopenia and lymphopenia (= stress response?)	Increased hematocrit value
Plasma/ biochemistry	Elevated enzyme concentrations (ALT, AP, LDH)	Hyperphospatemia

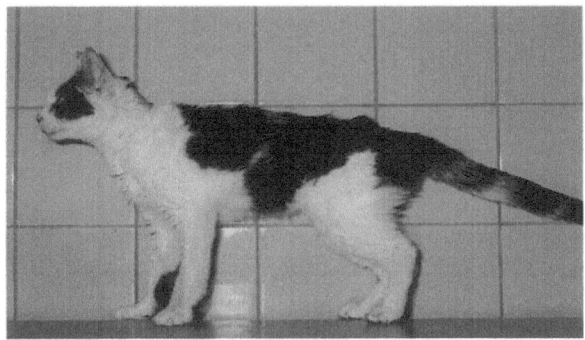 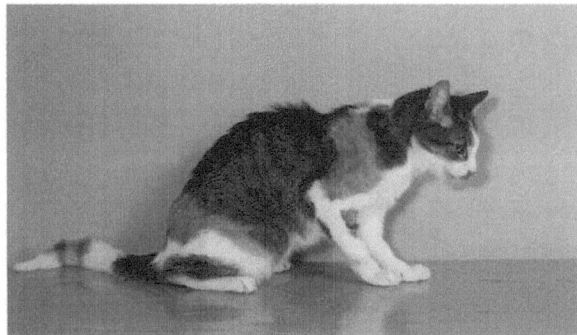

Fig. 3-22. Two spayed female cats, 15 (left) and 16 (right) years of age, with hyperthyroidism. Note the poor nutritional state and the "unkempt" coat of both cats. The open mouth of the right cat was due to panting.

aspects of the syndrome. First, the weight loss in combination with increased appetite and large volumes of somewhat fatty stools may be mistaken for pancreatic insufficiency and less likely for gastrointestinal lymphoma, as in the latter case there will be inappetence. Then of course the weight loss despite increased appetite, in combination with polyuria, may make one think of diabetes mellitus. However, routine urinalysis will immediately resolve this.

Diagnosis. When the suspicion of hyperthyroidism arises, the first step should be a careful (re)-palpation of the neck area by gently moving thumb and index finger along both sides of the trachea. The thyroids are only loosely attached to the surrounding tissues and therefore enlargement usually causes descent along the trachea, sometimes even as far as the thoracic inlet. They are usually easily movable along the trachea. Enlargement of one or both thyroid lobes can be found by an experienced examiner in up to 90% of cats with hyperthyroidism. However, it should be noted that occasionally thyroid enlargement is found without hyperthyroidism. In such cases the disease may develop with time and there is also some risk of malignancy. Rarely the thyroid enlargement arises from ectopic (sometimes intrathoracic) thyroid tissue.

A final diagnosis ought to rest on a direct measurement of thyroid function. For reasons explained earlier (3.3.1), measurement of plasma T_4 is of greater diagnostic value than that of T_3. In over 90% of cats presented with the syndrome of hyperthyroidism, the T_4 concentration in plasma exceeds the upper limit of the reference range (46

nmol/l). Plasma T_4 concentration fluctuates considerably over time and in cats with mild hyperthyroidism T_4 values may be in the high-normal range. In addition, concomittant non-thyroidal disease might cause lowering into the subnormal range. When the plasma-T_4 concentration falls within the reference range and the animal continues to be suspected of having the disease, the T_4 measurement can be repeated two and/or four weeks later.

One can also consider testing the suppressibility of plasma-T_4 concentration in a T_3-supression test (see also Fig. 3–21). Following seven 8-hourly oral doses of 15–25 μg T_3[a], the T_4 concentrations of healthy cats are suppressed to low values. Due to the autonomous (independent of TSH) character of the T_4 hypersecretion in hyperthyroid cats, the T_4 concentrations at 2–4 h after the last T_3 administration will remain practically unchanged.[21]

Although only available at some institutions, uptake studies with radioiodine (^{131}I, ^{123}I) may contribute to the diagnosis.[22] In hyperthyroid cats there is rapid uptake of the tracer to high values as compared to normal cats (Fig. 3–23). As explained in section 3.1 $^{99m}TcO_4^-$ is also taken up by the thyroid gland but is not organically bound. Nevertheless quantitations of $^{99m}TcO_4^-$ uptake can be valuable as it is usually higher than in healthy cats (Fig. 3–24).[23]

The main use of $^{99m}TcO_4^-$ is in the visualization of the thyroids, for which it has several advantages as compared to ^{131}I (rapid completion of the procedure and low radiation exposure). The

[a] Cytomel®, Smith Kline Beecham (5 and 25 μg liothyronine per tablet)

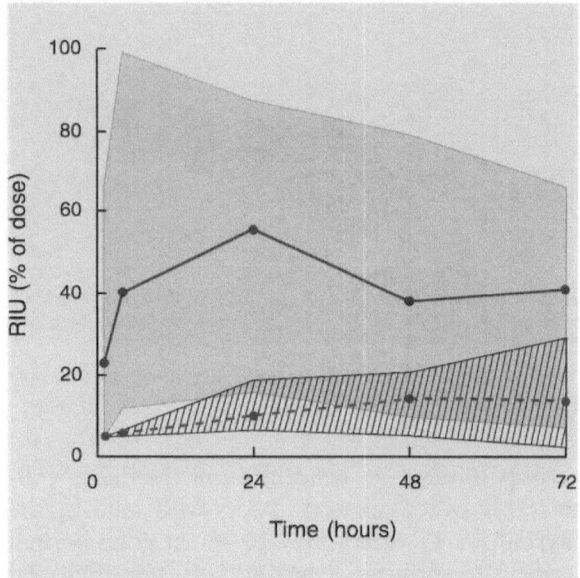

Fig. 3-23. Median curve and observed ranges (green) for thyroidal radioiodine uptake (RIU) in 20 hyperthyroid cats, compared with the data of 10 healthy house cats[22] (hatched area).

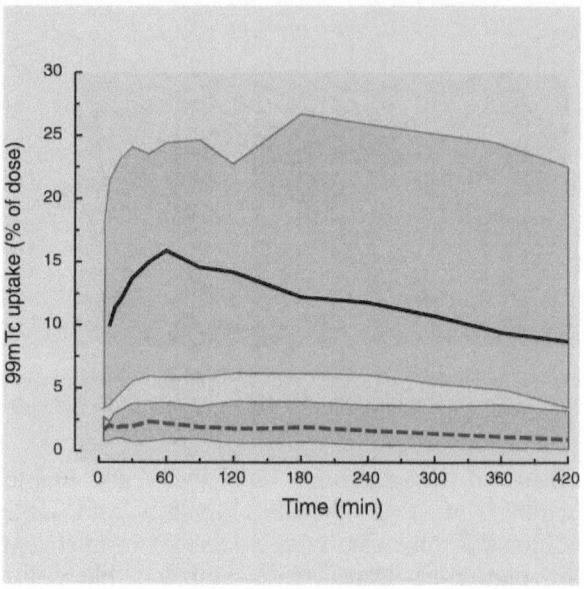

Fig. 3-24. Median and ranges for thyroidal $^{99m}TcO_4^-$ in 18 hyperthyroid cats (beige) as compared to the uptakes in 13 healthy cats[23] (blue area). (Adapted from Nap et al., 1994.[23])

increased uptake in the affected thyroid lobe becomes visible, whereas the non-affected thyroid tissue (contralateral lobe) is not visualized, because TSH secretion is suppressed by the T_4 excess (Figs. 3–21, Fig. 3–25). Thyroid scintiscanning is especially useful in hyperthyroid cats in which no thyroid enlargement can be palpated, in cases of recurrence of the disease following surgery (Fig. 3–24) and when there is suspicion of ectopic hyperfunctioning thyroid tissue or distant metastases, although both latter conditions are rare. The technique may also be used to establish whether there is bilateral involvement (more than half of cases!). However, when no scanning facilities are available and the animal will be treated by surgery anyway, bilateral enlargement can be identified during the surgical procedure.

Treatment. For the elimination of the source of the T_4 excess there are three options: (1) destruction with radioactive iodide, (2) surgery, and (3) antithyroid drugs. When the facilities are not a limiting factor, the first option is to be preferred. When this mode of treatment is not available, thyroidectomy is the best approach.

Thyroidectomy is performed by intracapsular

dissection from caudal to cranial. Thus the cranial parathyroid gland (occasionally two) usually can be preserved together with the associated part of the thyroid capsule containing the blood supply. It should be realized that it may be difficult to locate the parathyroid gland because of the anatomical changes due to the thyroid nodule.[24] It is advised to operate with the help of magnifying glasses. With this intracapsular approach it is possible to perform not only a unilateral but also bilateral thyroidectomy without a high incidence of hypoparathyroidism, although the results are highly dependent upon the available surgical skills. In cases of adenomatous hyperplasia arising in thyroid tissue in the ventral cervical or anterior mediastinal region (Fig. 3–26), the lesions can usually be reached via a caudal neck incision. By (careful!) exploration through the cranial thoracic inlet the anterior mediastinum can be reached sufficiently to find and to remove the lesion.[24]

If thyroid imaging is not available, a cat in which only unilateral enlargement was palpated, may be found at surgery to have enlargement of both lobes. Then the (experienced!) surgeon should proceed to perform a bilateral thyroidectomy. The alternative, to confine the procedure to the initial

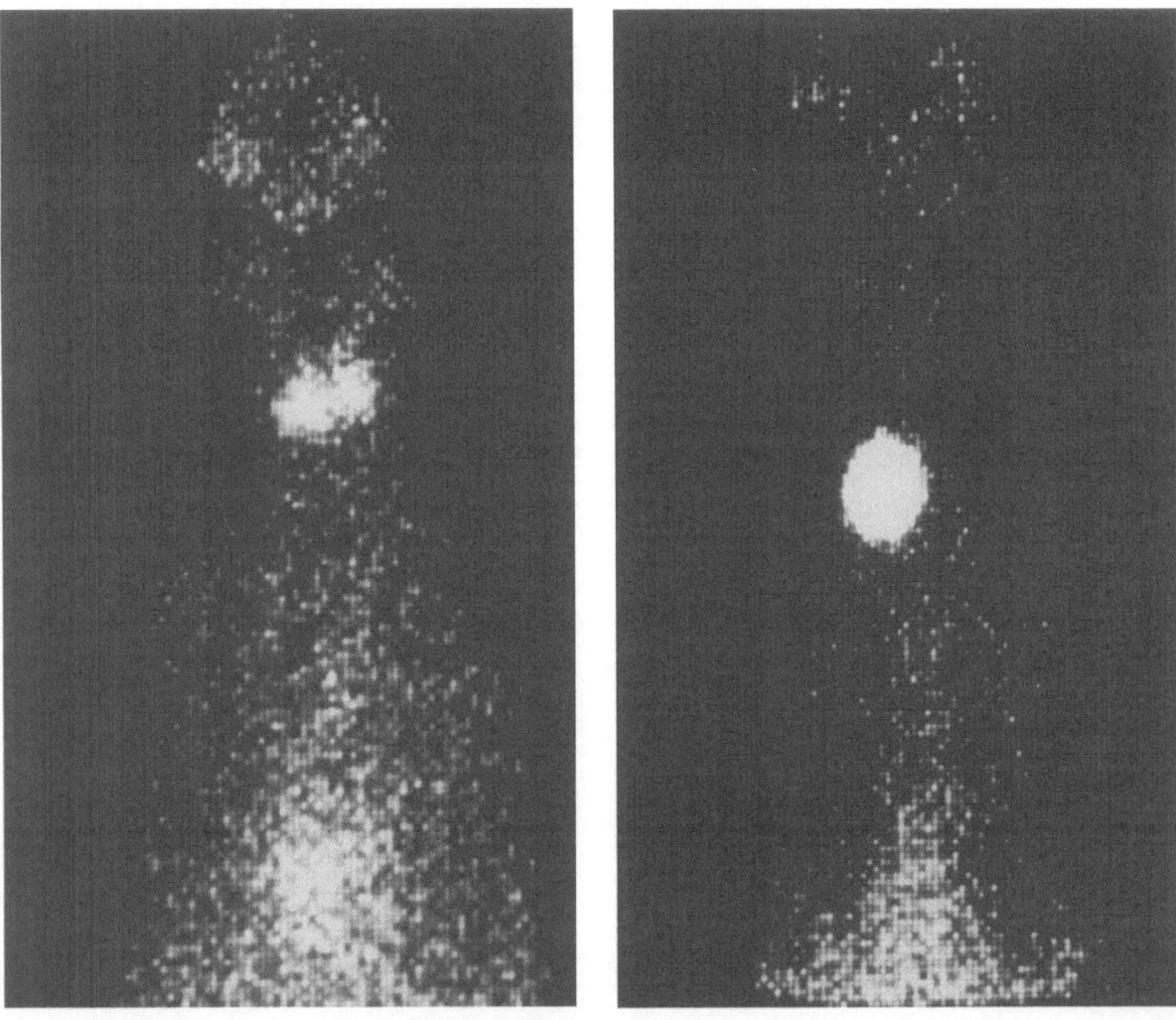

Fig. 3-25. Thyroid scintiscans made 30 min after intravenous injection of 0.5–0.8 mCi $^{99m}TcO_4^-$. In the normal cat (left) there is symmetrical and homogenous distribution of the radioactivity in the thyroid lobes and cranial to this the uptake in the salivary glands. In the scan of the hyperthyroid cat (right) with unilateral thyroid enlargement there is high uptake in the nodule and no visualization of the non-affected lobe.

plan for unilateral thyroidectomy and wait for the follow-up to see whether (mild) hyperthyroidism recurs, is less attractive as the disease may continue to exist right after surgery.

Cats in which the disease is complicated by cardiac abnormalities such as hypertrophic cardiomyopathy and congestive heart failure, are regarded as poor anesthetic and surgical risks. In these instances presurgical treatment is advised with antithyroid drugs for about four weeks. However, the risk of complications associated with the administration of these drugs is thereby introduced. (see below).

The most serious postoperative complication is hypocalcemia, which develops within 24–72 h after (bilateral) thyroidectomy. The signs may range from lethargy, anorexia, reluctance to move, and muscle tremors (face, ears) to tetany and convulsions. Tetany may become manifest especially when the cat is handled. Such a crisis will require the intravenous administration of 0.5 mmol Ca^{++}/kg body weight as calcium gluconate. However, this dramatic course can be prevented by measuring plasma calcium immediately after surgery and monitoring calcium concentrations in plasma once or twice daily. Mild hypocalcemia

54

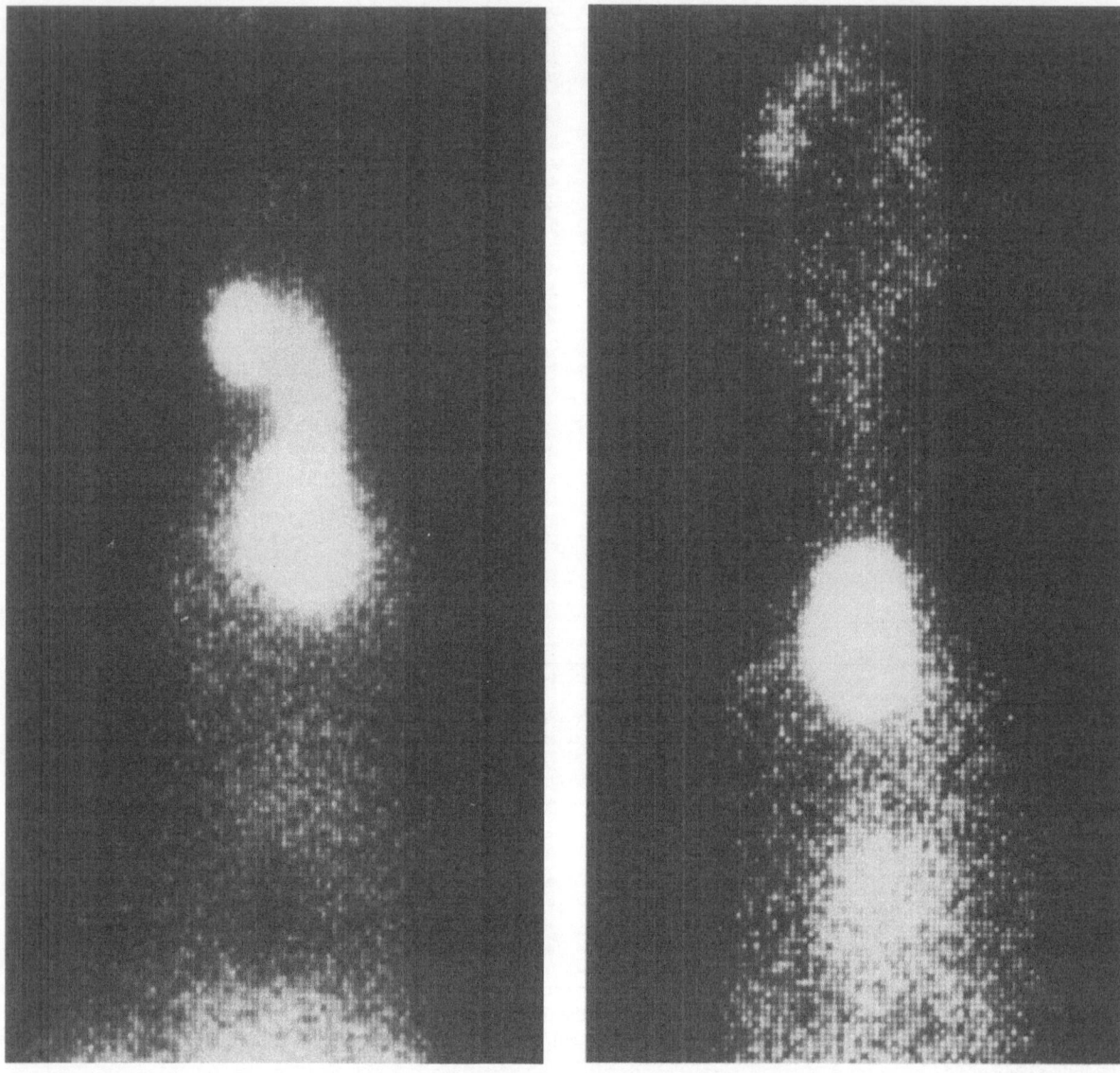

Fig. 3-26. Thyroid scintiscans of a 13-year-old castrated male cat with hyperthyroidism (plasma T_4 > 360 nmol/l). After removal of both thyroid lobes there was some improvement. Complete recovery was only achieved 2 months later, when the nodule at the thoracic inlet (right) was removed. (Courtesy M.E. Peeters)

not requiring treatment may occur, but when the calcium concentration in plasma is below 1.8 mmol/l supplementation is started with twice daily 50 mg calcium lactate or carbonate per kg body weight and twice daily 0.01 mg dihydrotachysterol[b] per kg body weight. The maximal effect is usually achieved after about three weeks and

[b] Dihydral®, Duphar, Amsterdam and Roxane Laboratories, Columbus OH (0.2 mg dihydrotachysterol per tablet)

commonly the dose of calcium lactate has to be lowered to prevent hypercalcemia. The hypoparathyroidism may be permanent, but spontaneous recovery from the parathyroid damage may occur within weeks to months. The cats that have undergone bilateral thyroidectomy should also be supplemented with thyroxine (twice daily 50 μg/kg body weight).

Radioiodine (^{131}I) by its β-radiation selectively destroys the hyperfunctioning thyroid tissue, thereby saving the unaffected (suppressed) thyroid tissue and the parathyroid tissue. Thus there is commonly no need for supplementation therapy. In principle the appropriate dose can be calculated from the uptake of tracer amounts of the radionuclide and the size of the tissue mass. However, with the pragmatic approach in many institutions of administering 4–5 mCi intravenously, little recurrence of hyperthyroidism and no permanent hypothyroidism has been observed.[25]

From a medical point of view radioiodine therapy is certainly the most attractive option. Complete cure is achieved with a non-invasive procedure that it is not associated with complications. The method is especially attractive in cases of bilateral involvement and in recurrences after surgical treatment, the latter being even at higher risk for postsurgical hypoparathyroidism than the former. However, the facilities are only available in licensed institutions. Apart from specific equipment, radiation safety precautions are required and the animals have to be hospitalized for over a week.

Of the available *antithyroid drugs* propylthiouracil (PTU) cannot be used in cats because of its serious side effects. It may cause not only anorexia, vomiting and lethargy, but more seriously it is also associated in a rather high incidence with autoimmune hemolytic anemia and immune-mediated thrombocytopenia.

What remains is the imidazol-derivative methimazole (Tapazole or Strumazol[c]) or the related compound carbimazole[d]. These drugs are given in a dose of 5 mg two to three times daily. Rarely a dose higher than 15 mg/day is needed to maintain control of hyperthyroidism. Dose adjustments should be based upon the clinical response and on (initially monthly) measurements of plasma T_4. Once a satisfactory therapeutic effect has been obtained, many cats can be maintained on once daily 5 or 10 mg methimazole, but a small proportion may need 15–20 mg/day.

As with PTU, gastrointestinal upsets are also seen, but they usually resolve with continuation of

therapy. Allergic skin reactions have also been observed. However, serious hematologic problems may also arise (agranulocytosis and thrombocytopenia), albeit in a much lower incidence than with PTU. In addition, signs of hepatic toxicity may be encountered. These reactions usually occur within the first three months of treatment and it is therefore advised in this period to perform a laboratory control examination every two weeks. Cessation of methimazole administration usually results in resolution of the drug reaction.[26]

Prognosis. In cats without severe complicating cardiac abnormalities the prospects for a return to a healthy condition are excellent after successful surgery. There may be recurrence after months or years, but this is usually the result of the new development of adenomatous hyperplasia in contralateral or ectopic tissue.[24] With radioiodine the prognosis is even better, for also in cases of bilateral involvement there is no risk of hypoparathyroidism and no need for supplementation with thyroid hormone. With methimazole the fate of the cat is in part dependent upon the (non) appearance of adverse reactions to the drug, although in the great majority of hyperthyroid cats the drug is effective.

3.4.2 Thyroid tumors and hyperthyroidism in dogs

Thyroid neoplasia accounts for about 2% of all canine tumors. Most benign canine thyroid tumors (adenomas) are small and commonly not detected during life. Only very occasionally they become cystic and thereby large enough to be detected by the owner. Another reason for detecting a benign thyroid tumor may be presentation of an animal with signs suggesting hyperthyroidism (Fig. 3–27). Careful palpation may reveal a small thyroid enlargement.

Over 85% of the canine thyroid tumors discovered clinically are rather large (diameter > 3 cm) malignant solid masses. Their malignant nature may already be evident during clinical examination, because of changes such as attachment to adjacent structures and metastases to regional lymph nodes and to the lungs.

Microscopic examination reveals most tumors to contain both solid and follicular patterns, with some largely composed of either type. Among the

[c] Strumazol®, N.V. Organon (10 or 30 mg thiamazol per tablet)

[d] Basolest®, Pharmachemie, Haarlem, The Netherlands; Neo-Mercazole®, Nicholas Laboratories, United Kingdom (5 mg carbimazole per tablet)

56

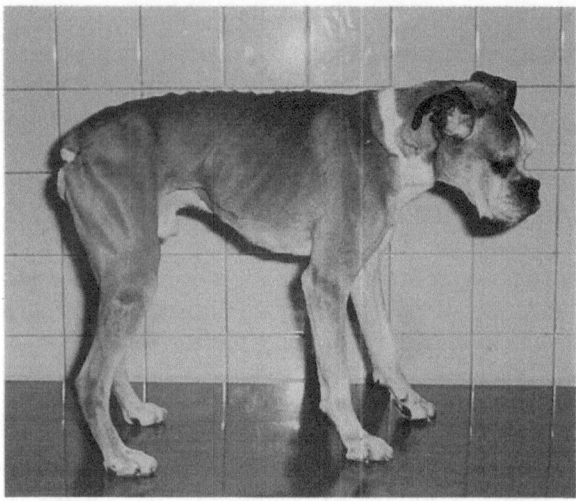 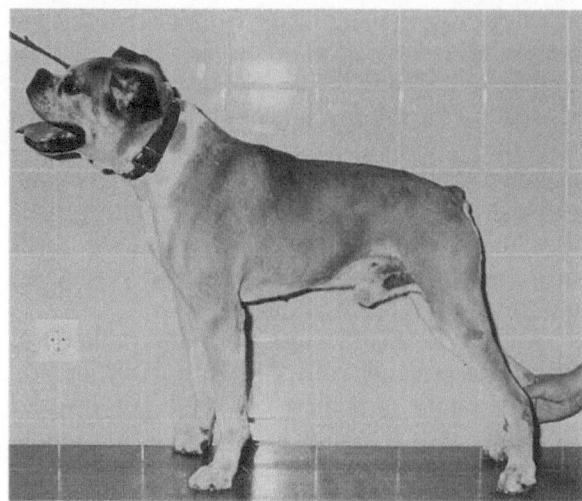

Fig. 3-27. A 9-year-old male Boxer dog in a very poor nutritional condition as a result of hyperthyroidism (left). Removal of a small thyroid adenoma resulted in resolution of the signs, including the severe polyuria. At a control examination after 5 months the dog had gained 10 kg in body weight (right). The dog had become so lively and strong again, that he was difficult to keep on the table for the photograph.

domestic animals thyroid cancer of the dog, and particularly the follicular type, most closely resembles human (follicular) carcinoma. These similarties concern not only the clinical behavior but also the pattern of circulating thyroglobulin levels[27] and the conservation of TSH receptors in the primary tumors (much less in metastases).[28] An intriguing difference with the disease in man has been found with respect to DNA ploidy, i.e., a high incidence of hypodipoidy in canine tumors[29].

The role of oncogenes and tumor-suppressor genes[30] in thyroid oncogenesis has not yet been studied in the dog.

Clinical features. For dogs presented with thyroid tumors the mean age is 9 years (range 5–15 years), with an overrepresentation of the Boxer dog. There is no sex predilection. The signs and symptoms fall into two categories: (1) thyroid enlargement, and (2) hypersecretion.

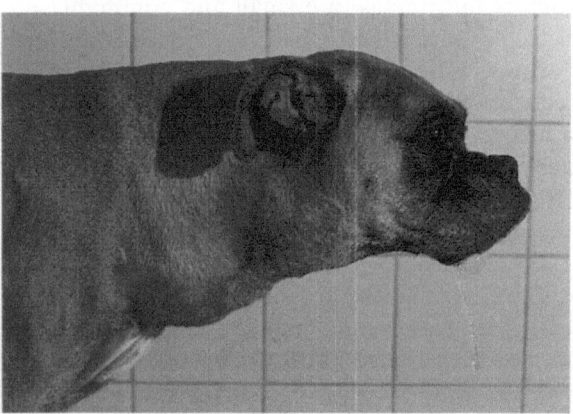 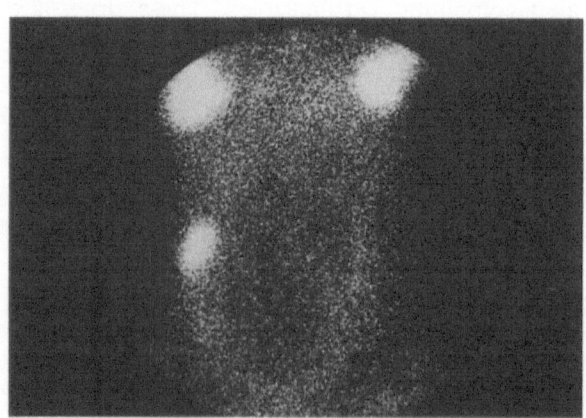

Fig. 3-28. A 9-year-old female Boxer dog (left) with an enormous thyroid tumor, that had caused tracheal obstruction and dysphagia (note the salivation). On the pertechnetate scintiscan (right) the mass appeared to be functionally inactive, i.e., did not concentrate pertechnetate. Such tumor tissues that are not visualized are referred to as being "cold". The tissue displacement is illustrated by the lateral position of the non-affected lobe that concentrated pertechnetate normally. In the upper part of the right figure the pertechnetate uptake by the salivary glands is seen.

Table 3-3. *Clinical manifestations in dogs with non-hyperfunctioning (euthyroid) thyroid tumors.*

System/organ	Euthyroid	
	Common	*Less common/ rare*
Thyroid	Unilateral (rather large) tumor	Bilateral tumor (with irregular shape). Palpable regional lymph nodes.
Metabolism		Weight loss
Respiratory/ Cardiovascular		Respiratory distress
Gastrointestinal/ renal		Dysphagia, anorexia
Neuromuscular		Painful neck

Table 3-3a. *Clinical manifestations in dogs with hyperfunctioning thyroid tumors.*

System/organ	Hyperthyroid	
	Common	*Less common/ rare*
Thyroid	Unilateral small or medium size tumor	
Metabolism	Weight loss despite good appetite	Intolerance to hot environment
Respiratory/ Cardiovascular	Panting	Tachycardia and forceful heart beat
Gastrointestinal/ renal	Polydipsia/ polyuria	Diarrhea
Neuromuscular	Weakness/ fatique and lethargy	Restlessness Muscle atrophy

Most thyroid tumors are discovered by the owners as a painless mass in the midcervical or ventrocervical region that causes no discomfort. However, with increasing size the tumors may give rise to pressure symptoms such as dysphagia, hoarseness, and tracheal obstruction (Fig. 3–28; Table 3–3). This may be especially true for the

masses that arise from thyroglossal duct remnants, which may involve the base of the tongue (Fig. 3–29). Masses originating from ectopic thyroid tissue at the base of the heart may give rise to arrhythmias, pericardial effusion and (anterior cervical) edema.

Hypersecretion of thyroid hormone is only ob-

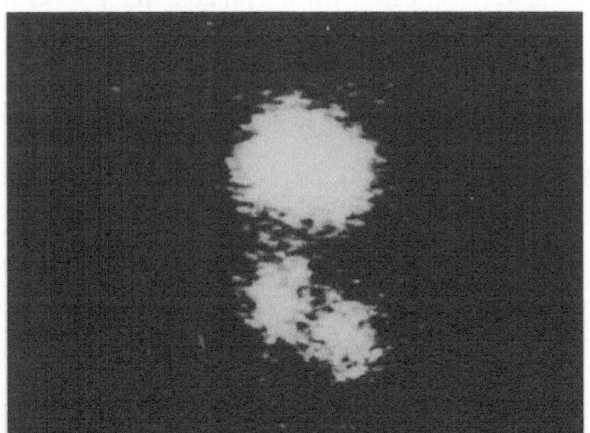

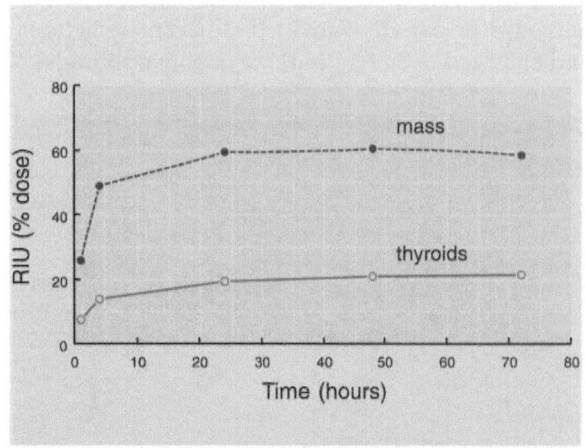

Fig. 3-29. Scintiscan (left) of a 9-year-old female miniature Poodle with a midline mass at the level of the hyoid bone, at 48 h after intravenous administration of 100 μCi [131]I⁻ . Both thyroids had a normal uptake but at the level of the mass there was even higher uptake. This is further illustrated in the figure on the right in which the radioiodide uptakes have been depicted separately for the thyroid area and the mass. Apparently the mass did not produce excessive amounts of thyroid hormone, for the dog was euthyroid (plasma T_4: 46 nmol/l) and there was no suppression of the unaffected thyroids. Biochemical studies of similar cases have revealed that such tumors produce an abnormal (albumin-like) iodoprotein and almost no Tg. In this dog the intravenous administration of 20 mCi [131]I⁻ made the tumor mass disappear completely and permanently.

served in about 10% of cases of thyroid tumor. This may give rise to the syndrome of hyperthyroidism, which in the dog is very similar to the condition in the cat, although often somewhat less pronounced (Table 3–3).

Only sporadically canine thyroid tumors arise from C-cells and this also may result in a hypersecretion syndrome, which may have diarrhea as the main characteristic.[31] These so-called medullary carcinomas may not only produce calcitonin but also other polypeptide hormones, such as somatostatin and vasoactive intestinal peptide, some of which may be responsible for the diarrhea.

Differential diagnosis. The differential diagnosis for a large cervical mass includes conditions such as inflammation (pharyngeal penetration by a foreign body), lymphoma, lipoma, and other tumors. In this respect it should be noted that very rarely thyroid tumors infiltrate the skin, giving the impression of an inflammation with much granulation tissue.

Diagnosis. The location and extension of the mass is judged by careful palpation of the ventral neck area with the animal sitting in a relaxed position and the head slightly tilted backward. Charateristically the smaller and medium sized tumors are easily movable along the trachea. The palpation may also reveal attachment to adjacent structures and enlarged deep (cranial) cervical lymph nodes.

When in doubt of whether the mass is of thyroidal origin, a pertechnetate or iodide scintiscan usually resolves the problem (Fig. 3–30). Fine needle aspiration and subsequent cytological examination may even be more informative as to the nature of the mass.

Measurements of plasma concentrations of T_4 are of limited use in the diagnosis of thyroid tumors, but a high T_4 will answer the question of whether the associated signs and symptoms can be ascribed to hyperthyroidism. T_4 measurements should also be performed in cases of bilateral thyroid tumor to establish whether the neoplastic expansion has caused hypothyroidism.

Treatment. As the great majority of the clinically detected tumors are malignant, the mass should be surgically removed without delay, provided radiography has not revealed lung metastases. The surgical excision of well-encapsulated thyroid carcinomas is often curative. Complete removal of all neoplastic tissue may be difficult if the tumor is large and invasive, aggressive approaches may result in laryngeal paralysis.

The surgical excision of ectopic carcinomas involving the base of the tongue poses specific problems because of their close attachments to the hyoid apparatus and the tongue, and because of the abundant neovascularization.[32] In these difficult surgical cases, when available, therapy with radioiodine may be a better alternative (Fig. 3–29), provided the scintiscan has not revealed "cold"

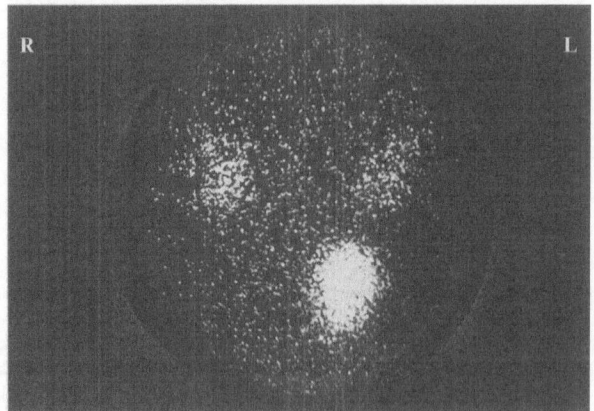

Fig. 3-30. Left: Scintiscan of a dog with a non-hyperfunctioning (also called "non-toxic") thyroid tumor. There was irregular distribution of radioactivity in the tumor mass (see also legend to Fig. 3–6). The contralateral lobe (on the right) could be visualized normally, i.e., was not suppressed. In contrast, the scintiscan (right) of the Boxer dog of Fig. 3–27 revealed a small hyperfunctioning ("toxic") tumor on the left with no visualization of the unaffected right lobe as a result of the suppression of pituitary TSH secretion.

areas in the tumor that may be solid/anaplastic tissue not accumulating radioiodine. However, in cases of mixed follicular/solid thyroid carcinoma and lung metastases, radioiodine therapy may be followed by temporary improvement.[33] Ectopic tumors originating from intrathoracic thyroid tissue may be resectable.[34]

When animals with bilateral thyroid tumor are treated by surgery, it is only occasionally possible to recognize and to save the parathyroid glands. If it is not, in addition to the full thyroxine replacement (see 3.3.1), treatment of hypoparathyroidism will be necessary (see 3.4.1 and 9.2).

Prognosis. The histomorphological grade of malignancy, taking into account cellular and nuclear polymorphism, capsular and vascular invasion, and the frequency of mitoses, appears to be the most important prognostic factor for canine thyroid tumors treated by thyroidectomy.[35] In addition, the size of the tumor is a critical factor.[31] In other words, in dogs with medium-sized or small well-encapsulated carcinomas surgical resection carries a good prognosis.

As carcinomatous thyroid cells do have TSH receptors, it is assumed that the prognosis can be influenced favourably by TSH-suppressive treatment with thyroxine. However, there is evidence that paracrine growth factors such as epidermal growth factor (EGF) and insulin-like growth factor-I (IGF-I) are more important for thyroid growth than TSH.[36] In addition, it should be remembered that metastases are associated with loss of TSH receptors. Although the debate over the therapeutic effectiveness of thyroid hormone in the prevention of recurrence of thyroid cancer continues, one may decide to supply thyroid hormone until such time as a definitive conclusion indicates otherwise.

4. Adrenals

4.1 Introduction

The adrenals are paired structures, situated craniomedial to the kidneys. Each consists of two functionally distinct endocrine glands of different embryological origin. The center of each gland, the medulla, comprises coalesced chromaffin cells of neuroectodermal origin that secrete epinephrine and norepinephrine. The surrounding cortex arises from mesoderm and histologically three zones can be distinguished: (1) zona glomerulosa (or arcuata), (2) zona fasciculata, and (3) zona reticularis (Fig. 4–1).

The zona fasciculata is the thickest layer. It consists of columns of cells extending from the inner reticularis zone to the zona glomerulosa. The cells are relatively large and contain much cytoplasmic lipid. The latter is removed during fixation, giving the cells a vacuolated appearance and therefore they are called "clear cells". In this zone glucocorticoids (cortisol and corticosterone) and androgens are produced.

The cells of the zona reticularis lay in anastomosing colums. They lack significant lipid content and contain densely granular cytoplasm and are therefore called "compact cells". This zone produces androgens such as androstenedione, but also glucocorticoids. It functions together with the zona fasciculata as one unit.

The zona glomerulosa lacks a well-defined structure. The small lipid-poor cells are scattered beneath the adrenal capsule. The zone produces mineralocorticoids (primarily aldosterone). It is deficient in 17α-hydroxylase activity (see below) and therefore cannot produce cortisol or androgens.

Synthesis and secretion of corticosteroids. The adrenal cortex is rich in receptors that internalize low density lipoproteins (LDL). From the LDL free cholesterol is liberated, which serves as the starting compound in steroidogenesis, although synthesis within the gland from acetate also occurs (Figs. 4–2, 4–3). Cytochrome P-450 enzymes are

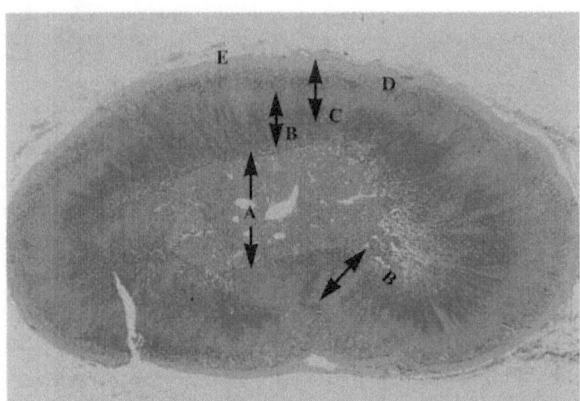
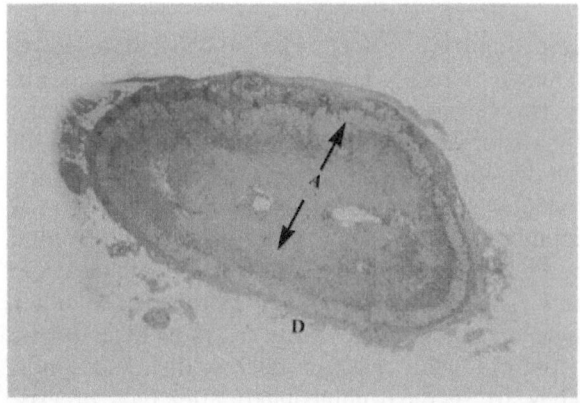

Fig. 4-1. Histological section of an adrenal gland of a healthy dog (left): A = medulla, B = zona reticularis, C = zona fasciculata, D = zona glomerulosa, E = capsule, B′ = zona reticularis of opposite cortex. Right: Similar section of a dog that had been treated with injections of progestagens. Their intrinsic glucocorticoid effect had caused suppression of endogenous ACTH secretion, which had led to complete atrophy of both the zona fasciculata and the zona reticularis, while the zona glomerulosa remained intact.

A. Rijnberk (ed.), Clinical Endocrinology of Dogs and Cats, 61–93.

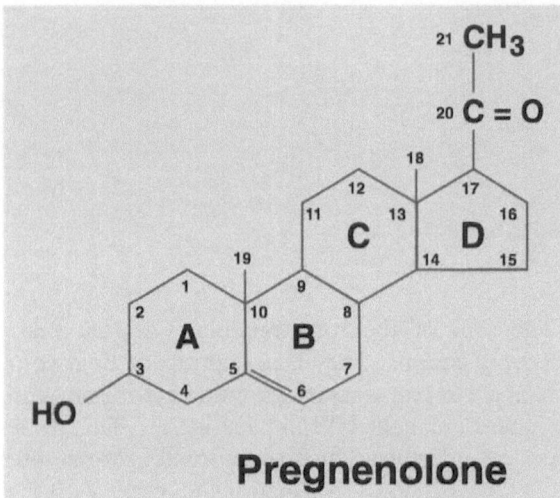

Fig. 4-2. Basic structure of adrenocortical steroids. In this pregnenolone molecule the four rings are identified by letters. Individual carbon atoms are numbered. [Recommendation of the International Union of Pure and Applied Chemistry, IUPAC-IUB 1967.[1]]

responsible for most of the enzymatic conversions from cholesterol to steroid hormones. These enzymes are membrane-bound hemoproteins that catalyze oxidation, including oxidative cleavage of the precursor molecule. They are named after a heme group they contain and that after reduction with carbon monoxide absorbs light at a wavelength of 450 nm.

The above-mentioned zonal difference in hormone production is due to selective presence of two different cytochrome P-450 enzymes.[2] The mitochondrial cytochrome P-450 aldosterone synthase, which converts deoxycorticosterone via corticosterone to aldosterone, is only found in the zona glomerulosa. The characteristic enzyme in the two inner zones is the microsomal cytochrome P-450$_{c17}$ (17α-hydroxylase/17,20-lyase), which catalyzes the 17α-hydroxylation of pregnenolone and progesterone as well as the side chain cleavage at C_{17} of 17-α-hydroxy C_{21} steroids. The other steroidogenic enzymes occur in all the three zones.

Steroidogenic cells cannot store their hormones. They are secreted immediately after biosynthesis. Cortisol, 11-deoxycortisol, corticosterone and 11-deoxycorticosterone are derived entirely from adrenocortical secretion, whereas the other steroids are derived from a combination of adrenocortical and gonadal sources. In dogs and cats the cortisol/corticosterone ratios found in adrenal venous blood range from about 3 to 7.

Transport and metabolism. Following secretion the adrenocortical hormones are largely bound to plasma proteins. Approximately 75% of cortisol in plasma is bound with high affinity to corticosteroid-binding globulin (CBG). Furthermore albumin and erythrocytes display low-affinity binding of an additional 10% of total cortisol in blood. Only the free fraction, in the dog estimated to range from 5 to 12%,[3,4] is biologically active. However, the amount of hormone that is potentially available to tissues is determined by the combination of free and bound fractions, because these fractions are in equilibrium. Higher CBG-

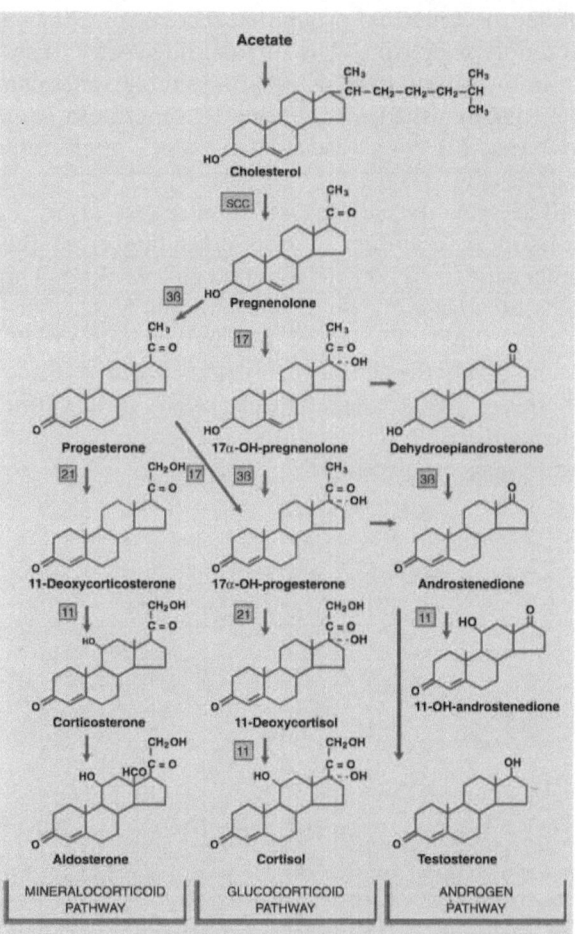

Fig. 4-3. Major biosynthetic pathways of adrenocortical steroid biosynthesis. scc = P-450$_{scc}$; 3β = 3β-hydroxysteroid dehydrogenase/Δ^{4,5}-isomerase; 11 = P-450$_{c11}$; 17 = P-450$_{c17}$; 21 = P-450$_{c21}$.

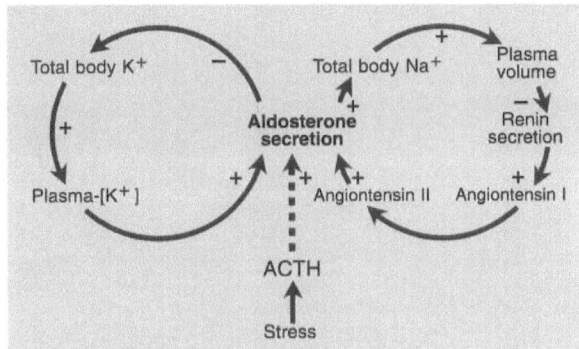

Fig. 4-4. Scheme of the physiologic control of aldosterone secretion, illustrating the interrelationships of the volume and potassium feedback loops on aldosterone secretion. ACTH has only a short-term effect on aldosterone synthesis. Thus the system is essentially volume and potassium driven, and pituitary-independent. The effects are mediated by binding of aldosterone to high-affinity type I or mineralocorticoid receptor proteins in target tissues.

binding capacities have been found in female dogs than in male dogs.[5] In rats sex differences in circulating CBG levels most probably relate to the sexual dimorphism of GH secretion.[6] Androgens and aldosterone are predominantly bound with low affinity to albumin. This explains the low plasma concentrations of these hormones.

The physiological role of the circulating binding proteins most probably lies in a buffering effect, preventing rapid variations of the plasma cortisol

level. They restrain the flux of active cortisol to the target organ and also protect it from rapid metabolic breakdown and excretion.

The metabolism of corticosteroids renders them inactive and increases their water solubility, as does their subsequent conjugation with glucuronide or sulfate groups. The liver is the major site of corticosteroid metabolism and conjugation. In several species including the dog most of these inactive conjugated metabolites are readily excreted by the kidney, whereas in the cat the excretion of glucocorticoid metabolites is largely biliary.[2]

Regulation of secretion. Synthesis and release of glucocorticoids (and androgens) by the two inner zones of the adrenal cortex is almost exclusively controlled by the pituitary hormone ACTH. The production of aldosterone in the zona glomerulosa is regulated by the volume and potassium status of the organism by a complex, multifactorial and almost exclusively extrapituitary control system (Fig. 4–4). The pituitary(ACTH)-glucocorticoid (cortisol) axis is clinically very relevant for dogs and cats and therefore the following paragraphs are devoted to the regulatory aspects of this system.

Glucocorticoid and especially cortisol secretion is directly dependent on the plasma concentration of ACTH or corticotropin (see also Fig. 1–8).

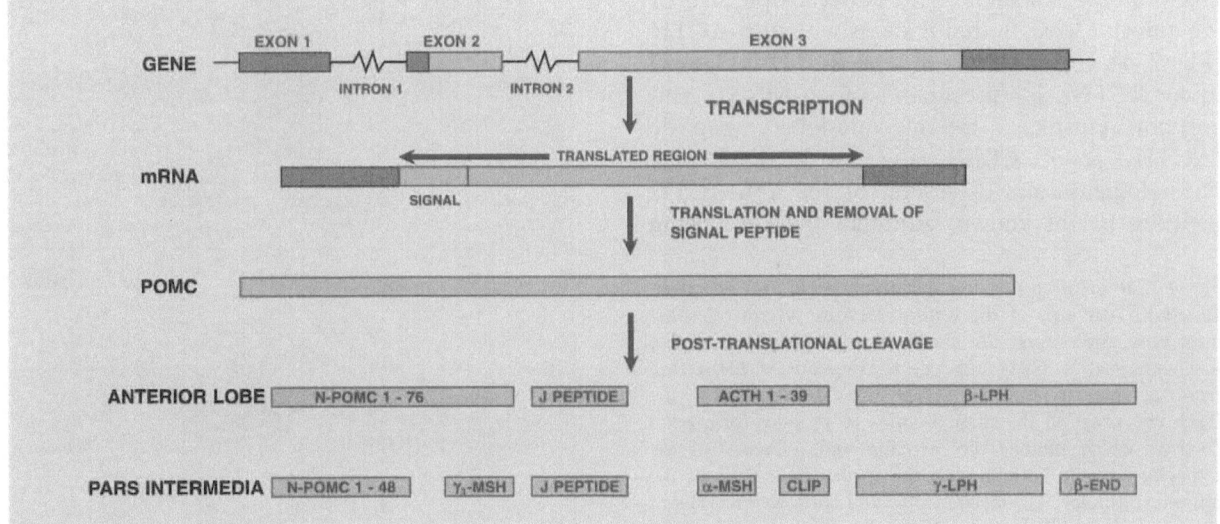

Fig. 4-5. Structure of the canine proopiomelanocortin (POMC) gene, its mRNA and the processing of POMC in the anterior lobe and in the pars intermedia. ACTH = adrenocorticotropic hormone; J PEPTIDE = joining peptide; LPH = lipotropin; MSH = melanocyte-stimulating hormone; CLIP = corticotropin-like intermediate lobe peptide, β-END = β-endorphin.

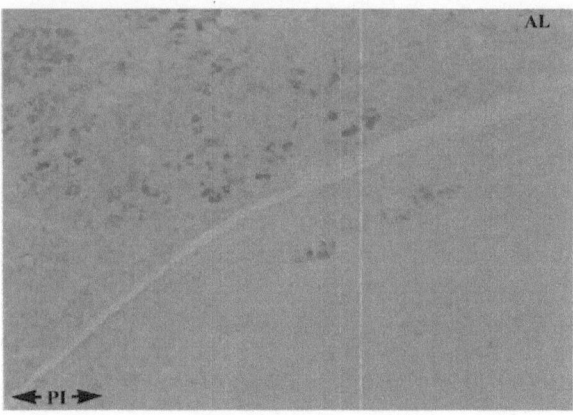
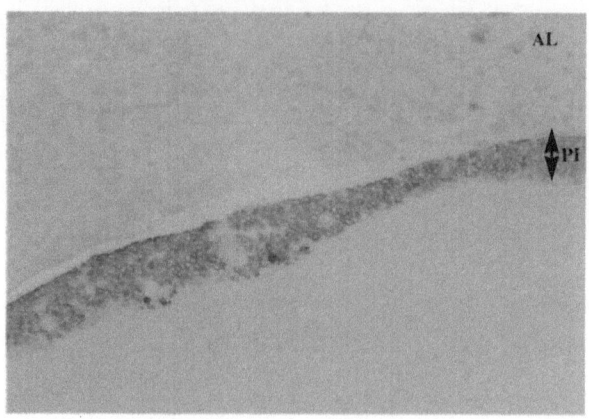

Fig. 4-6. Sections of the pituitary gland of a cat immunostained with anti-ACTH (left) and with anti-MSH (right). Compared to the anterior lobe (AL) and also compared to the pars intermedia (PI) of the dog (see Fig. 2–4) there are only few ACTH-positive cells in the PI. There is an abundance of MSH-positive cells in the cat's PI.

Chemically ACTH is a single-chain peptide comprising 39 amino acid residues. In the anterior lobe it is synthesized from a well-characterized precursor molecule pro-opiomelanocortin (POMC), which also gives rise to a number of other peptides that are co-released with ACTH (Fig. 4–5). Between species there is a strong amino-acid sequence homology for the ACTH molecule. Canine ACTH differs in the carboxy-terminal part of the molecule by only one amino acid from ACTH of other species.[7]

In dogs and cats the pars intermedia contains two cell types that also can synthesize POMC.[8] One cell type is similar to the corticotropic cells of the anterior lobe, in that it stains with anti-ACTH (Fig. 2–4). In the other cell type ACTH is cleaved into $ACTH_{1-14}$ (precursor of α-MSH) and corticotropin-like intermediate-lobe peptide ($ACTH_{18-39}$ or CLIP) (Figs. 4–5, 4–6). The physiological roles of several of the non-ACTH peptides is not known, although they are being

unraveled. For example, $N\text{-POMC}_{1-48}$ is now known to promote adrenocortical mitogenesis.

ACTH secretion by the anterior pituitary is regulated by the hypothalamus and central nervous system via neurotransmitters that cause the release of hypophysiotropic hormones such as corticotropin-releasing hormone (CRH) and

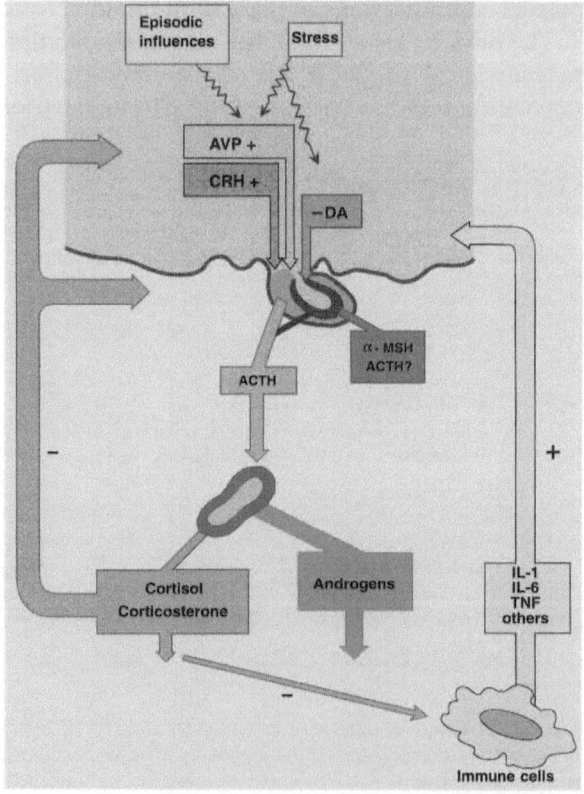

Fig. 4-7. Regulation of adrenal glucocorticoid and androgen secretion. Afferents of the central nervous system (episodic influences and stress) are mediated by hypophysiotrophic hormones such as CRH and AVP to stimulate ACTH release from the anterior pituitary. ACTH stimulates the cells of the inner two zones of the adrenal cortex to produce (primarily) cortisol, which inhibits the secretion and influence of the hypophysiotropic hormones on the corticotropic cells of the anterior pituitary. The melanotropic and corticotropic cells of the pars intermedia are largely under dopaminergic (DA) inhibitory control. The activation of the hypothalamus-pituitary-adrenocortical axis as evoked by challenges to the immune system is shown on the right.

arginine-vasopressin (AVP) (Fig. 4–7). In this neuroendocrine control four mechanisms can be distinguished: (1) episodic secretion and possible diurnal rhythm of ACTH, (2) response to stress, (3) feedback inhibition by cortisol, and (4) immunological factors (Fig. 4–7).[9]

Central nervous system events regulate both the number and magnitude of ACTH bursts, that range in the dog from 6 to 12 per 24-h period.[10] Unlike in man, studies of pulsatile ACTH secretion in dogs have revealed no increase in the number of episodes of secretion in the early morning hours. Although this equal distribution of the pulsatile ACTH release throughout the 24-h period denies a diurnal rhythm for dogs, there is some evidence that under different circumstances (sleep pattern, light-dark exposure and feeding times) different results may be obtained.[2] From some early work in cats it was suggested that in cats the highest cortisol levels occur in the evening, which was ascribed to the notion that the cat is a nocturnal animal. However, in a more recent study episodic fluctuations of plasma cortisol were found without evidence of a diurnal rhythm.[11]

ACTH and cortisol are secreted within minutes

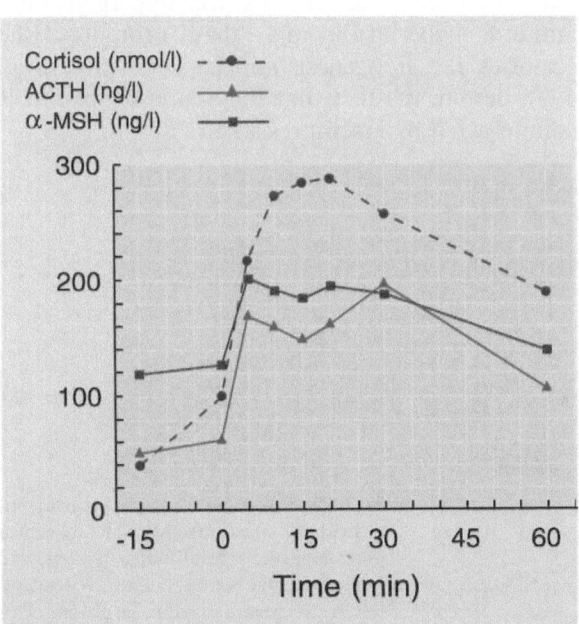

Fig. 4-8. Plasma concentration of cortisol, ACTH and α-MSH in 6 cats that underwent intradermal skin testing between t_0 and t_5 and reading of the skin reactions at t_{15}. Blood sampling was performed via previously placed jugular catheters. (Adapted from Willemse et al., 1993.[15])

following the onset of stresses such as surgery and hypoglycemia. Stress responses originate in the central nervous system and cause an increased release of the hypothalamic hypophysiotropic hormones such as CRH and AVP. These stress responses are reduced or totally abolished by prior high-dose glucocorticoid administration and also less pronounced in spontaneous hyperadrenocorticism.[12] In this context it should be noted that dogs and cats differ considerably in their responses to stress. In dogs several emotional or neurogenic stresses do not result in stimulation of ACTH secretion or MSH secretion[13]; only profound stress such as long-term immobilization uniformly causes elevations of plasma cortisol.[14] In cats, on the other hand, mild stresses such as handling and intradermal skin testing cause impressive increases in the plasma concentrations of cortisol, ACTH and α-MSH (Fig. 4–8). In contrast to dogs, cats appear to have an actively secreting pars intermedia that is strongly responsive to stress.[15]

The third major regulator of ACTH and cortisol secretion is that of feedback inhibition. The inhibitory action of glucocorticoids is exerted at multiple target sites, of which two have been unequivocally identified: neurons in the hypothalamus that produce corticotropin-releasing factors (CRH and AVP) and corticotropic cells in the anterior lobe. The feedback actions of glucocorticoids are exerted through at least two structurally different receptor molecules, i.e., a type I (mineralocorticoid preferring receptor, MR) and a type II (glucocorticoid preferring receptor, GR). There is evidence that the inhibition of the basal ACTH secretion by glucocorticoids is mediated via occupancy of the MR. The dog brain and pituitary contain very high quantities of MR, with highest levels in the septohippocampal complex and the anterior lobe of the pituitary.[16] The increasing basal activity of the pituitary-adrenocortical axis, observed with aging in several species including the dog, has been ascribed to neuronal degeneration and consequent loss of limbic MRs.[17] The GR is more evenly distributed in the brain with the amounts in the anterior lobe being about twice as high. The latter GRs are mainly involved in the feedback effect of glucocorticoids released as a result of stress-induced ACTH secretion.

Finally, challenges to the immune system by infections invariably activate the hypothalamus-pituitary-adrenocortical axis (Fig. 4–7). These responses are mediated by cytokines, a group of polypeptides released from colonies of activated immune cells. In this context interleukin-1 (IL-1) is of particular importance. It is released from activated macrophages in the periphery and produces marked increases in the release of ACTH and glucocorticoids.[9] The regulatory actions of the cytokines are exerted predominantly at the level of the hypothalamus, where CRH is the major mediator of the hypothalamic response.[18] These cytokine-mediated activations of the hypothalamus-pituitary adrenocortical axis are also subject to feedback regulation by glucocorticoids, not only by the impairment of the hypothalamic response to cytokine activation, but also by blockade of cytokine production in macrophages (Fig. 4–7). It has been suggested that in the cellular mechanism responsible for this blockade, the steroid-induced protein lipocortin is involved[9] (see also 4.3.3, Fig. 4–39).

Actions. Cortisol enters the target cell by diffusion, combines with the cytoplasmic GR and is transferred to acceptor sites on the chromosomes, resulting in changes of mRNA synthesis and subsequent protein synthesis. In addition, glucocorticoids have a high affinity for MR, but in some tissues a prereceptor modification inactivates these compounds. The widespread MR have equal affinity for aldosterone and the glucocorticoids cortisol and corticosterone, whereas the latter two hormones circulate at much higher concentrations than aldosterone. However, in the classical aldosterone targets (kidney, colon, salivary gland) the enzyme 11β-hydroxysteroid dehydrogenase converts cortisol and corticosterone (but not aldosterone!) to their 11-keto analogs. These analogs cannot bind to MR, thereby enabling aldosterone to occupy this receptor.[19]

Central in the metabolic effects of glucocorticoids is the synthesis of mRNAs leading to synthesis of key enzymes in gluconeogenesis, such as pyruvate carboxylase, fructose-1,6-diphosphatas and fructose-6-phosphatase. Especially in the fasted state glucocorticoids contribute to the maintenance of normoglycemia by gluconeogenesis and by the peripheral release of substrate. The latter is achieved via decreased glucose uptake and metabolism, and decreased protein synthesis leading to increased release of amino acids. In addition, in adipose tissue lipolysis is stimulated. However, in situations of glucocorticoid excess the latter may be overruled by the hyperglycemia-induced hyperinsulinemia that promotes the opposite, i.e., lipogenesis and fat deposition (Fig. 4–9), despite the fact that the action of insulin is counteracted by insulin resistance.[20]

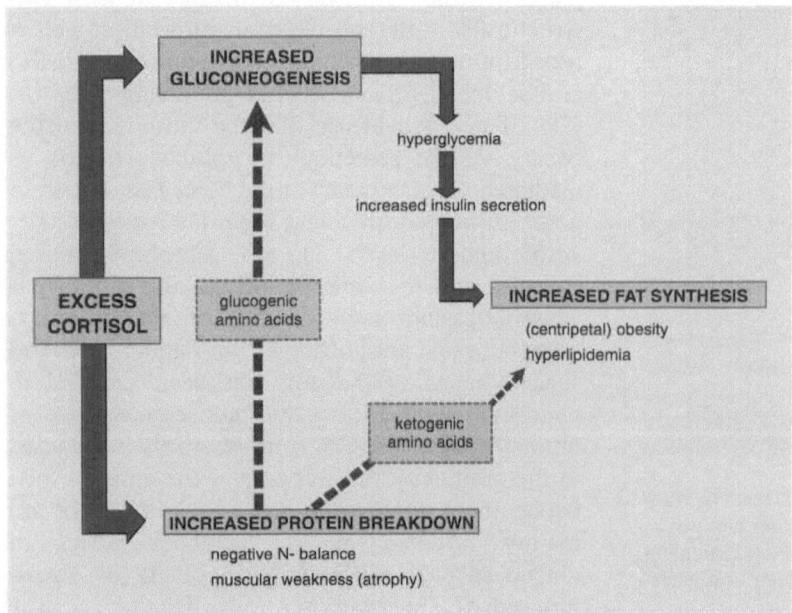

Fig. 4-9. Effects of cortisol excess on intermediary metabolism. The increased gluconeogenesis results in a tendency to hyperglycemia, which initially is controlled by increased insulin secretion. This hyperinsulinemia causes increased lipogenesis. Thus the final result of glucocorticoid excess is a catabolic effect on peripheral tissues such as muscles and skin for the delivery of substrate for the increased gluconeogenesis and lipogenesis.

Through these actions on intermediary metabolism and through other effects, glucocorticoids affect almost all tissues and in particular also blood cells and immunologic functions. Most of these effects are clinically relevant and will be mentioned in the following sections on adrenocortical disease.

The prinicipal effects of aldosterone are on maintenance of normal sodium and potassium concentrations and extracellular volume. This is accomplished by the stimulation of several (primarily renal) proteins that result in increases in (1) sodium permeability in the apical membrane exposed to the lumen of the distal tubules, (2) mitochondrial enzymes increasing cellular ATP and thus enhancing the action of Na^+/K^+-ATPase. These combined actions result in Na^+-reabsorption, whereby K^+excretion increases secondary to the Na^+/K^+ exchange.

4.2 Adrenocortical insufficiency

The term adrenocortical insufficiency (or hypofunction) comprises all conditions in which the secretion of adrenal steroid hormones falls below the requirement of the animal. Two forms can be distinguished:
1. Primary adrenocortical insufficiency, which results from lesions or disease processes located in the adrenal cortices.
2. Secondary adrenocortical insufficiency, which is due to insufficient ACTH release by the pituitary.

The conditions differ not only in pathophysiology, but particularly also in clinical presentation.

4.2.1 Primary adrenocortical insufficiency

Pathogenesis. Primary hypoadrenocorticism results from progressive destruction of the adrenal cortices, which must involve 90% or more of the glands before it causes signs and symptoms. In both the dog and the cat the often found atrophy (Fig. 4–10) is probably the end-result of an immune-mediated destruction. The condition is also named Addison's disease, after Thomas Addison, a physician who in 1856 first described the syndrome in man, which in those days was primarily the result of tuberculosis. In man it has been found that 21-hydroxylase ($P-450_{c21}$) is a major autoantigen in primary hypoadrenocorticism.[21] In the end there is an absolute deficiency of both glucocorticoids and mineralocorticoids together with high plasma levels of ACTH as a result of the strong feedback to the pituitary by the absence of cortisol. Rarely the destruction is confined to the two inner zones, although it may occur more often and remain unnoticed, as there is no mineralocorticoid deficiency, the main determinant of the signs and symptoms. As already indicated in Section 3.3.1, primary hypoadrenocorticism may be part of a polyglandular deficiency syndrome.

Other possible causes of primary adrenocortical insufficiency include (fungal) infections, hemorrhage and metastatic disease, but they seem to be extremely rare. Finally, a nowadays not un-

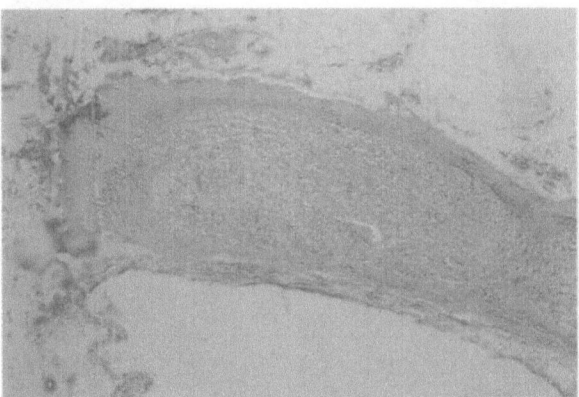 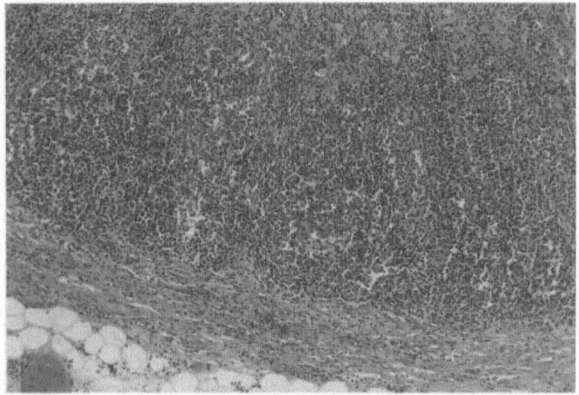

Fig. 4-10. Left: Section of an adrenal of a dog with primary adrenocortical insufficiency. The adrenal medulla is only bordered by the fibrous capsule. The three adrenocortical zones have completely disappeared. Right: Lymphocytic adrenalitis of the cortex (H & E, 10×); probably an autoimmune-mediated destruction of the adrenal cortex of which the end result may be the situation shown on the left.

common iatrogenic cause of the disease should be mentioned: chemotherapy with o,p -DDD for hyperadrenocorticism may deliberately or non-deliberately destroy the adrenal cortices to such an extent that hypoadrenocorticism ensues (see 4.3).

Clinical manifestations. Hypoadrenocorticism is an uncommon disease of primarily young to middle-aged dogs (mean 4 years) with a pre-dilection for the female. Familial occurrence has been described for Standard Poodles,[22] whereas recently a breed predilection for Bearded Collies was reported.[23] In the cat it is also a disease of young to middle-aged animals, although even more rare than in the dog.[24] In the limited number of cases reported so far, no sex predilection was observed.

Although glucocorticoid deficiency may cause some lethargy and weakness and this certainly will contribute to the clinical manifestations, Addison's disease is primarily a syndrome caused by mineralocorticoid deficiency. Many of the signs and symptoms can be related to the hypotonic dehydration due to the sodium losses. The hyperkalemia contributes to the problems by affecting neuromuscular function, particularly leading to conduction disturbances in the heart (Table 4–1; Figs. 4–12, 4–13).

As the disease usually is caused by a gradual autoimmune destruction of the adrenal cortices, one might expect an insidious onset of slowly progressive weakness, fatigue, anorexia and vomiting. Although this may be the case, more often the animal is presented as an emergency in a state of rather severe depression and hypotonic dehydration (Fig. 4–11). There may not have been mild signs initially or the these signs may have remained unnoticed by the owner and are only remembered in retrospect. Apparently the animal can cope with the hormone deficiencies for a long time until a critical threshold in the maintenance of fluid and electrolyte homeostasis is passed.

Thus the disease is usually seen in rather young, suddenly very sick animals, in which the history, physical examination and laboratory examination may reveal the changes listed in Table 4–1.

Differential diagnosis. For the cardinal features of the disease, i.e., rapidly worsening depression, weakness, anorexia and vomiting, there are only a

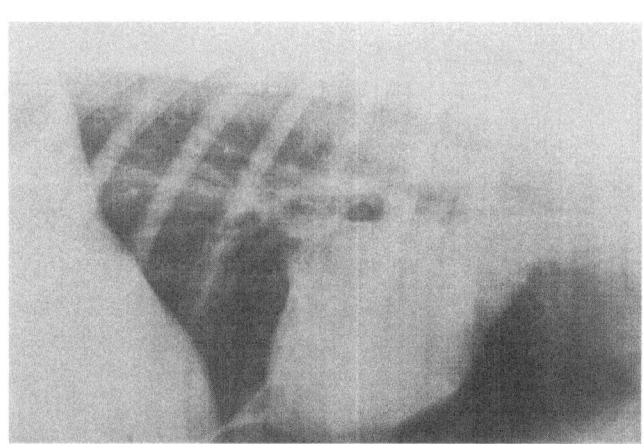

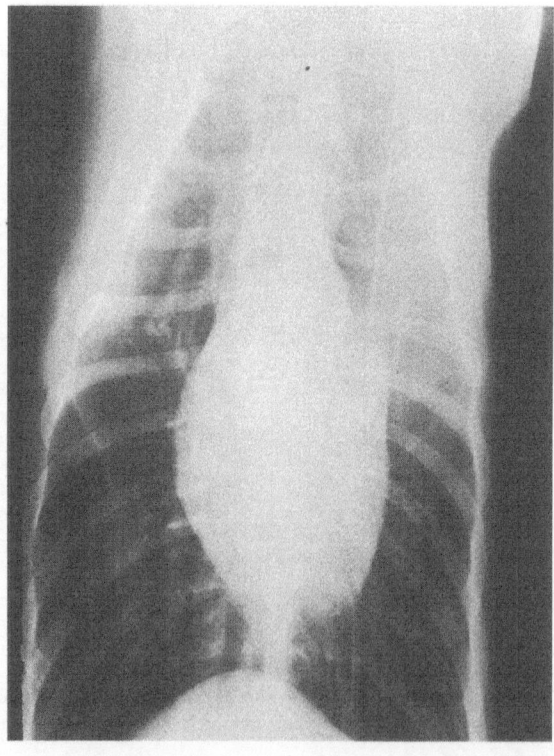

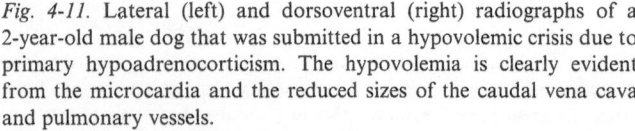

Fig. 4-11. Lateral (left) and dorsoventral (right) radiographs of a 2-year-old male dog that was submitted in a hypovolemic crisis due to primary hypoadrenocorticism. The hypovolemia is clearly evident from the microcardia and the reduced sizes of the caudal vena cava and pulmonary vessels.

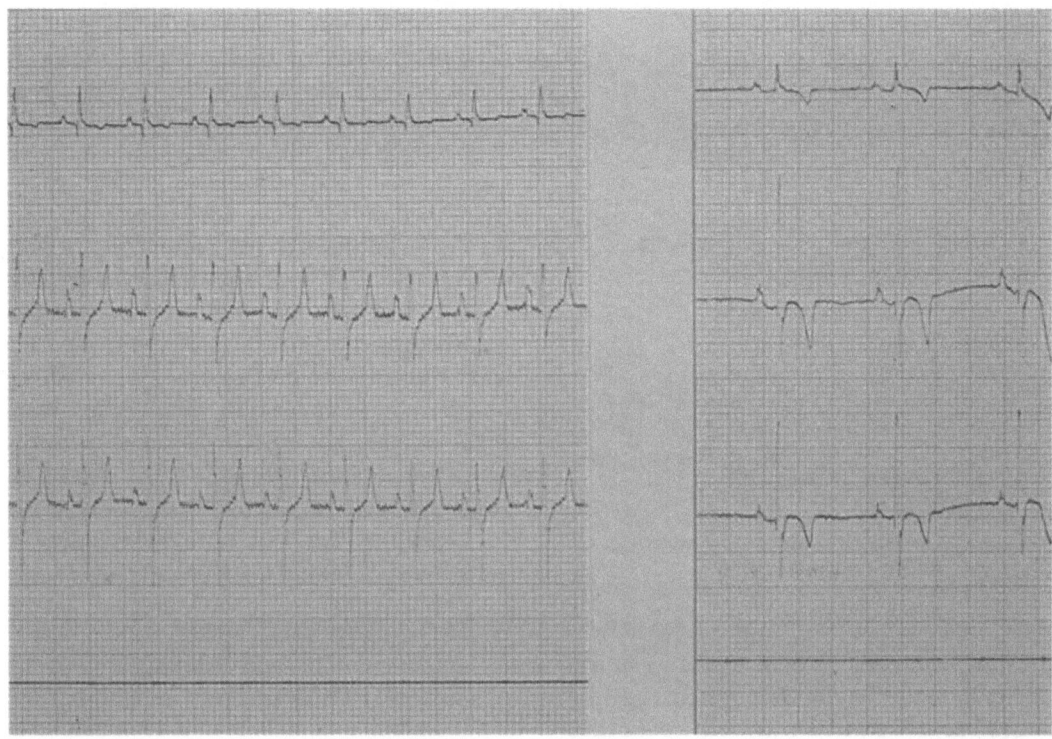

Fig. 4-12. ECG recordings (lead I, II and III) of a 3-year-old female Beagle dog with primary hypoadrenocorticism (calibration: 1 cm = 1 mV; paper speed 25 mm/s). Left: Before treatment (Na⁺ = 137 mmol/l; K⁺ = 6.8 mmol/l) the R-waves (lead II) had low amplitude with high spiked T-waves of about the same height. Right: After treatment the R-waves became normal and T-waves reversed.

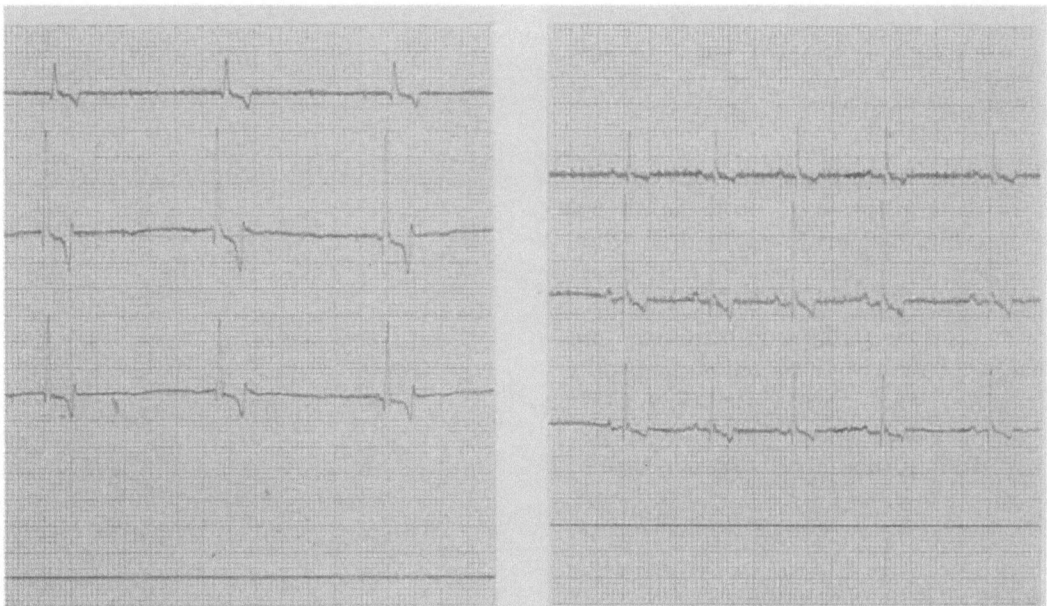

Fig. 4-13. ECG recordings of a 4-year-old mongrel dog with primary hypoadrenocorticism (see also legend to Fig. 4–12). Left: Before treatment (Na⁺ = 131 mmol/l; K⁺ = 8.7 mmol/l) there was extreme bradycardia with absence of P-waves. Right: Treatment more than doubled the heart the heart rate and P-waves reappeared. (Courtesy of A.A. Stokhof)

Table 4-1. Clinical manifestations of primary hypoadrenocorticism.

System	Common	Less common/rare
Metabolic	Anorexia and weight loss	Hypothermia
Neuromuscular	Lethargy / depression, weakness	shaking/shivering, fascicular muscle contractions, restlessness, (esophageal dilatation)
Cardiovascular	Dehydration (10-15%): hypovolemia (Fig. 4-11), hypotonic veins, weak pulse. In ECG (lead II) low R wave, spiked high T wave, wide P wave and QRS complex (Fig. 4-12)	Bradycardia. In ECG (lead II) P wave absent (K+ > 8.5 mmol/l) (Fig. 4-13). (Shock!)
Gastrointestinal	Anorexia and vomiting	Loose stools, (melena), (megaesophagus)
Renal + plasma biochemistry	Prerenal azotemia (urea/creatinine ratio >150), hyponatremia, hyperkalemia, hyperphosphatemia, acidosis	Relatively low urine specific gravity, hypoglycemia, hypercalcemia
Hematologic	Hypoplastic anemia (usually masked by hemoconcentration due to dehydration)	Lymphocytosis, eosinophilia

few syndromes that may have a similar picture. These are ileus, renal insufficiency, acute gastroenteritis and acute pancreatitis. (In countries where the rodenticide thallium sulfate is still used the animals intoxicated with this compound may also be presented with a similar picture). Initially the differentiation may pose problems, as the other conditions occasionally are associated with electrolyte disturbances as well. However, further diagnostic work-up and especially the favourable result of treatment in Addison's disease usually brings the clinician quickly on the right track.

Diagnosis. In cases with a characteristic routine biochemical pattern (prerenal azotemia, hyponatremia and hyperkalemia) and with a good response to treatment, there may be little doubt about the diagnosis. However, it is a diagnosis with as a consequence lifelong treatment and therefore also in these cases it should be secured by an endocrine test. Basal levels of cortisol, in either urine or plasma, are low in cases of complete primary hypoadrencorticism, but they may also be low for other reasons (see 4.2.2, 4.3.3). Therefore a test of adrencortical reserve capacity is necessary to establish the diagnosis, i.e., the ACTH-stimulation test (Chapter 13 and Fig. 4-14).

Treatment. Animals presented in hypovolemic shock and suspected of having Addison's disease

are treated without waiting for laboratory results. The main aims are to correct the hypovolemia by fluid therapy and to reverse the negative sodium balance by corticosteroid administration (Fig. 4–15). Via an intravenous catheter (preferably jugular vein) fluid therapy is started. Just prior to the start of the fluid administration, blood and urine are collected for routine laboratory work (Table 4–1). If later the diagnosis appears to be wrong, it is reassuring to know that the core of the protocol is the correction of the hypovolemia and that this and the corticosteroids certainly will not harm an animal that has been brought in hypovolemic shock. The *initial treatment scheme* for an *acute crisis* comprises the following:

1. *Fluid therapy*: Dehydration is corrected over a period of 4–8 h by intravenous administration of 0.9% NaCl to the total amount of 10–15% of body weight. The first quarter can be given within 30 min. After correction of the hypovolemia, fluid therapy is continued at a rate of 100 ml/kg body weight per 24 h. The

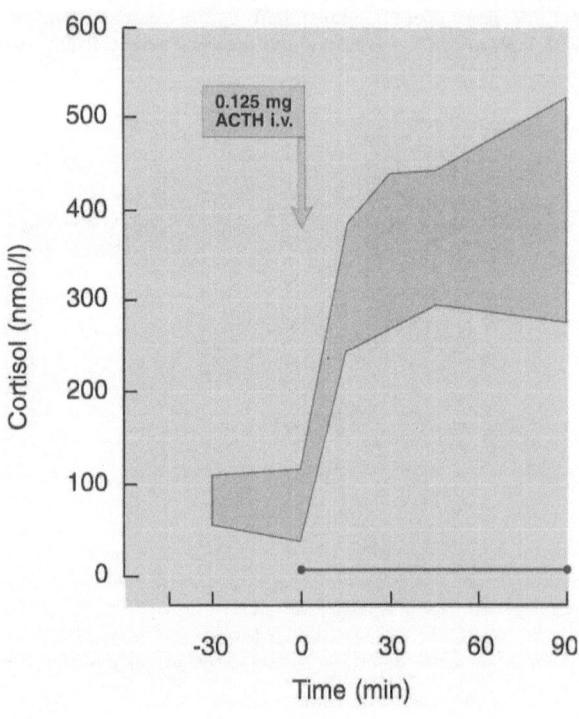

Fig. 4-14. Results of ACTH-stimulation tests in healthy cats (blue area) and in a cat with primary hypoadrenocorticism (uninterrupted line).

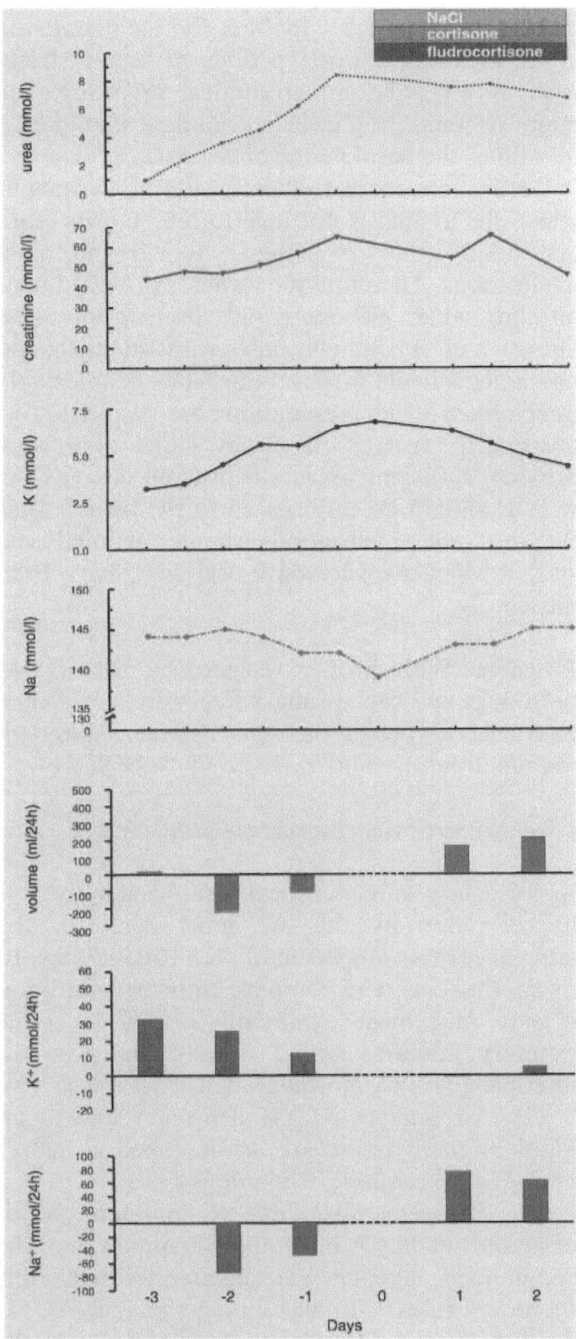

Fig. 4-15. Measurements of plasma concentrations of urea, creatinine, sodium and potassium together with fluid and electrolyte balances in a 6-year-old Cocker Spaniel that had recovered from an unrecognized primary hypoadrenocorticism with fluid therapy only. The dog was left without treatment from day —3 to day 0. The sodium and fluid loss together with potassium retention were compatible with primary hypoadrenocorticism. Treatment reversed these changes (days 1 and 2).

filling of the vascular bed is monitored by central venous pressure and urine production. This treatment will restore renal function, which also leads to correction of the hyperkalemia and the acidosis.

2. *Glucocorticoid therapy*: To the first infusion bottle about 5 mg/kg hydrocortisone succinate[a] is added. If not available, this can be replaced by prednisolone succinate[b] (1 mg/kg) or dexamethasone phosphate[c] (0.2 mg/kg), although these synthetic corticosteroids have the disadvantage of little or no intrinsic mineralocorticoid activity. Thereafter glucocorticoids are administered subcutaneously at 6-h intervals: 1 mg hydrocortisone[a]/kg or 0.2 mg prednisolone[b]/kg body weight.

3. *Mineralocorticoid therapy*: Especially if hydrocortisone or cortisone is used, sufficient mineralocorticoid activity is guaranteed, at least during the first 24 h. If appetite has not then been resumed so that oral medication cannot be started, either desoxycorticosterone acetate (DOCA,[d] once daily 0.1 mg/kg) or desoxycorticosterone pivalate[e] (DOCP, 2 mg/kg = depot for ≥ 20 days) are given, depending on the availability. The latter preparation releases the hormone at a rate of about 1 mg/day/25 mg suspension.[25]

Most dogs and cats with primary hypoadrenocorticism rapidly improve on this regimen. Usually dogs already are willing to eat again the next day, which enables starting oral maintenance therapy. In cats the signs of weakness, lethargy and anorexia may persist for 3 to 5 days despite proper management.[24]

The oral *maintenance therapy* consists of:
- Glucocorticoids: Cortisone acetate[f] is given at a daily dose of 1 mg/kg, or prednisolone at a dose of 0.1–0.2 mg kg body weight.
- Mineralocorticoids: A daily dose of 0.0125 mg fludrocortisone/kg body weight (= 1 tablet of 1/16 mg per 5 kg) is usually sufficient to

[a] Solu-Cortef®, Upjohn

[b] Solu-Medrol®, Upjohn

[c] Dexadreson®, Intervet

[d] DOCA, Veterinary Pharmacy, Yalelaan 6, Utrecht (fax: 31–30–532065)

[e] Percorten-V®, Ciba-Geigy

[f] Cortisoni acetas®, Genfarma (5 and 25 mg per tablet) or Kombivet b.v. (25 mg/tablet)

maintain normal electrolyte concentrations, when given with extra salt (see below). In regimens without salt the recommended dose of fludrocortisone[g] or Kombivet b.v. (0.0625 mg/tablet) is somewhat higher; up to 0.02 mg/kg body weight.[25] This regimen may be preferred in cats, as they tend to dislike the salt more than dogs and the requirements for mineralocorticoids may be somewhat higher than in dogs, although this may be just a matter of size, i.e., in dose rates per unit of body weight small individuals are underdosed per unit of metabolic body size. Alternatively, DOCP injections may be used (see above). The major disadvantages are the limited availability and the development of mild hypoalbuminemia in some dogs.[26]

– Sodium chloride: 0.1 g/kg body weight per day, which can be mixed with the food. In some dogs it causes vomiting right after the meal. This may be solved by adding the salt to the drinking water.

All these oral doses are divided into at least two administrations.

Client instruction and follow-up. At discharge the importance of accurateness in the administration of the substitution therapy is explained to the owner. The first follow-up examination is made 2 to 3 weeks later. Plasma Na and K are measured to find out whether the doses of fludrocortisone and salt need to be adjusted. These adjustments are carried out as follows:

– Slight elevations or decreases of Na in combination with normal K are corrected by adjusting the dose of salt alone.
– If Na is low and K is high, or the reverse, only the dose of fludrocortisone is changed.
– If Na is normal and K is abnormal, the dose of fludrocortisone is changed. In 2 to 3 weeks, Na and K are checked again to decide whether to change the dose of salt as well.

In the next months the cortisone dose may be further reduced to about 0.5 mg/kg, unless signs of hypocortisolism (lethargy, inappetence) appear.

It is recommended to increase the dose of cortisone during situations of stress such as fever, surgical procedures, injuries or gastroenteritis associated with fluid losses. A guideline is that the daily dose should be doubled during periods of minor sickness. During periods of major stress, such as intra-abdominal surgical procedures or major trauma, the glucocorticoid dose should be 2 to 4 times the basal maintenance dose.

During intercurrent illness or during periods in which the animal is not able to take tablets (e.g., anesthesia) it may be necessary to start injectable medications. Therefore the owner is provided with an injectable glucocorticoid preparation (see above) and if available also with an injectable mineralocorticoid preparation. When no injectable mineralocorticoid preparations are available, increasing the hydrocortisone by 4 to 6 times may provide sufficient mineralocorticoid activity as well. It should be emphasized to the owners that the injectable medications should definitely be started when two successive oral doses have been missed.

Prognosis. With proper replacement therapy in both dogs and cats, primary hypoadrenocorticism has a good prognosis. Once stable, follow-up examinations are undertaken only twice yearly.

4.2.2 Secondary adrenocortical insufficiency

In secondary adrenocortical insufficiency there is hyposecretion by the two inner zones of the adrenal cortices as a result of ACTH deficiency. In its spontaneous and complete form the condition is rare and most commonly caused by large pituitary tumors, which usually give rise to multiple pituitary hormone deficiencies (see also 3.3.2). An isolated ACTH deficiency due to an autoimmune hypophysitis, as described in man,[27] has not yet been reported in dogs or cats.

The iatrogenic form due to long-term corticosteroid therapy is much more common than the spontaneous disease. Via negative feedback this therapy causes chronic suppression of ACTH production and as a consequence atrophy of the zona fasciculata and reticularis (Fig. 4–1). Thus as in spontaneous cases these animals have two deficits, a loss of adrenocortical responsiveness to ACTH and a failure of pituitary ACTH release. Upon corticosteroid withdrawal these insufficiencies may continue to exist for several months before full recovery ensues. The condition will also be discussed in Section 4.3.3.

[g] Florinef®, Squibb (0.1 mg/tablet)

Another iatrogenic form of the disease and a more permanent one is of course ACTH deficiency due to hypophysectomy (see also 3.3.2).

Clinical manifestations. In secondary adrenocortical insufficiency the mineralocorticoid production is virtually unaffected, as it is primarily regulated via extra-pituitary mechanisms (see 4.1). Therefore there is not the tendency to hypotension and shock that gives primary adrenocortical insufficiency its dramatic features. On the contrary, although glucocorticoid deficiency may give rise to slight depression and anorexia, the abnormality may remain unnoticed for a long time. Nevertheless, the condition has to be regarded as potentially dangerous because of the animals' inability to cope with stress by activating their pituitary-adrenocortical system. Major (surgical) trauma might cause a crisis and/or non-recovery from anesthesia, if no extra glucocorticoids are given (see also 4.2.1).

Thus it may happen that the condition is found more or less incidentally during routine endocrine studies for problems such as lethargy or alopecia. On the other hand, it may occur that a pituitary tumor has been diagnosed and studies of pituitary function reveal ACTH deficiency.

Diagnosis. Suspicion of secondary adrenocortical insufficiency may be strengthened when the urinary corticoid/creatinine ratios (Chapter 13) are low in the absence of hyponatremia and hyperkalemia. In an ACTH-stimulation test (Chapter 13) low initial cortisol levels will be found, whereas after stimulation there may be (1) a normal or somewhat impaired cortisol response, or (2) no cortisol response. The former outcome excludes primary hypoadrenocorticism but not secondary hypoadrenocorticism, as the response might be seen soon after onset of the disease. In the case of an absent cortisol response there is the possibility of long-standing ACTH deficiency. However, there is also the exceptional possibility that there is still primary adrenocortical insufficiency with selective atrophy of the two inner zones and minimal or no involvement of the zona glomerulosa.[28]

For differentiation between these possibilities further studies are required, which should include measurements of plasma concentrations of ACTH, together with a CRH-stimulation test (Chapter 13). In dogs with primary adrenocortical insufficiency, basal ACTH concentrations are high and there is hyperresponsiveness to CRH. In dogs with secondary adrenocortical insufficiency ACTH levels are low and non-responsive to stimulation with CRH.[29]

Once there is biochemical certainty about the presence of secondary hypoadrenocorticism, visualization of the pituitary should follow in order to obtain some information on the morphology of the lesion that is causing the ACTH deficiency (see also 2.2.5, 3.3.2).

Treatment. The demonstration of a spontaneous form of secondary hypoadrenocorticism is alarming because of the possible underlying lesion rather than that there is a great need for treatment. Dogs seem to be able to live reasonably well with cortisol deficiency, although they may become more active and alert when oral cortisone (0.5–1.0 mg/kg) administration is begun or added to the medication for other deficiencies (see 3.3.2). The animals are especially at risk during stress, and in those situations the dose should be increased to prevent a crisis (see 4.2.1).

Prognosis. As in secondary hypothyroidism (3.3.2) the prognosis is highly dependent upon the development of the causative lesion.

4.3 Adrenocortical hyperfunction; Cushing's syndrome

As described in Section 4.1 the adrenal cortices produce mineralocorticoids, glucocorticoids and androgens. Thus in principle three distinct syndromes may arise in adrenocortical hyperfunction, in man known respectively as hyperaldosteronism or Conn's syndrome, Cushing's syndrome and adrenogenital syndrome. Until now in dogs and cats only the occurrence of a syndrome of glucocorticoid excess has been convincingly demonstrated, the condition being rather common in dogs and rare in cats.

Thus for dogs and cats hyperadrenocorticism can be defined as the physical and biochemical changes that are the result of chronic glucocorticoid excess, whatever its cause. Also in dogs and cats this syndrome is often named Cushing's syndrome, after Harvey Cushing, the neurosurgeon who in 1932 first described the syndrome in man. Apart from the exogenous form of the disease (see 4.3.3) there are two endogenous forms in both the dog and the cat: (1) ACTH-dependent, and (2) ACTH-independent.

In the ACTH-dependent form there is chronic ACTH hypersecretion, resulting primarily in hypersecretion of cortisol and in hyperplasia of the two inner zones of the adrenal cortices.[30] In this form, which accounts for about 85% of cases, the ACTH excess originates form the pituitary; an ectopic or paraneoplastic ACTH syndrome (see also Chapter 11) has not been recognized in dogs and cats so far. Thus for these two species the name for this category can be more specific: pituitary-dependent hyperadrenocorticism. ACTH-independent hyperadrenocorticism is due to autonomous glucocorticoid-secreting adrenocortical adenomas or carcinomas and comprises about 15% of cases. The simultaneous occurrence of both pituitary-dependent hyperadrenocorticism and autonomously hyperfunctioning adrenocortical tumor may also be observed.[31, 31a]

4.3.1 Pituitary-dependent hyperadrenocorticism

The pituitary lesions producing the excess of ACTH range from diffuse hyperplasia and small hyperplastic cell nests of corticotrophic (or melanotrophic) cells (Fig. 2–4) to adenomas (Fig. 4–16) and large tumors[32,33] (Figs. 2–21, 4–17), which exceptionally even may have characteristics of malignancy.[34] There is increasing evidence that in most cases pituitary tumors are the result of a process of tumorigenesis, that may be a multistep process requiring more than one mutation in the protooncogenes involved in hormone production and/or cell proliferation.[35] An inherited aberration may be the earliest step.[36] The process does not seem to be dependent upon continuous hypothalamic stimulation.[37]

In the introduction to this chapter (4.1) it was explained that in dogs and cats both the anterior lobe (AL) of the pituitary and the pars intermedia (PI) have cell types that can synthesize POMC, albeit with different posttranslational processing. Thus the ACTH excess may originate in both the AL and the PI. In about one-fourth to one-fifth of cases an adenoma in the PI is found, but tumors in both lobes may also occur.[32,38] This is of clinical interest not only because the PI tumors tend to be larger than the AL tumors,[32] but also because of the specific hypothalamic control of hormone synthesis in the PI. As mentioned briefly in Section 2.1, the PI is under direct neural control. This is principally a tonic dopaminergic inhibition,[39] which suppresses the expression of glucocorticoid receptors. This explains why cases of pituitary-dependent hyperadrenocorticism of PI origin are resistant to suppression by dexamethasone.[40]

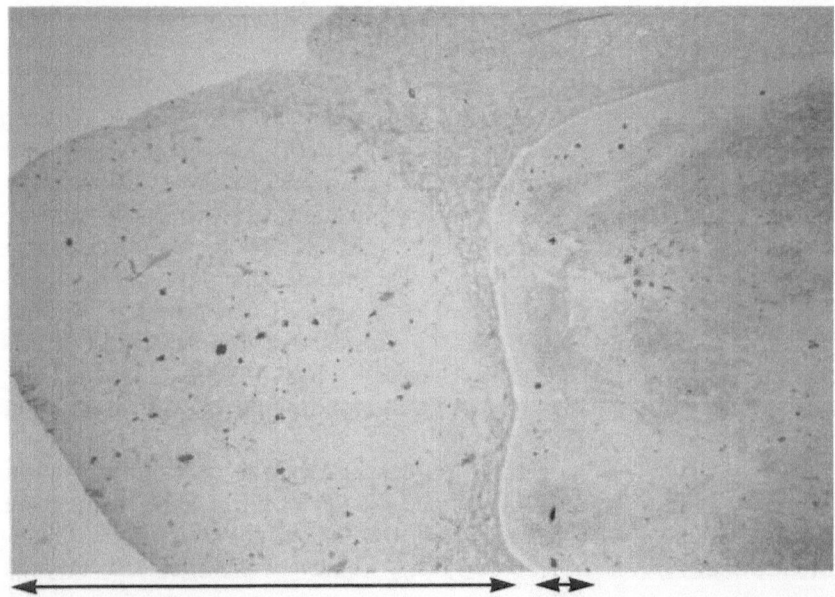

Fig. 4-16. Section of a pituitary of an 8-year-old female Miniature Poodle with pituitary-dependent hyperadrenocorticism due to an adenoma in the anterior lobe (PAS-Alcian Blue Orange-G stain).

AL   PI

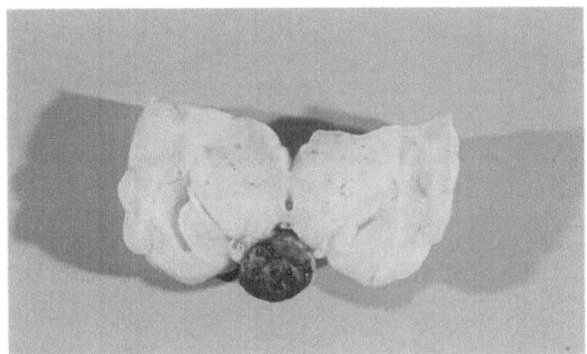

Fig. 4-17. Cross section of the ventral two-thirds of the brain of a 9-year-old male Boxer dog with pituitary-dependent hyperadrenocorticism. There was considerable pituitary enlargement with some compression of the hypothalamus, but not to the extent that it caused neurological signs.

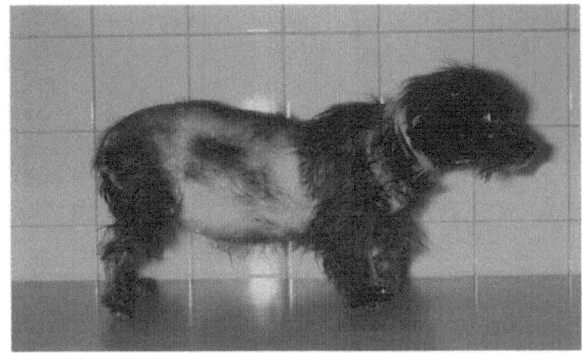

Fig. 4-18. A 10-year-old female mongrel dog with classical signs of hyperadrenocorticism: alopecia and truncal obesity, particularly of the abdomen.

However, this is not an absolute difference from AL lesions, as pituitary lesions causing hyperadrenocorticism may not maintain the regulation characteristics of the lobe of origin.[41] For example, corticotroph-cell adenomas in the AL tend to become less sensitive to the suppressive effect of glucorticoids than normal corticotrophic cells. Actually this is the functional hallmark of pituitary-dependent hyperadrenocorticism which is used to differentiate normal animals from animals with hyperadrenocorticism in the so-called low-dose dexamethasone suppression test (see below and Chapter 13). This loss of suppressibility seems to be a sliding scale, whereby a minority may become resistent even to high doses of dexamethasone, i.e., in the high-dose dexamethasone suppression test (see below and Chapter 13). On the other hand, in PI tumors the neoplastic transformation may be associated with loss of dopaminergic influence, resulting in derepression of the gene encoding the glucocorticoid receptor and thereby becoming suppressible by (high doses of) dexamethasone.

Clinical manifestations. In both dogs and cats pituitary-dependent hyperadrenocorticism is a disease of middle-aged and older animals, although in dogs very occasionally it may occur as young as one year of age. In dogs there is no pronounced sex predilection, whereas in cats the great majority of the reported cases are females.[11] The disease is seen in all dog breeds with possibly a slight predilection for small breeds such as Dachshunds and Miniature Poodles.[31a]

Many of the signs and symtoms can be related to the actions of glucocorticoids as presented in Section 4–1 and Fig. 4–9, that is, increased gluconeogenesis and lipogenesis at the expense of protein. In dogs the cardinal physical features are centripetal obesity and atrophy of muscles and skin with adnexa (Table 4–2, Figs. 4–18, 4–19, 4–20, 4–21). In addition polyuria and polyphagia are often dominating features. In dogs the polyuria is known to be due to both impaired osmoregulation of vasopressin release and interference of the glucocorticoid excess with the action of vasopressin.[42]

Table 4-2. Clinical manifestations of glucocorticoid excess in dogs and cats.

System	Common	Less common/rare
Metabolic	Polyphagia, obesity with abdominal enlargement and hepatomegaly	Weight loss (muscle wasting). Intolerance to hot environment
Skin and hair	Thin coat, alopecia, thin skin with keratin plugs in atrophic hair follicles	Hyperpigmentation, calcinosis cutis, full thickness skin defects (cats)
Respiratory/ Cardiovascular	Panting	Congestive heart failure Pulmonary embolism
Urinary	Polyuria and polydipsia Glycosuria (cats)	Urinary tract infection Glycosuria (dogs)
Neuromuscular	Lethargy, muscular weakness, muscular atrophy	Myotonia
Reproductive	Absence of estrus	Testicular atrophy
Hematologic + Plasma biochemistry	Eosinopenia, lymphopenia, hyperglycemia (cats!), elevated alkaline phosphatase (isoenzyme in dogs!), increased ALT, low thyroxine. Hypercholesterolemia, hyperlipidemia	Elevated hematocrit value. Hyperglycemia (dogs!), hypernatremia, hypokalemia.

76

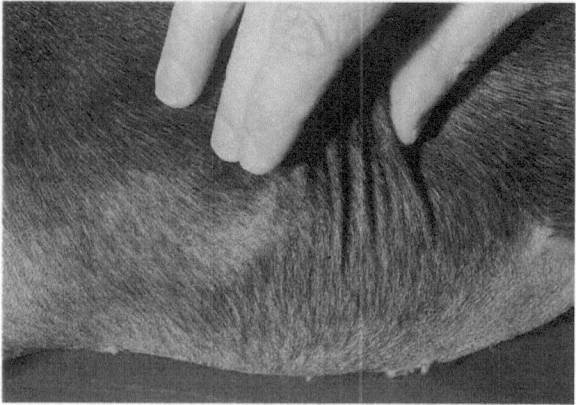
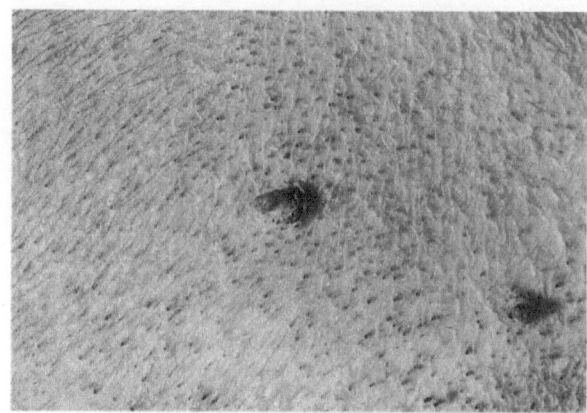

Fig. 4-19. Left: Enlarged belly of a 9-year-old female Dachshund with hyperadrenocorticism. The skin atrophy is shown by the thin coat and the thin skin folds. Right: Skin around the nipples of the same dog with keratin accumulation in atrophic hair follicles.

In cats the situation is somewhat different from that in the dog. The cutaneous manifestations are initially less pronounced than in the dog (Fig. 4–22). Furthermore glucocorticoid excess gives rise less readily to polyuria/polydipsia in this species than in dogs, and it may become obvious only when diabetes mellitus develops.[11] Cats seem to be much more susceptible than dogs to the diabeto-

genic effects of glucocorticoids. In the vast majority of the described cases of feline hyperadrenocorticism the disease was associated with diabetes mellitus and the suspicion of hyperadrenocorticism has often arisen specifically because of insulin resistance encountered in the treatment of diabetes mellitus. Only about 10% of dogs with hyperadrenocorticism develop overt diabetes mellitus.

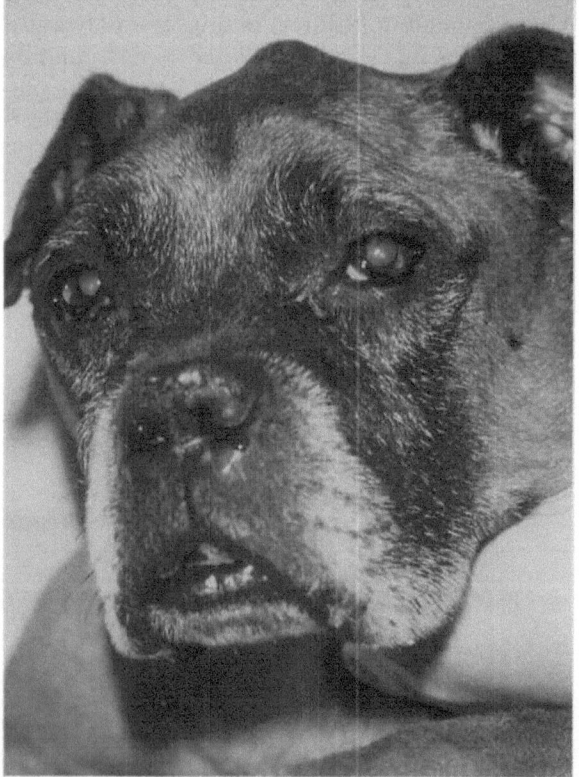
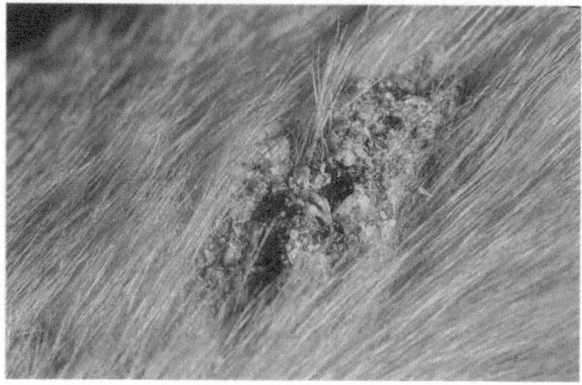

Fig. 4-20. Pictures of a 10-year-old male Boxer dog with pituitary-dependent hyperadrenocorticism. Left: pronounced atrophy of the temporal muscles. It made the owner think that a lumb had developed on the top of the skull, this being a normal anatomical structure (external occipital protuberance). There was also marked atrophy of the muscles of the thighs, back and shoulder/arm. Right: Calcinosis cutis along the dorsal midline. In this dog it was a hard plaque extending from the shoulder area to the lumbar area. These calcium depositions may also be found in the inguinal area. Only a little trauma may cause bleeding.

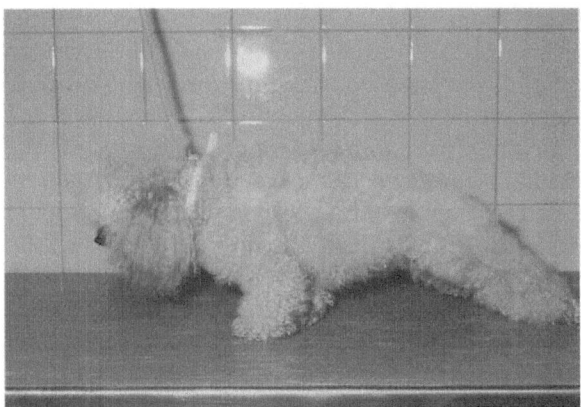

Fig. 4-21, Most commonly glucocorticoid excess results in muscular weakness (decreasing ability to climb, jump and walk) and muscular atrophy. Very rarely there is hypertrophy due to persistent muscle contraction. This myotonia is due to a degenerative myopathy. Affected dogs such as this 8-year-old female Poodle, are presented with a stiff gait, particularly in the hind legs. The continuous overextension may make walking very difficult.

Commonly the disease starts insidiously and progresses slowly, thereby developing the characteristic combination of signs and symptoms that may be recognized as the syndrome of glucocorticoid excess. However, especially in the beginning there may be only one or two presenting symptoms (Fig. 4–23). Very rarely dogs with the disease are presented in an emergency, such as respiratory distress. This may be due to the combination of intolerance to a hot environment and impaired ventilatory mechanics because of the physical changes (muscle wasting and enlarged abdomen). In situations of acute severe dyspnea one has to think of the possiblity that the disease is complicated by pulmonary embolism.

Other complications, although with less of an emergency character, may be abcesses (infected decubitus on elbow in large dogs), skin ulcers (full-thickness defects in cats),[43] urinary tract infections and congestive heart failure. For a description of the neurological signs associated with large pituitary tumor masses, the reader is referred to Section 2.2.5.

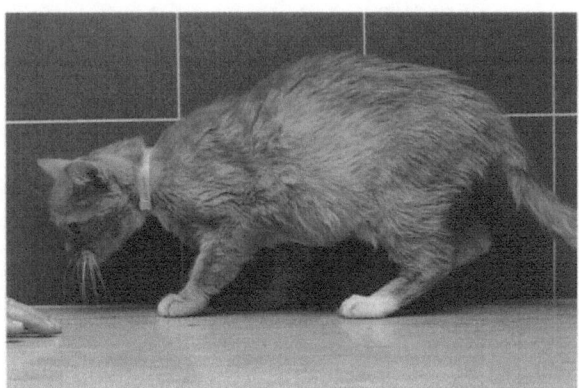

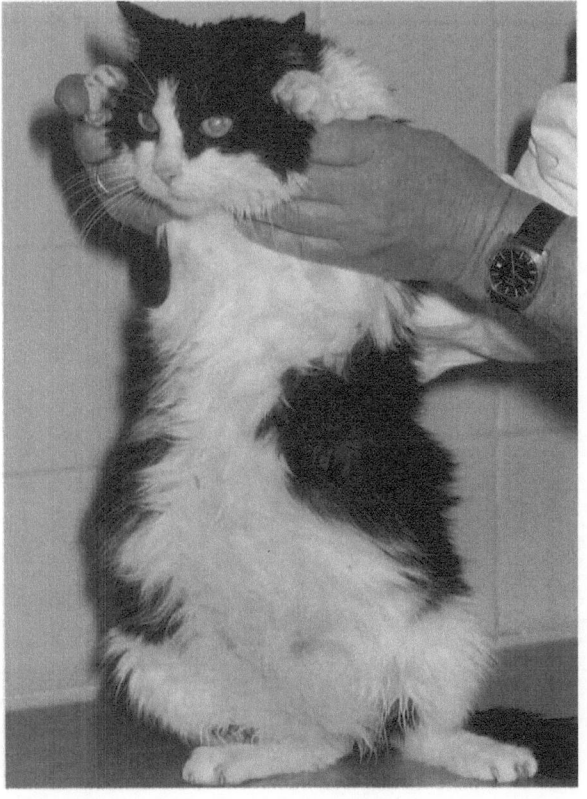

Fig. 4-22. Two spayed female cats, 13 years of age (left) and 8 years of age (right) with pituitary-dependent hyperadrenocorticism. There is some abdominal enlargement. The hair coats are somewhat unkempt and thin. At first sight the skin changes in hyperadrencorticoid cats seem to be less pronounced than in dogs. However, the skin may be very fragile and may tear during routine handling, leaving the cat with a full thickness skin defect.

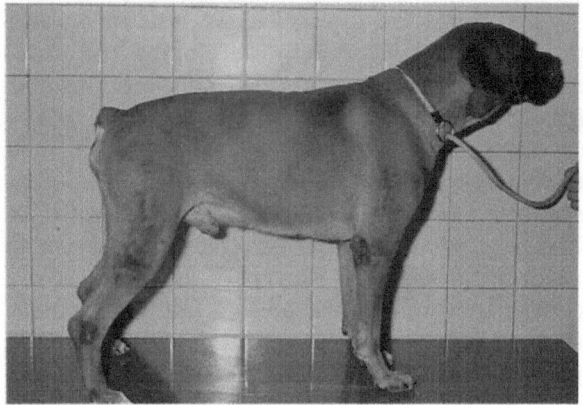

Fig. 4-23. As in most textbooks, in this book illustrations are included that depict pronounced features. It should be realized, however, that most diseases start as slight deviations of health and it may take several months before the classic muscle and skin changes become apparent. For example, this 9-year-old male Boxer dog with hyperadrenocorticism due to an adrenocortical tumor was presented with polyuria of 4 weeks duration as the only problem and no physical changes.

Among the routine laboratory data (Table 4–2) a consistent finding (in dogs only!) is an elevation of the plasma concentration of alkaline phosphatase (AP).[44] This is due to the induction of an isoenzyme which has greater stability at 65 °C than other AP-isoenzymes and is therefore easily measured by a routine laboratory procedure. It is also noteworthy that in the majority of dogs with hyperadrenocorticism decreased T_4 concentrations are found (Fig. 4–24), which seems to be a consequence of altered transport, distribution, and metabolism of T_4, rather than hyposecretion (see also Section 3.3.1).

Differential diagnosis. For the differential diagnoses concerning the two main clinical features, polyuria and alopecia, the reader is referred to Chapter 15, where algorithms for these problems are presented.

Diagnosis. In pituitary-dependent hyperadrenocorticism, feedback inhibition of ACTH (secreted from the pituitary adenoma) by glucocorticoids is impaired. Thus ACTH hypersecretion persists despite elevated cortisol secretion. However, measurement of plasma cortisol concentration has little diagnostic value, as the episodic secretion of ACTH results in variable plasma levels that may at times be within the reference range (see also Fig.

1–8). There are two ways to overcome this problem: (1) to test the integrity of the feedback system, and (2) to measure urinary corticoid excretion.

In the first approach the sensitivity of the pituitary-adrencortical system to suppression is tested by administering a synthetic glucocorticoid in a dose that discriminates between healthy animals and animals with hyperadrenocorticism. A potent glucocorticoid such as dexamethasone is used in order that the administered compound may be given in such small amounts as not to contribute significantly to the steroids to be analyzed. In this so-called dexamethasone screening test or low-dose dexamethasone suppression test (LDDST), 0.01 mg dexamethasone per kg body weight is administered intravenously in the morning. Blood for cortisol measurement is collected 8 h after dexamethasone administration. In

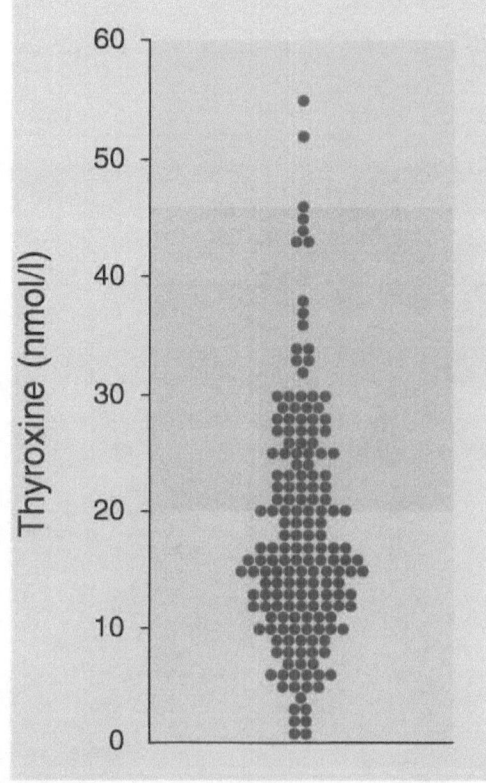

Fig. 4-24. Plasma T_4 concentration in 174 dogs with hyperadrenocorticism. The reference range is indicated by the blue zone. Although in some dogs with pituitary-dependent hyperadrenocorticism the pituitary tumor may interfere with TSH release (Section 3.3.2), in the majority of cases the low T4 values are the result of the glucocorticoid excess per se.

healthy animals the plasma cortisol concentrations are still depressed at this time, whereas in animals with hyperadrenocorticism they have remained high or may have escaped from initial suppression. This test is described in detail in Chapter 13.

This LDDST is increasingly replaced by the second approach, i.e., the measurement of urinary corticoids. In this way an integrated reflection of the corticoid production is obtained, thereby adjusting for fluctuations in plasma levels. The urinary corticoids (largely cortisol) are measured by radioimmunoassay and related to the creatinine concentration. This test requires little time from the veterinarian, is not invasive (no blood collection), has a high diagnostic accuracy and easily allows follow-up examination.[45,46] In addition the test procedure, as described in Chapter 13, has the advantage of combining a test for basal adrenocortical function and a dynamic test for differential diagnosis (see below).

Once the diagnosis of hyperadrenocorticism has been made it is necessary to distinguish between pituitary-dependent hyperadrenocorticism and hyperadrenocorticism due to adrenocortical tumor. Despite a decreased sensitivity to suppression by glucocorticoids, the ACTH secretion of most animals with pituitary-dependent hyperadrenocorticism can be suppressed with a 10-fold higher dose of dexamethasone, resulting in a decreased cortisol secretion. The autonomous hypersecretion by adrenocortical tumors will not be influenced by the high dose of dexamethasone. (see also Figs. 1–5 – 1–7). Two procedures are used, one employing plasma cortisol as a reflection of adrenocortical secretion and the other urinary corticoid/creatinine ratios (Chapter 13). In both, a greater than 50% decline from baseline values is regarded as diagnostic for pituitary-dependent hyperadrenocorticism.

When suppression is less than 50%, the hyperadrenocorticism may be due to either an adrencortical tumor or a pituitary ACTH excess that is extremely resistent to dexamethasone suppression. For the differentiation between these two forms, measurements of endogenous ACTH are necessary. In the great majortiy of the dogs with adrenocortical tumor the basal ACTH values are completely suppressed and much lower values (< 35 ng/l) are found than in the cases of pituitary-dependent hyperadrenocorticism (Fig. 4–25).

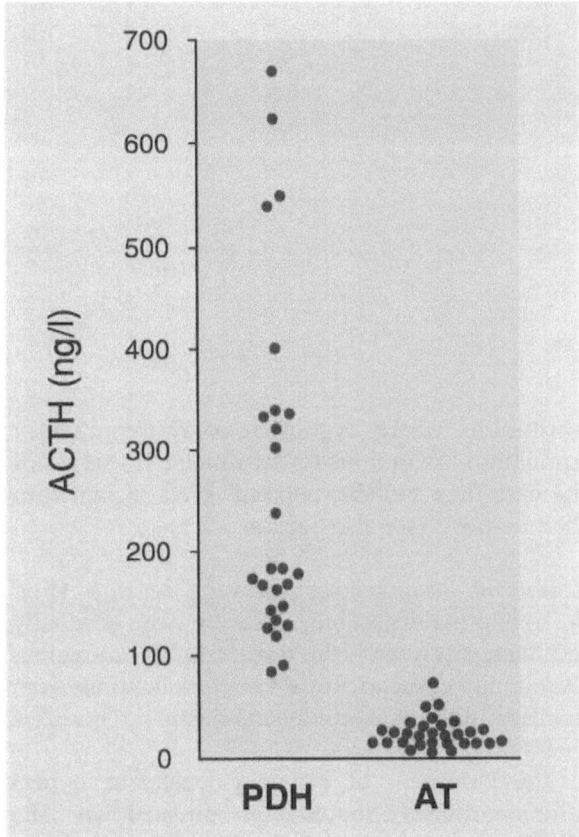

Fig. 4-25. Plasma concentrations of ACTH in hyperadrenocorticoid dogs with dexamethasone resistance, i.e., dogs with less than 50% suppression of the elevated urinary corticoid/creatinine ratios by three 8-hourly administrations of 0.1 mg dexamethasone/kg. In almost all dogs with pituitary-dependent hyperadrenocorticism (PDH) the ACTH values were considerably higher than in the dogs with adrenocortical tumor (AT).

In the situation of questionable ACTH values, which for example might be due to the simultaneous occurrence of both entities[31,31a], further studies are required. These may include a CRH-stimulation test[40,47] (Chapter 13) and visualization of the adrenal glands and the pituitary. It may also be helpful to measure plasma concentrations of α-MSH. High values may be found especially in cases of intermediate lobe tumors, which tend to be dexamethasone resistent and rather large (see also the introduction of this section).

Once the biochemical work-up indicates the presence of pituitary-dependent hyperadrenocorticism, the pituitary is visualized if possible (Fig. 2–27). This visualization is imperative in

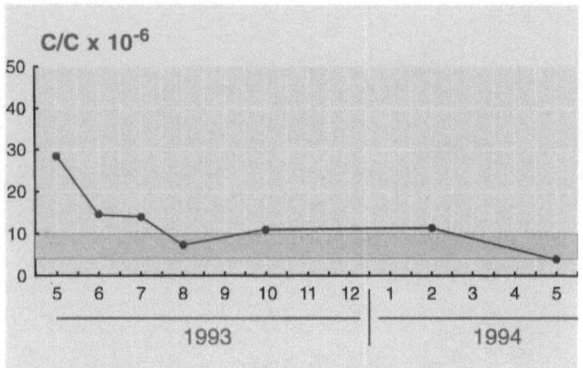

Fig. 4-26. Urinary corticoid/creatinine ratios (averaged duplicate measurements on 2 consecutive days) in a 7-year-old castrated male Dachshund presented with alopecia, lethargy and some weight gain (orange band = reference range). Especially because the signs and symptoms were rather mild, the owners decided to postpone treatment and to follow the course of the disease by measuring urinary corticoids. The dog gradually recovered, became more lively, and lost some weight and by May 1994 the hair coat had fully regrown. Such exceptional cases have been observed in man and could be ascribed to spontaneous necrosis of a pituitary corticotroph adenoma.[88]

institutions where hypophysectomy or pituitary irradiation are options for treatment. If this is not the case then visualization still gives insight into the prognosis (see also Section 2.2.5).

Treatment. Spontaneous recovery is rare (Fig. 4–26) and life expectancy in severe cases is usually less than one year if the disease is left untreated. Death may ensue as a result of complications such as heart failure, thromboembolism or diabetes mellitus.

The treatment of pituitary-dependent hyperadrenocorticism should be directed at the elimination of the stimulus for the augmented production of cortisol, i.e., the pituitary lesion causing the excessive ACTH secretion. Particularly because there is increasing evidence that these lesions are of primary pituitary origin (see above) and not the result of increased hypothalamic stimulation,[35–37] hypophysectomy is being revisited (Fig. 4–27). The transsphenoidal approach was introduced for clinical use in the 1960s,[48] but there were at least three problems that prohibited general use: (1) uncontrollable bleeding from a venous sinus surrounding the pituitary sometimes necessitated premature ending of the surgery, (2) for reasons of anatomical orientation the operation was difficult to perform in brachycephalic breeds, (3) complete removal of larger lesions was often not succesful.[49,50] In the

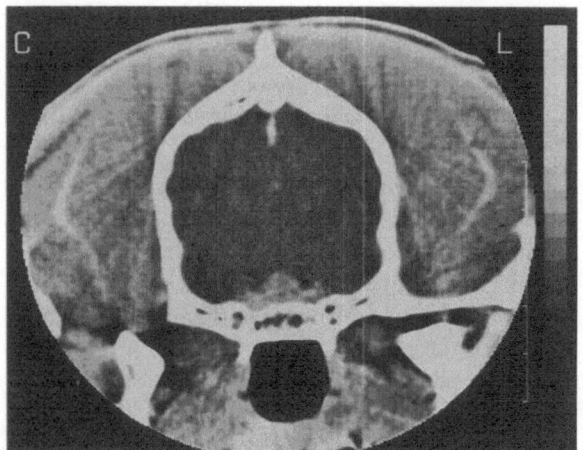
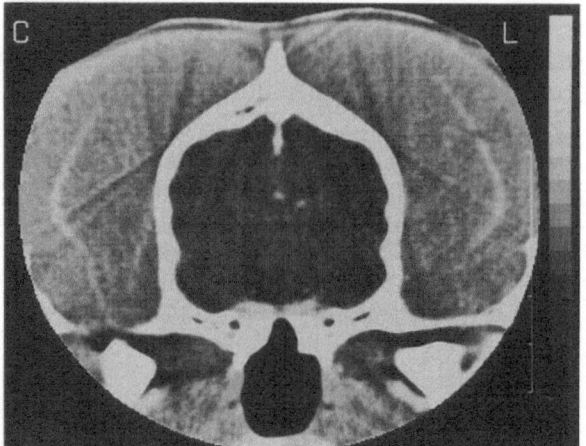

Fig. 4-27. Transverse CT images of the head of a 9-year-old female Bouvier-cross with pituitary-dependent hyperadrenocorticism, before (left) and three months after hypophysectomy (right). Prior to surgery contrast enhancement revealed a pituitary tumor with a height of 7.3 mm and a width of 8.3 mm, whereas after surgery no pituitary tissue could be visualized. In this dog the condition was characterized as dexamethasone-resistent because the urinary corticoid/creatinine ratios after dexamethasone suppression (23×10^{-6}) had decreased less than 50% as compared with the average of the ratios of the two preceding control days (33×10^{-6}). The high basal plasma ACTH values (238 and 240 ng/l) indicated pituitary-dependency, whereas the high α-MSH concentrations (185 and 235 ng/l) suggested that the tumor had originated from melanotropic cells of the pars intermedia. After surgery the urinary corticoid/creatinine ratios in two consecutive morning urines were < 0.5 and 1.1×10^{-6}. (Courtesy of B.P. Meij.)

meantime visualization techniques have become available that enable presurgical insight into the size and expansion of the lesion. This in combination with improved surgical and anesthetic techniques now permits removal of rather large tumors (Fig. 4–27). Also because in this approach the causative lesion is removed, this may become the method of choice in dogs and cats, as it is in man. The animals need lifelong replacement therapy with thyroxine (see 3.3.1) and cortisone (see 4.2.1). In addition there may be transient diabetes insipidus, requiring treatment for some time (see 2.3.1). Dogs with microadenomas are regarded as good candidates for hypophysectomy. Their prognosis is said to be excellent,[51] although so far there are no reports on series with long-term follow-up.

Other approaches are directed at the elimination of the glucocorticoid excess, either by bilateral adrenalectomy or by chemotherapy. With total adrenalectomy the cure is 100% and the prognosis with glucocorticoid and mineralocorticoid replacement (4.2.1) is good, unless the expansion of the pituitary lesion gives rise to neurologic signs (see 2.2.5). Details on the peri- and postoperative medication are given in section 4.3.2. Probably because of the effectiveness and relative convenience of chemotherapy with o,p'-DDD, bilateral adrenalectomy is hardly used in dogs. As o,p'-DDD in cats does not give satisfactory results, in this species bilateral adrenalectomy has been used most often to treat pituitary-dependent hyperadrenocorticism. It is often succesful but from the experience with the few cats that have been operated it has been concluded that long-term prognosis is guarded.[52] As in dogs, hypophysectomy may become a more attractive approach.

Currently the most common form of treatment of pituitary-dependent hyperadrenocorticism in the dog is still the administration of the adrenolytic drug o,p'-DDD.[h] Many schedules aim at the selective destruction of the adrenal cortices, i.e., the destruction of the zona fasciculata and zona reticularis, while sparing the zona glomerulosa. However, in 5–6% of the dogs the zona glomerulosa is destroyed to such an extent that iatrogenic hypoadrenocorticism occurs.[53] In more than half of cases there are one or more relapses of

[h] Lysodren®, Bristol Laboratories

hyperadrenocorticism during treatment.[53]

In order to circumvent these complications a treatment schedule has been introduced that is aimed at the complete destruction of the adrenal cortices and substitution therapy for the induced adrenocortical insufficiency:[54]

– 50 to 75 mg o,p'-DDD/kg per day is given for 25 days. This daily dose should be divided into three or four portions and administered with food (Fig. 4–28).
– On the third day, supplementations begins (see also 4–2-1):
Cortisone, 2 mg/kg per day
Fludrocortisone, 0.0125 mg/kg per day
Sodium chloride, 0.1 g/kg per day
All doses are divided into at least two administrations.

After 25–30 days, a follow-up examination is made. The cortisone dose is reduced to 0.5–1.0 mg/kg per day. Fludrocortisone and/or salt are adjusted according to the results of measurements of Na and K in plasma (see also 4.2.1).

Owner compliance is imperative for good results; an example of written instructions for owners is given in Chapter 14. During the first month the owner is requested to report by telephone at least once a week and as often as questions or problems arise. The owner is also instructed very clearly to stop o.p'-DDD admin-

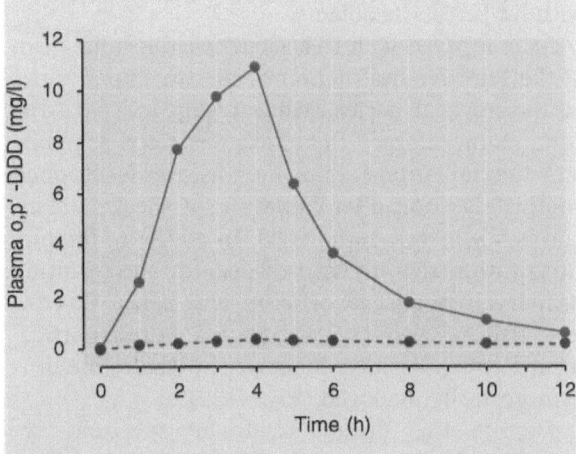

Fig. 4-28. Mean o,p'-DDD concentrations in plasma of 6 dogs given the drug as intact tablets without food (blue line) and with food (red line). The figure clearly illustrates that systemic availability of this lipophylic drug is very poor when intact tablets are administered without food. Ordinary dog food seems to contain sufficient fat to allow good absorption.[89]

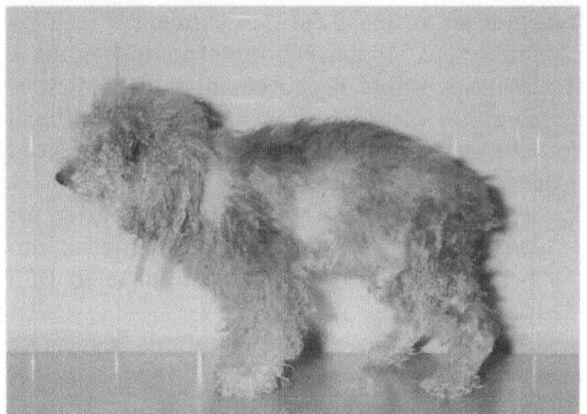 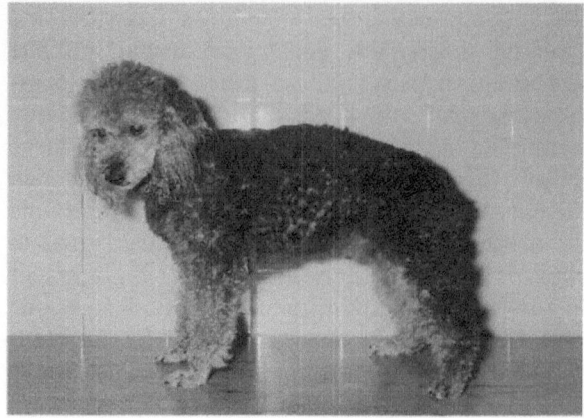

Fig. 4-29. Eight-year-old male miniature Poodle with pituitary-dependent hyperadrenocorticism and diabetes mellitus before (left) and 6 months after (right) destruction of the adrenal cortices with o,p'-DDD. In addition to the recovery of hyperadrenocorticism, the insulin demand decreased considerably and remained stable at a low level.

istration when partial or complete inappetance develops, but with equal emphasis, to continue adrenocortical hormone substitution. If this measure is taken, the owner should also contact the veterinarian, who may increase the cortisone substitution temporarily. When a reduction in appetite is neglected and the o,p'-DDD treatment is continued the dog may start to vomit, refuse substitution therapy, and develop a hypoadrenocorticoid crisis. However, with good instructions this is rare and usually the o,p'-DDD administration can be resumed after a few days without further problems.

As compared with treatment schedules that aim at the selective destruction of the two inner zones of the adrenal cortex, while trying to spare the zona glomerulosa,[53] the above described schedule has the advantage that the disease is stopped completely soon after initiation of the treatment and is not merely suppressed. In addition, lifelong substitution therapy is provided for the resulting primary hypoadrenocorticism and hence there is less risk of sudden, unexpected adrenocortical insufficiency. Finally, concurrent diabetes mellitus is more easily managed (Fig. 4–29).

Despite this drastic treatment schedule, recurrences do occur in about 20–30% of cases within one year. The owner may call because the animal's appetite and water intake have increased. Omitting the cortisone substitution may ameliorate the signs temporarily, but the possible recurrence should be investigted by asking the owner to send urine specimens for measurements of corticoid/creatinine ratios. Two morning urine samples are collected at an interval of 4 to 5 days, each time omitting the cortisone and fludrocortisone administration on the preceding evening. Ratios exceeding the upper limit of the reference range indicate glucocorticoid excess, and o,p'-DDD therapy is then started for another 25 days, followed by once weekly administration of o,p'-DDD for 8 weeks. Substitution therapy and follow-up examinations are carried out as in the first course. In the rare case of a second recurrence, this procedure is repeated and the weekly o,p'-DDD dose is continued for half a year.

Another therapeutic option, although an expensive one, could be the inhibition of adrenocortical steroidogenesis by ketoconazole,[i] a synthetic imidazole analogue used as a broad-spectrum antifungal agent. Its therapeutic properties result from binding to yeast and fungal cytochrome P-450. At high concentrations, ketoconazole also affects certain cytochrome P-450 enzymes in microsomal and mitochondrial fractions of mammalian cells.[55] This drug has been used in dogs in the treatment of both pituitary-dependent hyperadrenocorticism and hyperadrenocorticism due to adrenocortical tumor. The initial dosage is 5 mg/kg twice daily for 7 days and then 10 mg/kg twice daily. Several dogs require 15 mg/kg twice daily to maintain control of the

---

[i] Nizoral®, Janssen (200 mg/tablet; 20 mg/ml suspension)

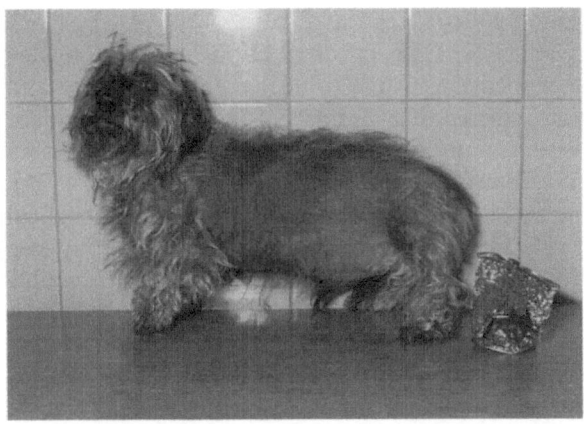 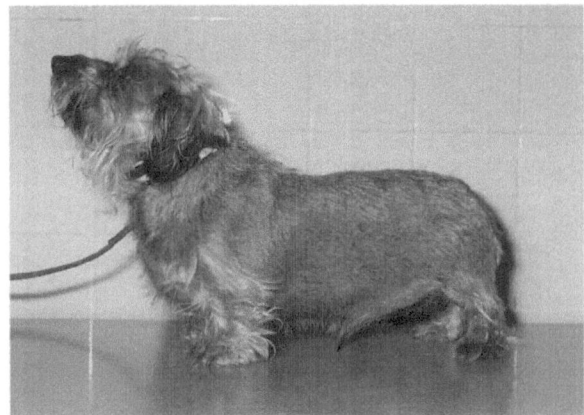

Fig. 4-30. Nine-year-old castrated male Dachshund with pituitary-dependent hyperadrenocorticism (basal urinary corticoid/creatinine ratios 42 and 48×10^{-6}; after three 8-hourly oral doses of 0.1 mg dexamethasone/kg: 6×10^{-6}). In this case it was particularly the dog's ravenous appetite that concerned the owner; as an illustration, he brought the empty can which the dog had tried to eat (left). Following destruction of the adrenal cortices with o,p'-DDD and substitution for the thus induced primary hypoadrenocorticism the dog and owner resumed a normal life (right, photograph 7 month after initiation of treatment).

hyperadrenocorticism. The major limitations in using ketoconazole in dogs are (1) the need for continuing twice daily administration, (2) the expense, and (3) the failure of some dogs to respond.[56] In cats the results have been unpredictable and variable.[26]

Finally, two treatment options should be mentioned that so far have been used infrequently. First there is radiation therapy for pituitary macroadenomas. This may lead to some decrease in the tumor mass and peritumoral edema, but concurrent adrenocortical suppression treatment is needed[57] (see also 2.2.3, 2.2.5). Cats not amenable to bilateral adrenalectomy may be treated with Metyrapone.[j] This drug reduces cortisol synthesis by inhibiting $P-450_{11}\beta$ (11β-hydroxylase), thereby blocking the conversion of 11-deoxycortisol to cortisol (Fig. 4–3). It is advised for controlling the harmful effects of hypercortisolemia, in cats prior to surgery,[43] although it may be effective in long-term treatment as well.[58]

Prognosis. With the above schedule for dogs, that aims at the destruction of the adrenal cortices, the hyperadrenocorticism can be satisfactory controlled. The dogs can live a healthy life for several years (Fig. 4–30), provided there is no expansion of the pituitary lesion to such an extent that it

causes neurological signs. As mentioned above, following succesful bilateral adrenalectomy cats still have a guarded prognosis.

4.3.2 Hyperadrenocorticism due to adrenocortical tumors

When there is resistence to suppression by dexamethasone, either in the HDDST or in the corticoid/creatinine ratios (see Chapter 13), there is about equal chance of adrenocortical tumor or (dexamethasone resistant) pituitary-dependent hyperadrenocorticism. It may be tempting to try to decide upon basis of the physical changes and/or the results of the suppression test(s) whether there is an an adrenocortical tumor or pituitary-dependent hyperadrenocorticism.

One could for example think that adrenocortical tumors more easily produce large amounts of hormone than hyperplastic adrenal cortices, so that in the former the physical changes would be most severe. This is not the case (Fig. 4–31). In many dogs with adrenocortical tumor the hormone excess and as a consequence the signs and symptoms are rather only moderate. It may even happen that the corticoid production as measured by corticoid/creatinine ratios is just around the upper limit of the reference range, but that the suspicion of the disease especially arises because of the lack of suppressibility. Thus despite the fact that adrenocortical tumors usually greatly

[j] Metopirone®, CIBA

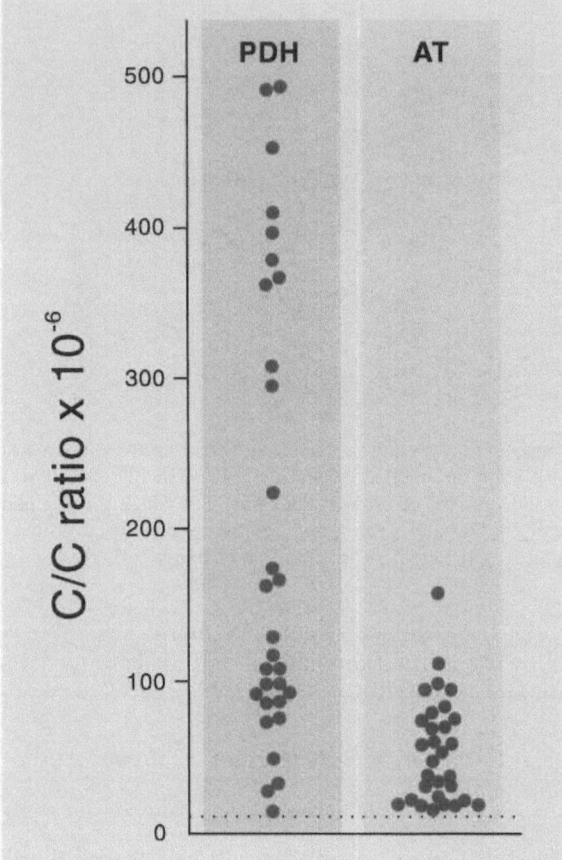

Fig. 4-31. Urinary corticoid/creatinine (C/C) ratios in dogs with hyperadrenocorticism and resistence to suppression of these values (< 50% suppression) by three 8-hourly admin-istrations of 0.1 mg dexamethasone/kg body weight. Final diagnoses of pituitary-dependent hyperadrencorticism (PDH) and adrenocortical tumor (AT) was secured by measurements of plasma ACTH and visualization of the adrenals. Note that in several AT cases the C/C ratios were only moderately elevated and that the highest ratios were found in dogs with PDH.

exceed the size of the normal gland, the tumor tissue is only moderately active, i.e., the neoplastic transformation results in a decreased degree of function per unit of volume.

As far as suppressibility by dexamethasone is concerned, in dogs with adrenocortical tumors dexamethasone administration may cause a para-doxical rise in both the corticoid/creatinine ratios and the plasma cortisol values. On the other hand in dogs with pituitary-dependent hyperadreno-corticism there may still be some suppressibility. However, there is insufficient consistency in these observations to allow differentiation between

these two forms of the disease.

Thus for the differentiation between hyper-adrenocorticism due to adrenocortical tumor and non-suppressible forms of pituitary-dependent hyperadrenocorticism, measurements of plasma ACTH are still required (see 4.3.2 and Fig. 4–25). However, in many instances an adrenocortical tumor is readily detected by ultrasonography (see below). Therefore in cases of non-suppressible hyperadrenocorticism it is common practice to measure plasma ACTH and to perform ultra-sonography of the adrenals. When an adreno-cortical tumor is found it is still useful to have ACTH measurements, as ACTH levels ought to be low and if not, further studies are warranted, as there might be a co-existent pituitary-dependent hyperadrenocorticism.

Pathology. Adrenocortical tumors causing hyper-adrenocorticism occur in both the dog and the cat.[31,59] Most are unilateral solitary lesions. The left and the right adrenal glands are affected about equally. Bilateral tumors occur in about one out of 10 cases.[31,60] Histological types range from small well-encapsulated adenomas (Fig. 4–32) to large carcinomas (Fig. 4–33) with liver and lung metastases. However, it should be noted that miscroscopic examination of a seemingly benign looking tumor may reveal expansion of tumor tissue into vessels.[31] Especially the larger carcino mas may contain necrosis and hemorrhage. The

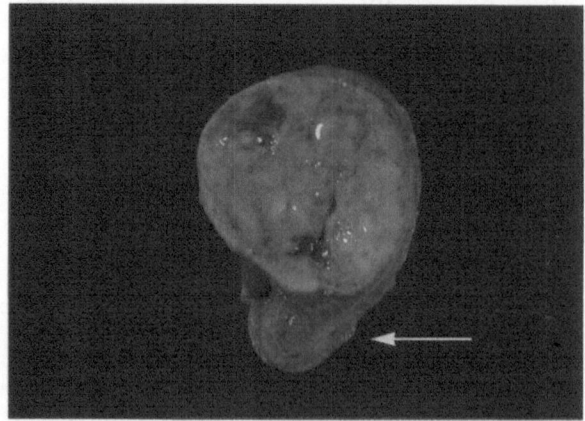

Fig. 4-32. Cut surface of a small adrenocortical tumor in the cranial pole of the left adrenal gland. The tumor was surgically removed from a 10-year-old female Miniature Schnauzer with hyperadrenocorticism. Note the atrophic adrenal cortex, which is visible as a small rim surrounding the adrenal medulla at the caudal pole (arrow).

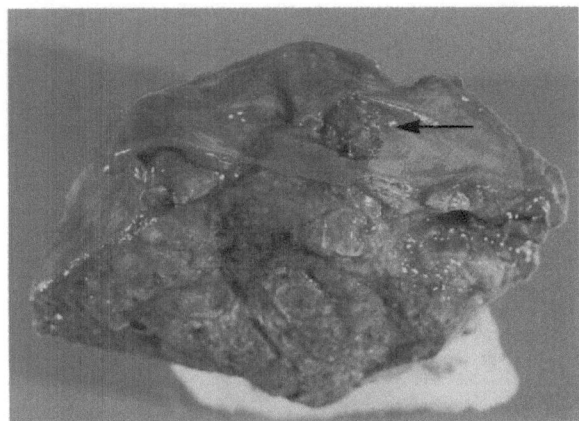

Fig. 4-33. Large adrenocortical tumor of a 9-year-old male Boxer dog with hyperadrenocorticism. The tissue was removed at autopsy. Tumor tissue (arrow) protrudes into the longitudinally opened vena cava.

latter may also become apparent clinically; the animal may be presented as an emergency with hypovolemia due to hemo(retro)peritoneum.[61.62.] Another interesting feature of adrenocortical tumors is that it is not uncommon for them to be associated with pheochromocytoma (see also 4.4),[31] although so far the co-existence of these tumors has remained clinically undetected.

Diagnostic imaging. The preferred procedure for visualization of the adrenals is computed tomography (CT) (Fig. 4–34).[63] However, the equipment is expensive and anesthesia is required.

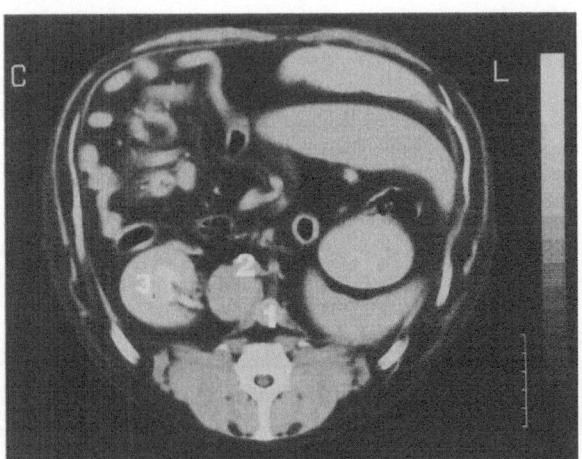

Fig. 4-34. Contrast-enhanced CT image of the abdomen of a 9-year-old male German Shepherd with a well-demarcated mass between the aorta (1), the caudal vena cava (2), and the right kidney (3).

Ultrasonography is a less expensive procedure, the examination time is shorter and it can be performed without anesthesia. Therefore ultrasonography is now the first choice for the visualization of adrenal glands, although it is more difficult to perform and to interpret than CT. The technique allows good estimates of the size of the tumor and may reveal information about its expansion (Fig. 4–35).[64] In individual cases it may be difficult to distinguish between macronodular hyperplasia and adrenocortical tumor. In these instances additional visualization with CT may be needed, and especially in these cases the observations should be interpreted in conjunction with the results of the biochemical studies,[65] i.e., basal plasma ACTH concentrations and if necessary extended by a CRH test (Chapter 13). It should be added that an experienced radiologist may be able to localize adrenocortical tumors by survey radiography in about half of cases,[63] but because of this low detection rate it is not used as a routine.

Once the presence of an adrenocortical tumor has been established, the possibility of distant metastases should be considered. During the abdominal ultrasonography for the identification of the adrenals the liver can also be investigated for metastases. In cases of suspicion of liver metastases an ultrasound guided biopsy can be performed to test this this supposition. In addition thoracic radiographs should be made.

Treatment. When the preoperative investigations reveal that it is likely that there is a resectable unilateral tumor, it should be treated by surgery, because the succesful removal of the tumor will result in complete recovery without the need for continuing medication. Because of the atrophy of the contralateral adrenal, due to the longstanding glucocorticoid excess, glucocorticoid substitution is needed initially. At the time of anesthesia, when intravenous fluid administration is started, 5 mg hydrocortisone-succinate[a]/kg body weight is added to the first bottle and this amount is administered over a period of 6 h (see also 4–2-1). Subsequently 0.5 mg hydrocortisone[a]/kg is administered at 6 h intervals until oral medication is possible. This will consist of 1 mg cortisone/kg body weight twice

[a] Solu-Cortef®, Upjohn

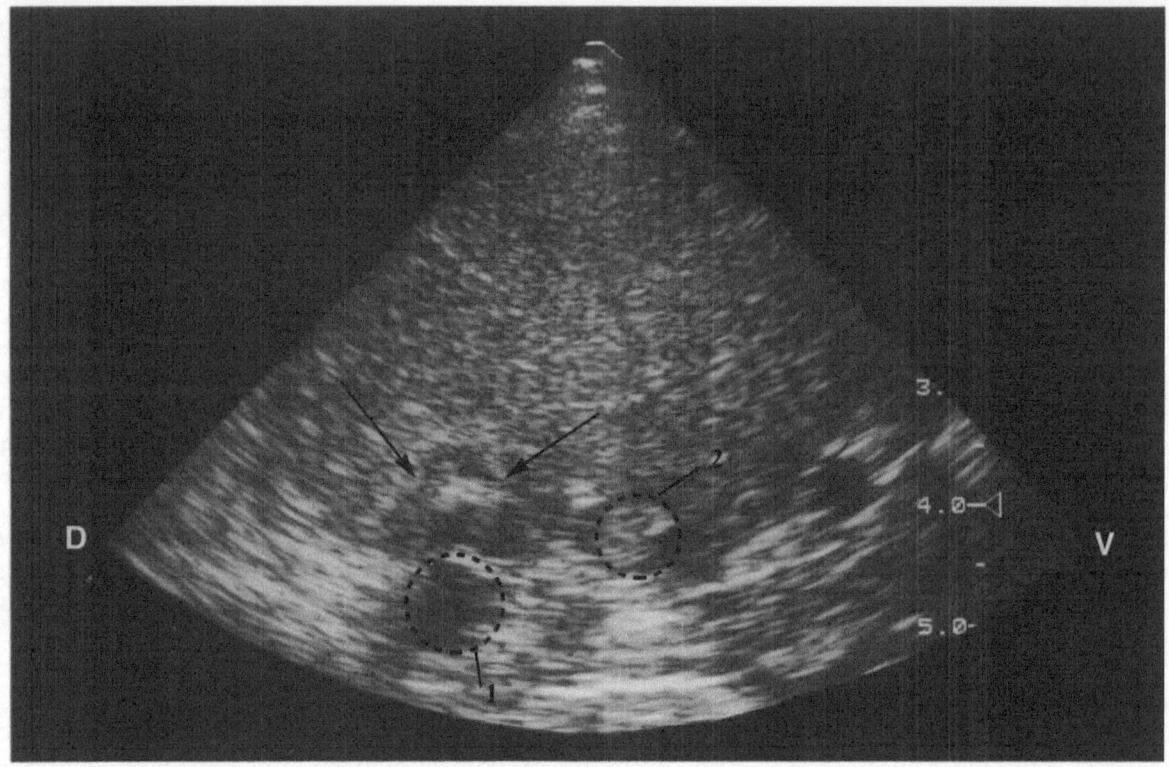

Fig. 4-35. Tranverse ultrasonogram from the right lateral intercostal region, immediately cranial to the righ kidney, of an 8-year-old Miniature Poodle (D = dorsal, V = ventral). Lateral to the aorta (1) and dorsal to the caudal vena cava (2) an adrenocortical tumor is visualized (arrows). The lumen of the caudal vena cava is echogenic due to the presence of a tumor thrombus.

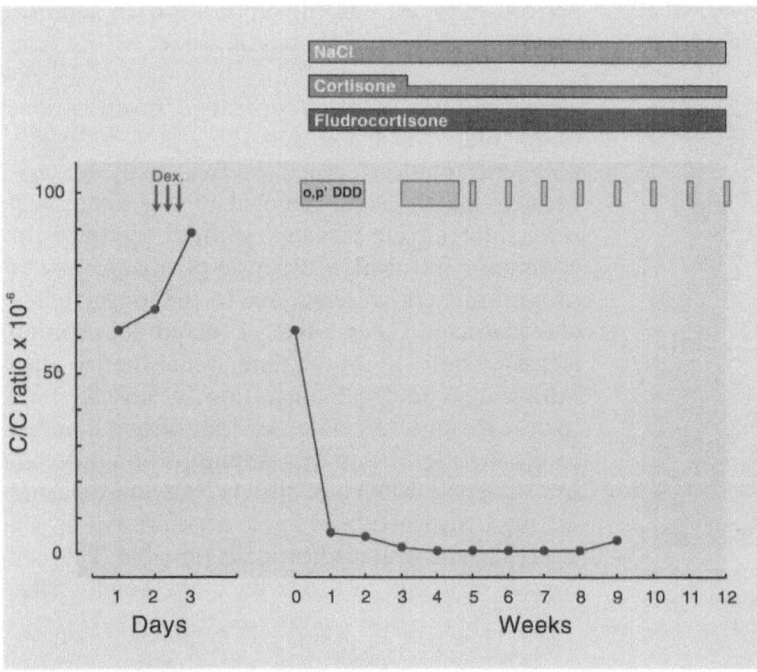

Fig. 4-36. Results of measurements of urinary corticoid/creatinine (C/C) ratios of an 11-year-old female mongrel dog (24.8 kg). On the left are the ratios on three consecutive days, i.e., on two control days and on the day following three oral doses of dexamethasone of 0.1 mg/kg each. Treatment with o,p′-DDD (500 mg 3 times daily) was monitored by weekly measurements of C/C ratios, cortisone and fludrocortisone being withheld the evening before urine collection. The owner had to discontinue the initial o,p′-DDD course for a few days because of the dog's inappetence. After completion of the 25-day course, the daily dose was given once a week for three months. At the time of writing (1 year after the start of o,p′-DDD therapy) there were no signs of recurrence of hyperadrenocorticism.

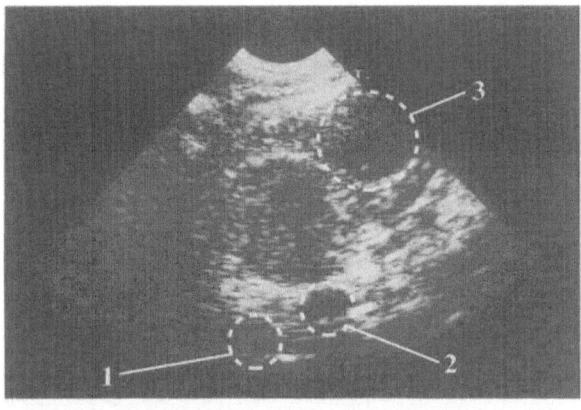 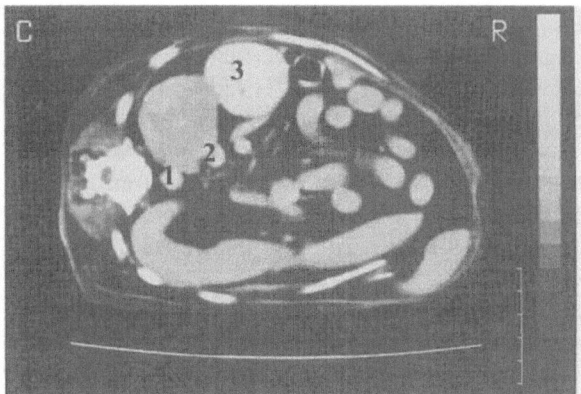

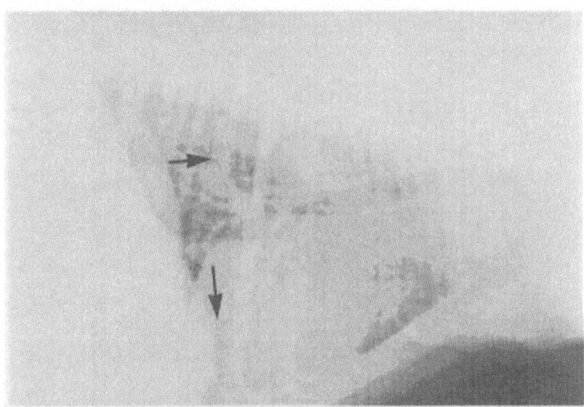 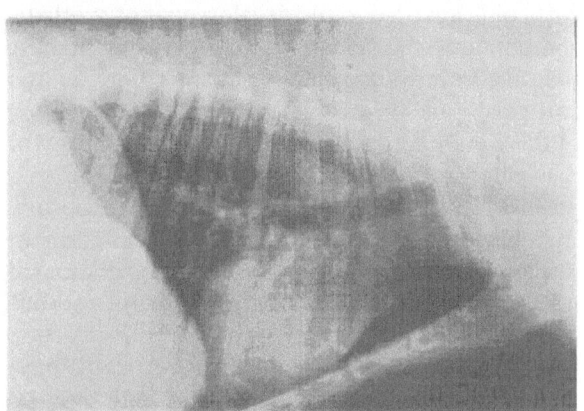

Fig. 4-37. Results of diagnostic imaging in a 10-year-old castrated female Miniature Pinscher (8 kg) with hyperadrencorticism due to a tumor of the right adrenal cortex. For comparison with the ultrasonogram (upper left) the CT can (upper right) was made in lateral recumbency. A large tumor of the right adrenal gland was visualized between the aorta (1), caudal vena cava (2), and right kidney (3). One year after surgical removal of the tumor (microscopically there was expansion into blood vessels), the dog was presented with recurrence of the hyperadrenocorticism. The expiratory radiograph of the thorax of this obese dog revealed several nodular densities (arrows), indicative of pulmonary metastases (lower left). The dog was treated for 35 days with 125 mg o,p'-DDD four times daily and substituted for primary hypoadrenocorticism. Thereafter the daily o,p'-DDD dose was administered once a week for 1 year. At the time of writing (2 years after the start of o,p'-DDD) there was no evidence of recurrence of hyperadrenocorticism or lung metastases (lower right).

daily, which is gradually decreased and then stopped 6–8 weeks after surgery.[31]

After bilateral adrenalectomy desoxycorticosterone acetate[d] (DOCA, once daily 0.1 mg/kg) or desoxycorticosterone pivalate[e] is also given. Mineralocorticoid substitution is continued orally with fludrocortisone as indicated earlier for spontaneous primary hypoadrenocorticism (4.2.1).

Dogs with irresectable tumor or recurrence of disease after adrenalectomy can often be treated

successfully with o,p'-DDD, thereby initially employing the same schedule as for pituitary-dependent hyperadrenocorticism (see 4.3.1). After 25 days of daily administrations of 50–75 mg o,p'-DDD/kg, this chemotherapy is continued for at least three months by once weekly administrations of the same daily dose. This approach often leads to complete and permanent cure of the hyperadrenocorticism (Fig. 4–36), and ultrasonographic examinations may reveal that the size of the tumor has decreased considerably.[46] Even lung metastases may disappear (Fig. 4–37), although it may also happen that this tumor dissemination cannot be affected.

[d] DOCA, Veterinary Pharmacy, Yalelaan 6, Utrecht (fax: 31–30–532065)

[e] Percorten-V®, Ciba-Geigy

Prognosis. Complete surgical resection of a unilateral tumor that has not metastasized has an excellent prognosis. This holds also true for bilateral tumor, although here maintenance therapy for the induced hypoadrenocorticism will be needed. Dogs with irresectable tumors and recurrence of the tumor may be treated succesfully with o,p'-DDD according to the above schedule.

4.3.3 Iatrogenic hypercorticism and iatrogenic secondary hypoadrenocorticism

Alterations in the chemical structure of the glucocorticoids have led to the development of synthetic compounds with greater glucocorticoid activity than the natural hormones cortisone, cortisol and corticosterone (Fig. 4–38). The increased activity of these compounds is due to increased affinity for the glucocorticoid receptor (GR) and delayed plasma clearance, which increases tissue exposure. In addition, the pharmaceutical formulation of injectable preparations plays a role. Esterified microcrystalline suspensions are slowly resorbed from the subcutaneous or intramuscular injection site. Many of these synthetic glucocorticoids have negligible mineralocorticoid effects and thus do not result in sodium retention and hypokalemia (Table 4–3).

Table 4-3. Actions of commonly used glucocorticoid preparations.

Name (+ duration of action)	Glucocorticoid potency	Mineralocorticoid activity
Short-acting		
Cortisol (hydrocortisone)*	1	Yes
Cortisone	0.8	Yes
Prednisone	4	No
Prednisolone	4	No
Intermediate-acting		
Methylprednisolone	5	No
Triamcinolone	5	No
Long-acting		
Betamethasone	25	No
Dexamethasone	30	No

*) The glucocorticoid potency of cortisol has been set arbitrarily at 1.

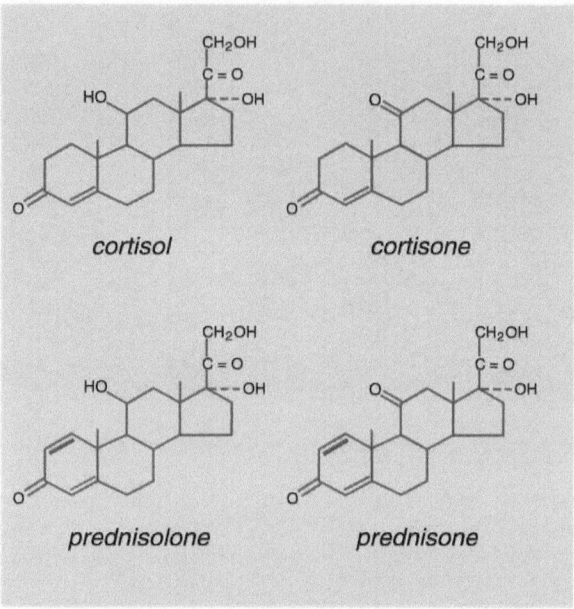

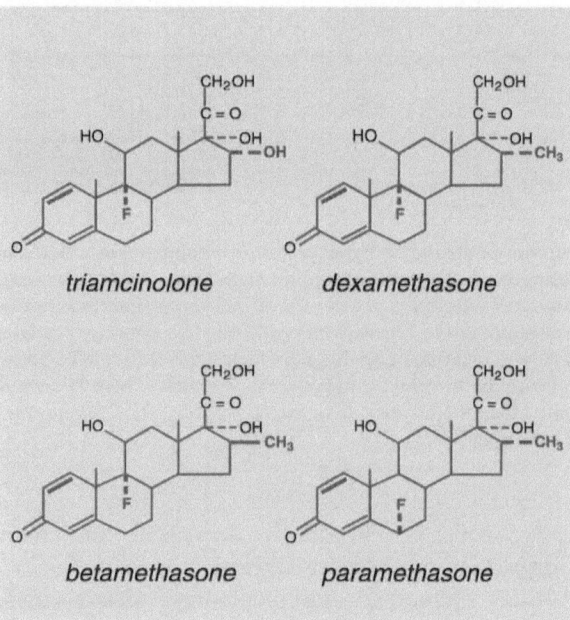

Fig. 4-38. Structures of commonly used glucocorticoids. The chemical modifications introduced to enhance glucocorticoid activity are indicated (green).

However, it should be realized that the duration of action of a glucocorticoid is not solely determined by its presence in the circulation. The molecules bind to specific intracellular receptor proteins (see Chapter 1). This corticosteroid-receptor complex modifies the process of DNA

89

transcription, thereby altering – via RNA translation – the rate of synthesis of specific proteins. By this modification of the phenotypic expression of the genetic information the glucocorticoid may continue to exert an effect after it has disappeared from the circulation.[66]

For glucocorticoid activity hydroxylation at C-11 is required (see also Figs. 4–2, 4–3). Prednisone and cortisone are 11-ketocompounds (Fig. 4–38) and therefore conversion to cortisol and prednisolone is needed for glucorticoid activity. This conversion occurs predominantly in the liver and is only moderately impaired in the presence of liver disease. Thus, topical application of prednisone is ineffective. Cortisone and prednisone are only used for systemic therapy. All glucocorticoid preparations marketed for topical use are 11β-hydroxylcompounds, obviating the need for biotransformation.[66]

Glucocorticoids as pharmacologic agents. Glucocorticoids are used in clinical endocrinology for substitution in adrenocortical insufficiency (see 4.2) and for the diagnosis and differential diagnosis of hyperadrenocorticism (4.3.2). However, this constitutes only a small part of their application in practice, where they are widely used as pharmacologic agents for the treatment of a variety of allergic, autoimmune, inflammatory and neoplastic diseases.

There is no simple mechanism of action underlying the many effects of glucocorticoids on inflammatory and immune responses. Probably the most important anti-inflammatory effect of glucocorticoids is the ability to inhibit the recruitment of neutrophils and monocyte-macrophages to an inflammatory site. This process of initiation of inflammatory response is mediated by interleukines. Glucocorticoids inhibit the transcriptional and postranscriptional expression of interleukines (see also Fig. 4–7).

Glucocorticoids also inhibit prostaglandin and leukotriene synthesis by inhibiting the conversion of membrane phospholipids into arachidonic acid (Fig. 4–39). This inhibition is mediated by lipocortin, a glucocorticoid-induced protein that inhibits phospholipase A$_2$, thereby inhibiting not only the production of leuktrienes but also of thromboxanes and prostaglandins. In contrast, nonsteroidal anti-inflammatory drugs such as salicylates inhibit only the path to prostaglandins and thromboxanes.

With regard to the well-known effects on lymphocytes and malignant lymphoma, it should be added that this loss of cells is probably caused by so-called apoptosis or programmed cell death. In normal life apoptosis plays an important role in the maintenance of tissue structure and function. It is highly regulated by a variety of hormones including glucocorticoids, so that a discrete population of cells is eliminated at a particular point in time. Glucocorticoids promote endonuclease activity, causing an irreversible process of DNA cleavage at susceptible internucleosomal linker

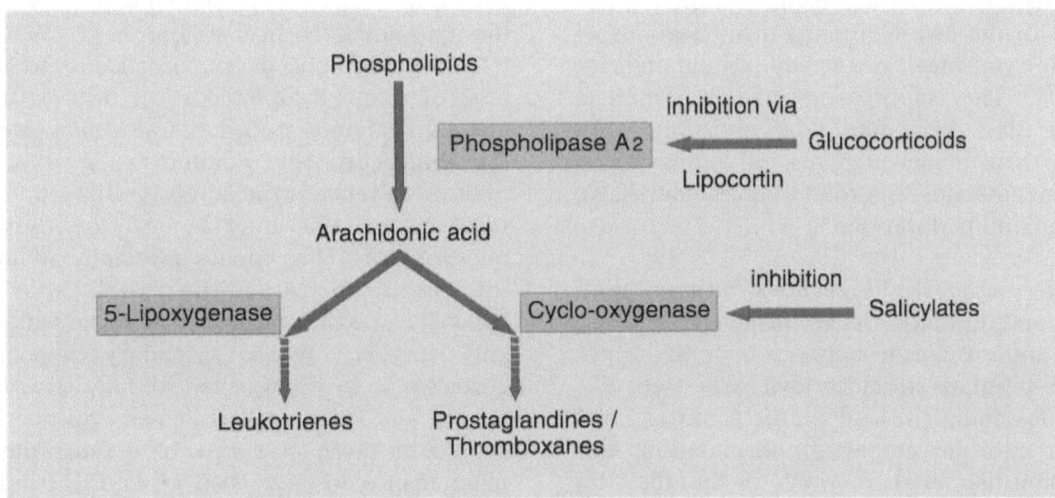

Fig. 4-39. Action points of glucocorticoids and nonsteroidal anti-inflammatory agents (salicylates) in the synthesis of derivatives of arachidonic acid.

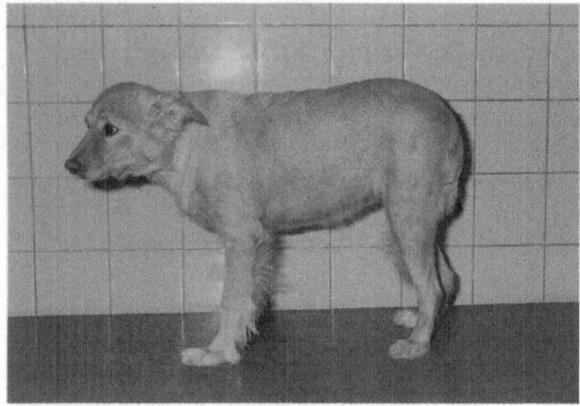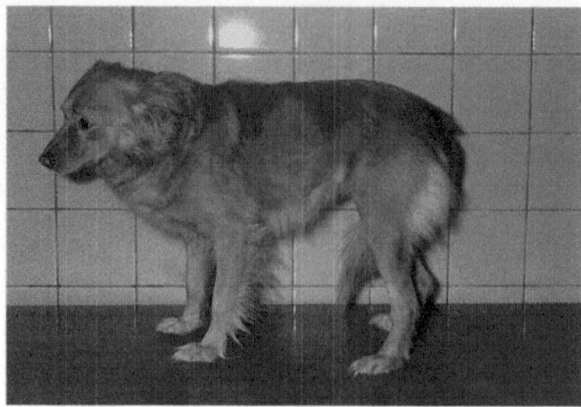

Fig. 4-40. A 3-year-old female mongrel dog that had been treated for half a year with injections with 9F, 16-Methylprednisolone and 6-Methylprednisolone for pruritus due to (underestimated) flea infestation (left). Note the obesity and the thin coat. With antiparasitic treatment and omission of the corticosteroids the dog regained a normal shape and a thick hair coat (right).

regions.[67] This DNA degradation precedes cell death.

Iatrogenic hypercorticism. As in spontaneous hyperadrenocorticism, the development of signs and symptoms of glucocorticoid excess depends on the severity and duration of the exposure. The effects vary among individual animals and (initially) seem to be less pronounced in cats. Within days after the start of glucocorticoid administration polyuria/polydipsia and polyphagia may develop. After several weeks of ongoing glucocorticoid therapy, the classic physical changes such as centripetal obesity, muscular weakness and skin atrophy may develop (Fig. 4–40).

The side effects of glucorticoid therapy are not confined to the just mentioned manifestations of Cushing's syndrome, which may include diabetes mellitus.[68] The suppression of the immune response may precipitate fatal infections.[69] In addition there is increased risk of complications such as pancreatitis, gastrointestinal hemorrhage, ulceration and perforation.[70]

Iatrogenic secondary hypoadrenocorticism. Both systemic and topically applied corticoids[71-73] cause prompt and sustained suppression of the hypothalamus-pituitary-adrenocortical axis (see also 4.2.2). Depending on the dose, the continuity, the duration and the preparation/formulation, this suppression may exist for weeks or months after cessation of the corticosteroid administration[74] (Fig. 4–41).

The animals may look healthy during corticosteroid therapy. Nevertheless it should be realized that they lack the ability to increase cortisol secretion sufficiently in response to stress. If stressed, they may develop signs of acute adrenocortical insufficiency, such as hypotension, weakness, anorexia and vomiting. For example, they may not recover from surgery if left without extra glucocorticoid supplementation. Similar long-lasting suppressions of the hypothalamus-pituitary-adrenocortical system occur in dogs treated with progestins.[75] Also in cats, where progestins are used for the treatment of a variety of dermatologic and behavioral disorders, the glucocorticoid actvity inherent to these compounds may cause a similar suppression of the pituitary-adrenocortical system.[76]

During prolonged glucocorticoid treatment, tests of pituitary-adrenocortical reserve function (see 4.2.2) are not needed. A test is indicated when the glucocorticoid administration has been reduced to replacement levels or stopped, and the recovery of the integrity of the system is questionable. This applies especially to animals that need an increase in the corticosteroid supply to cover a stressful event such as general anesthesia and surgery. When secondary hypoadrenocorticism is to be expected or has been demonstrated and the animal is at risk, glucocorticoids should be given at a rate of 4 times the basal maintenance dose (see also 4.2.1), i.e., 1 mg cortisone/kg body weight 4 times daily or an equivalent dose of another glucocorticoid (Table 4–3).

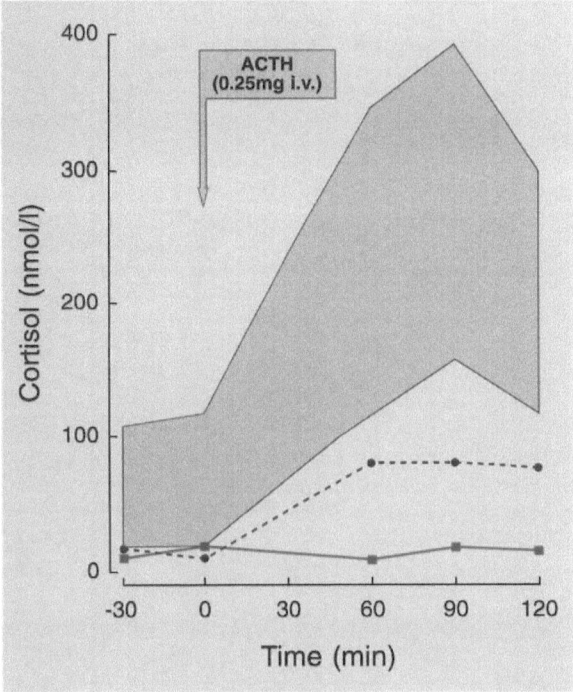

Fig. 4-41. Results of ACTH-stimulation tests in a reference population of dogs (blue area), compared with the results of the dog presented in Fig. 4–40: at first admission (red line), and 3 weeks after cessation of corticosteroid therapy (blue line).

Withdrawal from glucocorticoids. The consequences of the decision to discontinue glucocorticoid therapy may not only lead to an exacerbation of the disease that is being treated. It may also cause signs of corticosteroid withdrawal syndrome and as mentioned above the patient (if not supplemented) may even develop secondary adrenocortical insufficiency.

The features associated with glucocorticoid withdrawal include anorexia, lethargy and weight loss. The lethargy may be the result of what people experience following glucocorticoid withdrawal: myalgia, arthralgia, headache and postural hypotension. These symptoms may occur in patients in which the dose has been tapered to a normal glucocorticoid maintenance dose. They are explained by the sudden cessation of the glucocorticoid-induced inhibition of prostaglandin production (see also Fig. 4–39). Many of the features of the corticosteroid withdrawal syndrome can be produced by prostaglandins.[66]

Therefore the glucocorticoid dosage should be tapered gradually, similar to the transition from spontaneous hyperadrenocorticism to normo-corticism (see 4.3.1, 3.3.2), where also initially at least twice the maintenance dose is given. The recovery of pituitary-adrenocortical function is not promoted by the use of ACTH. It is not the ACTH secretion but rather the hypothalamic hypophysiotropic stimulation that recovers last[77] and injections of ACTH will retard this recovery and that of the pituitary corticotrophic cells.

Alternate-day glucocorticoid therapy. In alternate-day glucocorticoid therapy a short-acting gluco-corticoid (prednisone or prednisolone) is given once every 48 h. The aim of this approach is to minimize the adverse effects while retaining the therapeutic benifits. Thus it is an attempt to prevent the development of Cushing's syndrome and of secondary hypoadrenocorticism while providing therapeutic benefit. Although it is not definitely known whether alternate-day admin-istration yields a better overall risk-benefit ratio than a (steadily decreasing) morning dose,[78] it is common practice to use the alternate-day schedule when corticosteroids are used for a prolonged period of time.

For the induction of remission of a fulminant (autoimmune) inflammatory process, treatment is usually begun with a regimen of glucocorticoids once every day. By the time there are signs of improvement, attempts are made to reduce the dose. As an example the following schedule is given for oral administration of prednisolone:
– Day 1–3: 2 to 4 mg/kg;
– Day 4–6: 1 to 2 mg/kg;
– Day 7–14: 1 to 2 mg/kg every 48 h.

The dose is lowered further at weekly intervals if there are no exacerbations of the disease. Usually the final dose cannot be lower than about 0.5 mg/kg every 48 h. In some diseases it may be necessary to administer a higher dose or even to resume (temporarily) full daily doses.

4.4 Adrenal medullae

4.4.1 Introduction

The adrenal medullae are an integral part of the sympathochromaffin (sympathoadrenal) system and can be regarded as sympathetic postganglionic

92

neurons without axons. However, whereas the vast majority of sympathetic postganglionic neurons release the catecholamine norepinephrine (noradrenaline), the adrenal medullae release epinephrine (adrenaline) predominantly, although they also release some norepinephrine. The adrenal medullae release their products such as epinephrine directly into the circulation and thus function in an endocrine fashion. In contrast, sympathetic postganglionic neurons release norepinephrine into synaptic clefts, thereby having direct access to target tissues.[79]

Epinephrine, norepinephrine and dopamine are called catecholamines, because they share the dihydroxyphenyl ("catechol") ring structure. The catecholamines are synthesized from the amino acid tyrosine (Fig. 4–42). Tyrosine hydroxylase, the enzyme that converts tyrosine to dihydroxyphenylalanine (DOPA), is the rate-limiting enzyme in catecholamine biosynthesis.

The sympathoadrenal system is an efferent limb of the nervous system and events take place in seconds compared with the minutes or hours that characterize the time course of action of other hormones. Catecholamines influence virtually all tissues and many functions. Those clinically most relevant are the hemodynamic and metabolic effects. These are the result of catecholamine occupancy of α- and β-adrenergic receptors. Catecholamines increase the rate and force of myocardial contraction (β_1) and produce vasoconstriction (α) in most vascular beds (skin, mucosae and kidney), although vasodilatation (β_2) occurs in other vascular beds such as those of skeletal muscle. The metabolic effects are the result of both direct and indirect actions. Catecholamines directly stimulate hepatic glucose production,[80] whereas through the limitation of insulin secretion (α_2) they indirectly promote a glycemic response.

In line with the rapid induction and the quick dissipation of the effects of catecholamines, they are cleared rapidly from the circulation with half-times of 1–2 min. Clearance is largely via extrarenal degradation; less than 5% appears unaltered in the urine. Released catecholamines are degraded via catechol-O-methyltransferase (COMT), which converts them into metanephrines (Fig. 4–42). Ultimately 3-methoxy-4-hydroxy-mandelic acid (vanillylmandelic acid, VMA) is

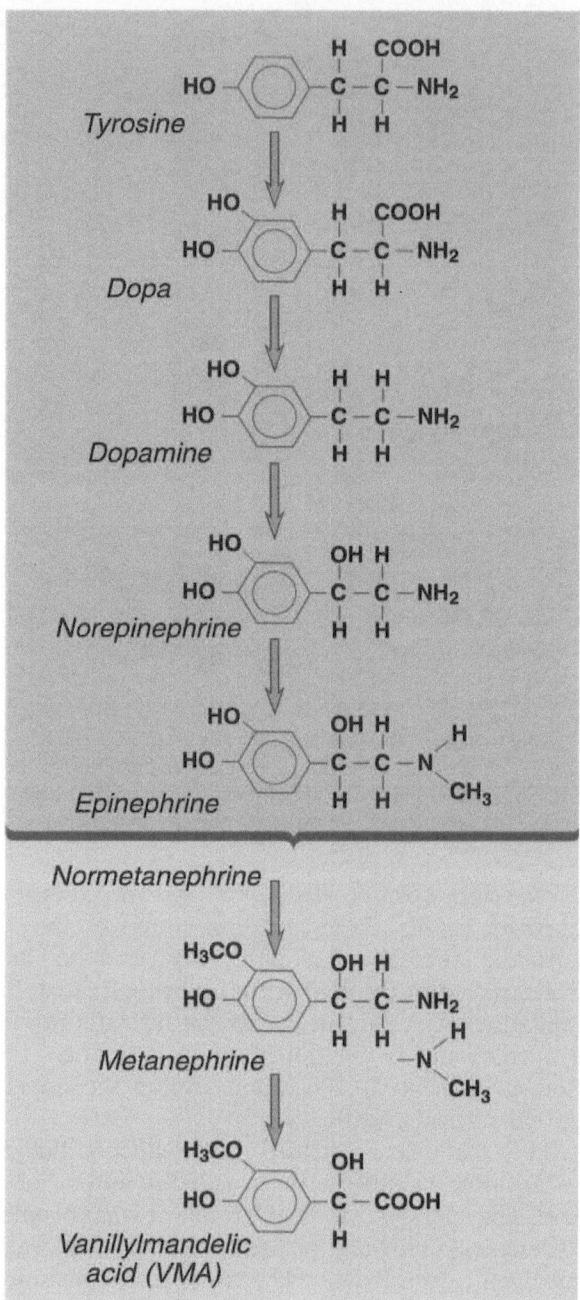

Fig. 4-42. Catecholamine biosynthesis (upper panel) and metabolic degradation (lower panel). The degradation scheme is confined to the metanephrine pathway, as this is the main route for catecholamines that are released into the circulation. Catecholamine degradation within sympathochromaffin cells occurs via monoamine oxidase (MAO) to dyhydroxymandelic acid, that subsequently is also converted to VMA.

formed, which is the major end product of catecholamine metabolism.[79]

4.4.2 Pheochromocytoma

Pheochromocytomas are catecholamine-releasing tumors, most commonly arising from adreno-medullary chromaffin cells. Tumors arising from extra-adrenal chromaffin cells are called extra-adrenal pheochromocytomas or paragangliomas.[81] Pheochromocytomas are rarely clinically recognized tumors, but do occur in both dogs and cats. Unfortunately they are often an unexpected finding at autopsy or surgery.[31] The tumors can be benign as well as malignant.

Clinical features. Partly because in almost all of the few reports on adrenal medullary pheochromocytomas the clinical features had to be assembled in retrospect,[82,83] the knowledge of the syndrome is limited. In addition it seems from what is now known that the clinical signs are aspecific (anorexia, depression, weakness) and intermittent. Excessive production of catecholamines should be considered in the differential diagnosis of episodic weakness, panting, tachycardia, polyuria and hypertension. Especially the latter is an important lead for the disease in man, and with increasing use of blood pressure measurements in dogs and cats the possibilities for detection of pheochromocytomas may increase. In addition, the wider use of abdominal imaging by ultrasonography and computed tomography may disclose adrenal masses that on further examin

ation may turn out to be pheochromocytomas.

Apart from the clinical features resulting from the catecholamine excess, there have been descriptions of illness and death due to the tumor mass itself. Malignant tumors may metastasize and in addition the animals may be presented in an emergency because of intra-abdominal hemorrhage due to rupture of the tumor.

Diagnosis. In man, biochemical screening of catecholamine hypersecretion is mostly carried out by measurements of metanephrines in 24-h urine samples. If clinical suspicion is high, then epinephrine, norepinephrine, dopamine and VMA measurements may be added to the 24-h studies.[84] Plasma catecholamine, particularly norepinephrine, levels are also increased substantially in the majority of patients.[79] These methods still need to be introduced for clinical use in dogs and cats, although there is a start.[85,86]

Treatment. Following biochemical diagnosis and anatomical localization by ultrasonography and/or computed tomography, treatment can be considered. When the tumor appears resectable from the diagnostic imaging, surgery is the treatment of choice. In order to prevent intraoperative hypertensive and postoperative hypotensive crises, the patients should be treated with great care prior to surgery by combined α- and β-adrenergic blockade.[84] Very recently there have been reports on the succesful removal of adrenal pheochromocytomas in dogs[86] and in a cat.[87]

5. Endocrine pancreas

5.1 Introduction

In both the dog and the cat the pancreas is a V-shaped organ. The angle points forward and lies caudomedial to the pylorus. The left lobe is somewhat shorter and thicker than the right lobe. Two pancreatic ducts discharge exocrine secretions into the duodenum (Fig. 5–1). Scatterred throughout the exocrine tissue there are numerous clusters of cells called islets of Langerhans (Fig. 5–2). In young animals the islets comprise about 5% of the volume of the pancreas and in adults 1–2%.

Each islet is a highly vascularized cluster of

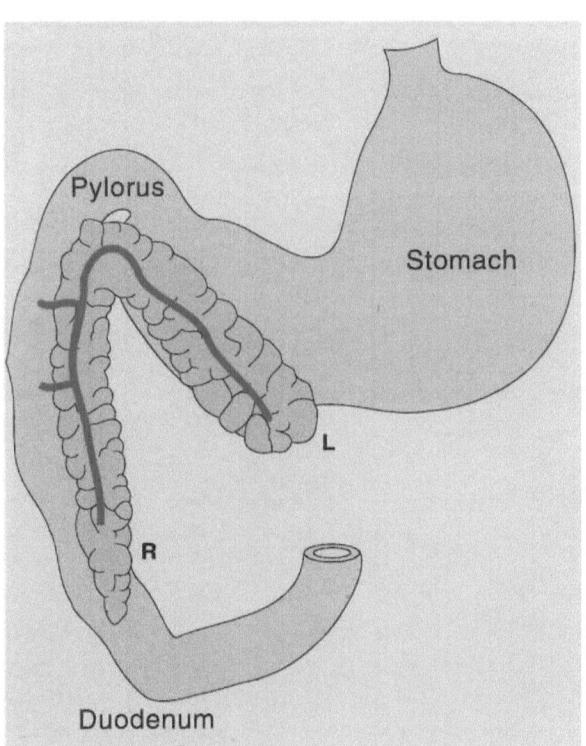

Fig. 5-1. Schematic drawing of the ventral aspect of the pancreas with its left (L) and right (R) lobe.

several types of cells. Four cell types are common to all species: B (β) cells produce insulin, A (α) cells produce glucagon, D (δ) cells produce somatostatin, and F (PP) cells produce pancreatic polypeptide. The cells have a consistent pattern of organization, with the D, A, or PP (non-B) cells occurring as a discontinuous mantle of one to three cells thick around a central core of B cells.[1] Apart from these secretory products of the endocrine pancreas, immunocytochemical techniques have revealed the presence of a number of other peptides such as gastric inhibitory polypeptide (GIP), cholecystokinin (CCK), secretin, corticotropin, and TRH. As yet, it is unclear what physiological role, if any, these peptides have in the islets.

Insulin synthesis and secretion. Insulin is a protein consisting of 51 amino acids contained within two peptides chains: an A chain, with 21 amino acids and a B chain with 30 amino acids (Fig. 5–3). The insulin molecule has been highly conserved during evolution. One practical implication of this conservation of structure is that heterologous insulins can be used therapeutically without being strongly immunogenic. The structure of insulin of pigs and dogs is identical and the structure of insulin of cats differs from that of dogs at three positions in the A-chain.[2] Insulin is synthesized according to the usual pathway for peptide hormones (Fig. 1–3). Following synthesis, the precursor molecule (preproinsulin) is cleaved to proinsulin (MW about 9,000), which is converted into insulin and a smaller connecting peptide (C-peptide) by proteolytic cleavage at two sites (Fig. 5–3). In contrast to the insulin itself, the C-peptide displays considerable species variation.

Insulin and C-peptide are secreted by the B-cells in equimolar amounts, together with about 3%

A. Rijnberk (ed.), Clinical Endocrinology of Dogs and Cats, 95–117.
© 1996 *Kluwer Academic Publishers.*

96

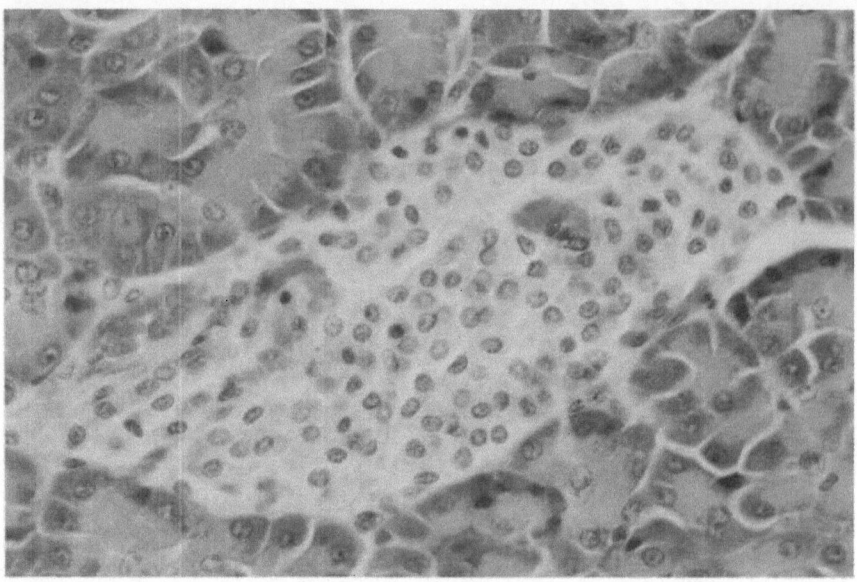

Fig. 5-2. Photomicrograph of a section of the canine pancreas, showing an islet of Langerhans surrounded by acini of the exocrine tissue (H & E stain, 40×).

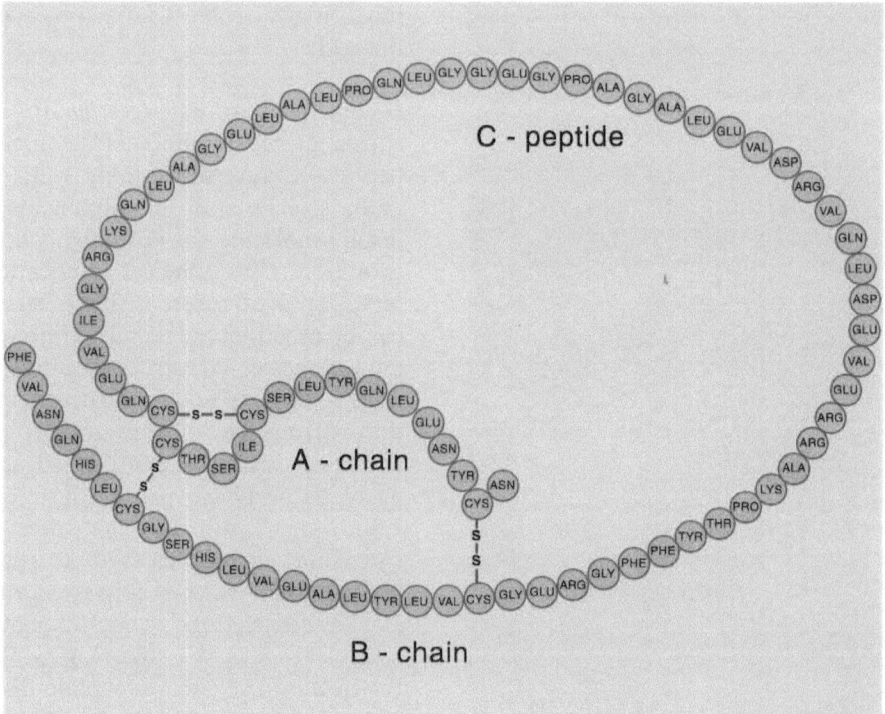

Fig. 5-3. Structure of canine proinsulin. The amino acids of the insulin sequence are represented by blue circles and the amino acids of the connecting peptide (C-peptide) by beige circles. The insulin molecule consists of two peptide chains linked by two sulfhydryl bridges. Conversion of proinsulin to insulin involves the removal of the C-peptide. Feline insulin differs from canine insulin at three positions in the A-chain: A8(Ala), A10(Val) and A18(His)[2]; the B-chain is identical and the composition of the C-chain is unknown.

unaltered proinsulin. Via the portal circulation the peptides reach the liver, where more than half of the insulin is retained, while C-peptide passes through the liver completely. Insulin circulates unbound to plasma proteins and in the fasted state its concentration is usually below 20 U/l. C-peptide circulates in much higher concentrations. This not only because of the hepatic extraction of insulin but also because its half-life is 5–6 times longer (half an h vs 3–5 min) than that of insulin. C-peptide has not yet been demonstrated to have bioactivity, but measurements of its concentration in plasma may give a better impression of B-cell function than measurements of insulin.

Regulation of insulin secretion. Glucose is the most potent stimulant of insulin release, but other sugars (fructose and mannose) and amino acids such as leucine may also stimulate insulin release. The mechanism of glucose-stimulated insulin release is not well understood but it is thought to involve the metabolism of the sugar rather than direct recognition by a "glucoreceptor".[3]

Factors other than these direct stimulants, that are involved in the regulation of insulin secretion include (1) amplifiers, and (2) inhibitors. The amplifier substances are gastrointestinal hormones such as GIP, CCK, secretin, and gastrin. These hormones are released upon food intake and therefore the insulin response to orally administered substrate is greater than the response after intravenous administration. In addition to these hormonal amplifiers there are neural influences, the greatest being β-adrenergic stimulation. Inhibition of insulin release is of less significance and is due to effects of catecholamines and somatostatin.

For understanding of the role of the latter hormone, the paracrine interaction of islet hormones will be discussed briefly, including the role of glucagon. Pancreatic glucagon is a single-chain polypeptide consisting of 29 amino acids. Its secretion is probably directly inhibited by glucose, whereas its release is stimulated by many amino acids, catecholamines, gastrointestinal hormones, and glucocorticoids. Glucagon makes energy available between meals, when ingested food is no longer available for absorption. It stimulates the breakdown of stored glycogen and maintains gluconeogenesis and ketogenesis.

Pancreatic somatostatin is identical to the hypothalamic peptide that inhibits GH release (see Section 2.2). Almost all stimulators of insulin release also promote somatostatin release from D-cells. Somatostatin acts in several ways to restrain the movement of nutrients from the intestinal tract into the circulation. It prolongs gastric emptying, decreases gastric acid and gastrin production, diminishes pancreatic exocrine secretion, and decreases splanchnic blood flow.

The paracrine effects of the B- and D-cells on the adjacent A-cells are of considerable importance. Even small increases in insulin secretion suppress glucagon secretion. Conversely, insulin secretion is directly stimulated by small changes in the secretion of glucagon. In addition, the response of somatostatin, which largely parallels that of insulin, acts to inhibit glucagon secretion.

Thus glucose stimulates B- and D-cells to release insulin and somatostatin respectively, both of which inhibit A-cells (Fig. 5–4). Amino acids stimulate the release of glucagon as well as insulin. The type and amounts of islet hormones released during food intake depend on the ratio of ingested carbohydrate to protein. The higher the carbohydrate content of the food, the less glucagon secretion is stimulated by amino acids. Conversely, feeding largely protein will result in relatively greater glucagon secretion. Thus the islets form a unit for finely tuned regulation of fuel metabolism.

Insulin action. Insulin exerts its effects on target cells after binding to specific plasma membrane receptors. This binding results in autophosphorylation at specific sites in the receptor molecule. The insulin-receptor complex becomes internalized by the cell and insulin is subsequently degraded. The phosphorylated receptor activates intracellular proteins. These proteins may move to the cell surface and facilitate transport of nutrients (glucose, amino acids) into target cells. Insulin-facilitated transport increases the entry of glucose into the cell by a factor of 20. This occurs in target tissues such as muscle and adipose tissue, but not in the brain and in the liver. Here the glucose transfer across the cell membrane is primarily dependent upon diffusion.

Chronically elevated levels of circulating insulin may decrease the number of insulin receptors. This so-called "down-regulation" of receptors is prob-

98

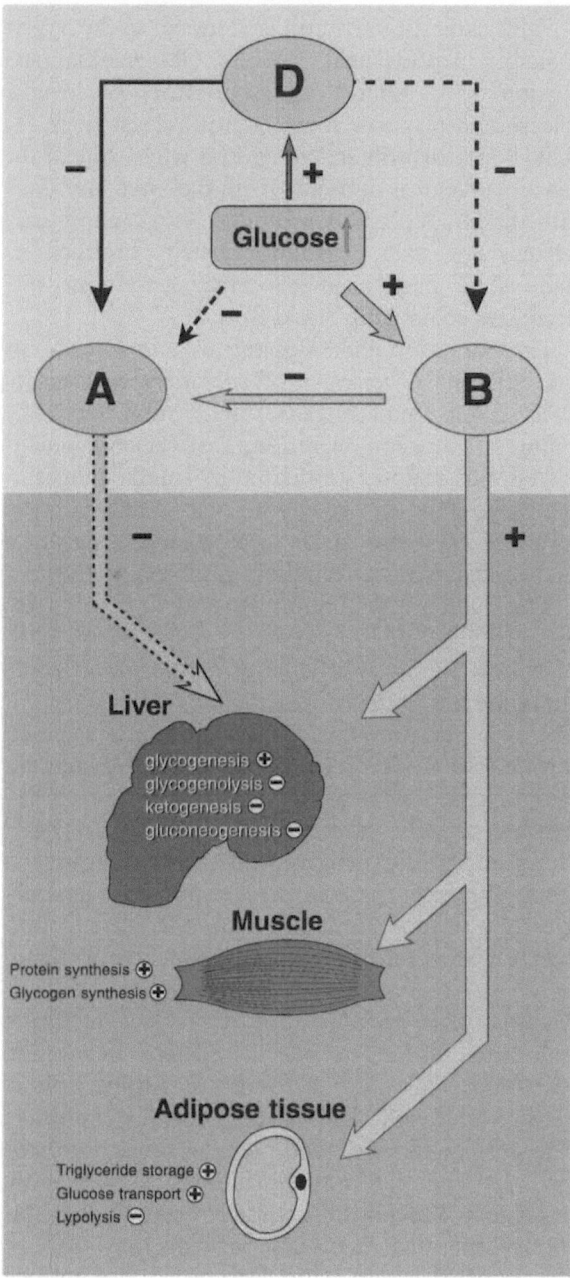

Fig. 5-4. The upper part is a schematic illustration of paracrine communication in the pancreatic islet. A rise in plasma glucose will cause the B-cells to release insulin, which inhibits glucagon secretion from the A-cells. In addition, there may be a direct inhibitory effect of glucose on glucagon secretion. Glucose also promotes somatostatin release from the D-cells, which inhibits glucagon release and has a modulating inhibitory influence on the insulin response. In the lower part of the figure the effects of insulin secretion (in combination with low glucagon secretion) on the three major tissues for energy storage are shown.

Insufficient insulin secretion will increase glucagon secretion. The resulting high [glucagon]:[insulin] ratio reverses hepatic carbohydrate metabolism as well as the metabolism in muscle and adipose tissue, i.e., — changes into ⊕ and the reverse.

receptor, although it is not clear whether this is an effect of the hormone itself or largely the consequence of the increased insulin secretion counteracting the increased gluconeogenesis (see also Section 4.3; Fig. 4–9).

Generally speaking, the major action of insulin is the promotion of storage of nutrients, in which three target organs play a central role: liver, muscle, and adipose tissue (Fig. 5-4). In the liver insulin is anabolic, promoting synthesis of glycogen, protein, and fat (triacylglycerols, VLDL). In addition, insulin inhibits the catabolic events of the postabsorptive (glucagon-dominated) state: glycogenolysis, ketogenesis and gluconeogenesis (Fig. 5–4). In muscle insulin increases protein synthesis by promoting amino acid transport and by stimulating ribosomal protein synthesis. Furthermore, glycogen synthesis is promoted to replace glycogen stores expended by muscle activity. In adipose tissue insulin promotes triacylglycerol storage in adipocytes by (1) inducing endothelium-bound lipoprotein lipase, which leads to hydrolysis of triacylglycerols from circulating lipoproteins, thereby making fatty acids available for uptake into fat cells, (2) increasing the availability of α-glycerol phosphate, which participates in the esterification of free fatty acids to form triacyglycerols, and (3) decreasing lipolysis of stored triacylglycerols by inhibiting intracellular lipase.

5.2 Diabetes mellitus

Diabetes mellitus is a heterologous disorder of carbohydrate metabolism with multiple etiologic

ably the result of increased intracellular degradation. On the other hand, when insulin concentrations are low, receptor binding is up-regulated. With high intake of carbohydrates and obesity the relatively high insulin levels reduce binding to insulin receptors. Conversely, with fasting and exercise the low insulin concentrations are associated with increased binding. Glucocorticoid excess decreases insulin binding to the factors that involve absolute or relative insulin deficiency or insulin resistance or both. All causes ultimately lead to hyperglycemia, which is the hallmark of the syndrome. This somewhat complicated definition will be considered a little further by paying attention to the classification problem and to some general metabolic pathophysiology and its clinical consequences.

Classification. In veterinary medicine there has been a tendency to follow the classification in man,[4,5] where there is first of all a distinction between Type I, or insulin-dependent diabetes mellitus (IDDM), and Type II, or non-insulin dependent diabetes mellitus (NIDDM). Type-I disease usually develops prior to or during early adulthood as a result of autoimmune destruction of B-cells. There is little or no insulin secretion, which leads to marked hyperglycemia and ketosis. The patients are entirely dependent upon exogenous insulin. Type-II diabetes usually develops later in life ("maturity onset diabetes"), and the endogenous insulin production is sufficient to prevent diabetic ketoacidosis. The patients are not dependent on exogenous insulin for immediate survival. This classification does not seem to be completely satisfactory as it combines etiologic aspects (islet lesions) and pathophysiological states (insulin dependency), which do not necessarily run parallel. For example, a person with autoimmune diabetes (Type-I) may pass through a period of NIDDM as long as the B-cell destruction is incomplete. When insulin dependence appears, the classification would change into IDDM. Conversely, in patients with Type-II diabetes (NIDDM) islet function may deteriorate and eventually they may become dependent on insulin (IDDM).

In the dog and maybe to a lesser extent in the cat, the great majority of cases of diabetes mellitus do not develop along the lines of Type-I and Type-II disease of man. More recently the classification of diabetes mellitus in dogs and cats has been confined to a division in the pathophysiologic states (IDDM and NIDDM).[7] This is certainly justified, as both situations may be encountered in the dog and more so in the cat. However, as explained above, this is only a description at the moment, without taking into account the pathogenetic aspects. Especially in the dog there are

Table 5-1. Causes of diabetes mellitus in dogs and cats.

1.	**(Primary) pancreatic disease**	
	1.	Endocrine pancreas
		(Autoimmune) destruction of islets (dogs) Islets amyloidosis (cats)
	2.	Exocrine pancreas
		Pancreatitis Neoplasia
2.	**Secondary diabetes mellitus**	
	1.	Overproduction of counterregulatory hormones
		Progestin-induced GH excess (dogs) Hyperadrenocorticism Pituitary GH excess (cats)
	2.	Drugs
		Glucorticoids Progestins $\Rightarrow$ GH excess (dogs) Progestins $\Rightarrow$ glucocorticoid effect (cats)
	3.	Obesity

unique pathogenetic aspects with regard to counterregulatory hormones, that have important diagnostic and therapeutic consequences. Therefore these attempts to classify diabetes mellitus in dogs and cats in terms of human disease are avoided here. Instead a pathogenetic division is presented that may fit in with our present understanding of diabetes mellitus in dogs and cats (Table 5–1).

A main division is made into (1) a (primary) destruction of B-cells, and (2) secondary diabetes mellitus that results from peripheral insulin resistance at receptor and/or postreceptor level. In both the dog and the cat the secondary forms of diabetes mellitus and specifically those due to excess of counterregulatory hormones are frequently observed. They may be presented in any stage, from only mild hyperglycemia to the severe (final) stage with severe hyperglycemia and ketoacidosis.

In the second category catecholamine excess (pheochromocytoma) and overproduction of thyroid hormone (hyperthyroidism) have not been listed (Table 5–1). Although thyroid hormone is regarded as one of the insulin counterregulatory hormones and experimentally induced hyperthyroidism in cats is associated with impaired glucose tolerance and hyperinsulinism,[8] in spontaneous cases apparently this does not occur to the extent that it leads to manifest diabetes mellitus. The same seems to hold true for pheochromocytoma, as the reported cases have not been associated with diabetes mellitus (see also Section 4.4.2).

On the other hand there is reason to include obesity, as it has been demonstrated that in both dogs[9] and cats[10] obesity is associated with impaired glucose tolerance. Therefore, as in man, obesity may be regarded as a contributing factor in the development of diabetes mellitus. As mentioned above, the decreased sensitivity, to the effect of insulin is ascribed to reduced receptor binding. In addition, coexisting postbinding defects in insulin action have been demonstrated.[11]

Metabolic pathophysiology. Lack of insulin and the associated increase in glucagon secretion initiate several biochemical changes with a subsequent pattern of progressive pathophysiological changes and clinical manifestations. Central are the disturbed glucostatic function of the liver and the decreased peripheral utilization of glucose (see also Fig. 5–4). Extracellularly and intracellularly the consequences are the opposite: there is hyperglycemia and intracellularly there is lack of glucose.

The elevated glucose concentration in plasma leads to glycosuria when it exceeds the renal threshold of about 10 (dog) or 14 (cat) mmol/l. The resulting osmotic diuresis causes polyuria and loss of electrolytes (Table 5–2), although hypokalemia and hypophosphatemia[12] may only become apparent when insulin treatment is started and acidosis is corrected (see below). Especially when the polyuria is insufficiently compensated by water intake, the extracellular volume may contract and hypotension with renal insufficiency may develop. This limits renal glucose excretion and contributes to the rise in plasma glucose. The high plasma osmolality may cause intracellular dehydration, which will be most noticeable in the brain and lead to coma.

Then there are less immediate life-threatening consequences of hyperglycemia, that nevertheless after some time may cause complications. The mechanisms involved are glycation of proteins and sorbitol formation. Enzymatic glycosylation is a normal post-translational process that greatly expands the structural and functional repertoire of proteins. However, when a protein is exposed to

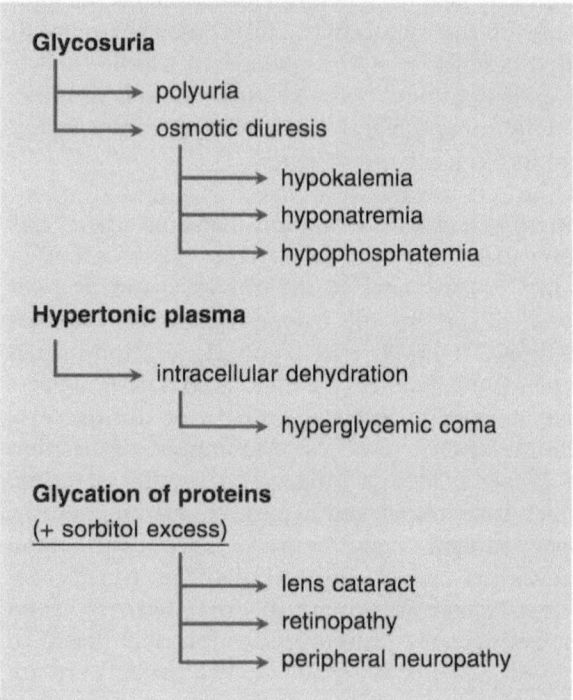

Table 5-2. Consequences of extracellular glucose excess (hyperglycemia > 10-14 mM).

high glucose concentrations, unregulated glycation may occur. This may alter structure and function of the protein. Apart from proteins in the circulation such as hemogloblin, red blood cell membranes and immunoglobulins, increased glycation of proteins has been found outside the circulation, i.e., lens, glomerular basement membrane, arterial walls, and nerves.[6]

Glucose may be reduced to sorbitol under the influence of aldose reductase. This enzyme is present in tissues that are frequently damaged in diabetes, such as retina, kidney and Schwann cells. In the lens sorbitol may cause osmotic swelling. It is not clear how and to what extent the sorbitol formation interacts with glycated proteins in the pathogenesis of cataracts (Fig. 5–5), retinopathy, nephropathy, and neuropathy.

The lack of intracellular glucose causes the peripheral tissues to switch from glucose utilization to utilization of fatty acids (Table 5–3). However, the high [glucagon]:[insulin] ratio decreases the hepatic capacity for reesterification of the mobilized fatty acids to triacylglycerols that are normally transported back to the plasma as

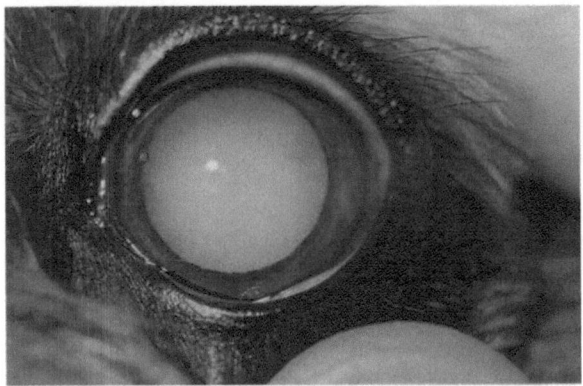

Fig. 5-5. Left eye of a 9-year-old female dog with diabetes mellitus, that had led to mature cataract. (Courtesy of F.C. Stades.)

VLDL. Instead the hepatic oxidation of fatty acids is activated, and incoming fatty acids are preferentially shunted into ketone body production. Unfortunately the released ketone bodies cannot provide much energy as the entry into most cells (not in the brain!) is insulin dependent.

The high concentration of keto acids causes acidosis, with a shift of intracellular potassium and phosphate to the extracellular space. When severe, the acidosis may become manifest by the

Table 5-3. Consequences of intracellular lack of glucose.

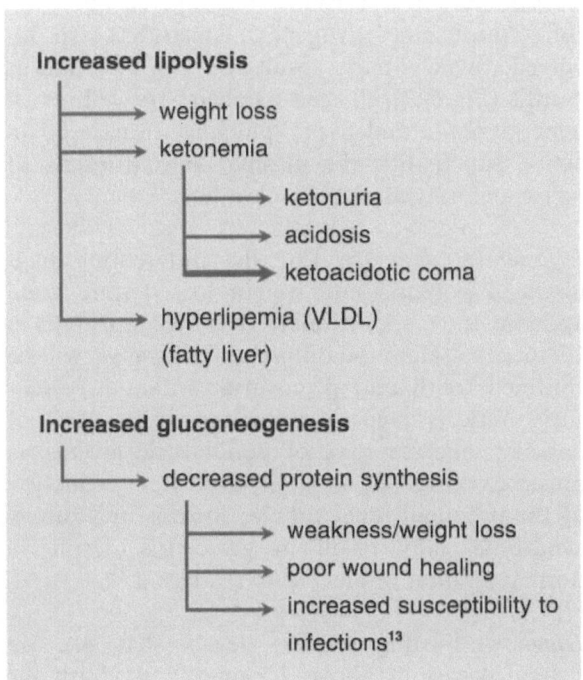

respiratory compensation, i.e., deep respiration. Despite the change into the oxidative pathway with decreased reesterification, the increased mobilization of fatty acids is associated with hyperlipemia (VLDL), largely because the endothelium-bound lipoprotein lipase is almost inactive in the absence of insulin (see also Section 5.1).

5.2.1 Diabetes mellitus in the dog

Pathogenesis. Of the primary forms (Table 5–1) the autoimmune mediated destruction of islets with fully insulin-dependent diabetes mellitus at a young age, appears to be rare. Nevertheless, the occurrence of diabetes mellitus as part of polyglandular failure syndrome[14] (see also 3.3.1) and the presence of circulating anti-B-cell antibodies in some diabetic dogs,[15] indicate that autoimmune mechanisms may affect islet cell function. This and a genetic susceptibility[16] may be determinants for an individual dog whether (later in life) environmental factors (e.g., drugs) or endogenous counterregulatory hormone excess will precipitate diabetes mellitus.

Although also uncommon, inflammatory disease of the exocrine part of the pancreas may progress to such an extent that it is accompanied by insulin deficiency. In these situations the signs and symptoms of pancreatitis may precede those of diabetes mellitus, but it also happens that the dog is presented with a somewhat atypical and puzzling picture due to the presence of both diseases.

Especially in countries where the bitches are not spayed at a young age, secondary diabetes is the most common form of the disease. Exogenous or endogenous progestins (see also 2.2.3, 7.6) may give rise to excessive GH release of mammary origin. In addition, there is the possibility that diabetes mellitus develops as a result of glucocorticoid excess, either endogenous or exogenous. Both hormones induce peripheral insulin resistance.[17] Initially this is compensated by increased insulin secretion (see also Fig. 2–23), but finally the islet cells may undergo hydropic degeneration[18] resulting in what is called "atrophy from exhaustion". Then there is insulin-dependent diabetes mellitus that is not reversible upon elimination of the insulin resistance (= the counterregulatory hormone excess), although this intervention will decrease the insulin demand and thereby facilitate regulation. As explained in Section 4.1, the diabetic effect of glucocorticoid excess is not only due to insulin resistance but also to increased gluconeogenesis.

Clinical manifestations. Diabetes mellitus is a disease of middle-aged dogs with a peak incidence around 8 years of age. Females are affected more often than males, which can be explained by the GH-inducing effects of progesterone or the use of progestins for estrus prevention. As long as the plasma glucose concentrations do not exceed the renal threshold values (see previous section), there will be no signs of diabetes mellitus. However, dogs with, for example, pancreatitis or exposure to glucocorticoid or GH excess should be regarded as candidates for the development of diabetes mellitus. The clinical features will be confined to those of the primary disease, but by laboratory examination mild hyperglycemia may be found.

Once the plasma glucose concentrations exceed the renal threshold, which may initially only happen shortly after meals, the cascade as outlined in Table 5–2 starts. Usually the energy loss via the glycosuria is insufficiently compensated by increased food intake and consequently the dog loses weight. The classic picture is that of a middle-aged bitch presented in the late metestrus or thereafter with polyuria, polydipsia, and some weight loss (Fig. 5–6). In most of these cases the findings by physical examination are not remarkable, although there may be signs of acromegaly (see also 2.2.3). In cases without such a characteristic pathogenetic history and therefore especially in male dogs, history and physical examination should be directed at the other possiblities of secondary diabetes mentioned in Table 5–1, e.g., hyperadrenocorticism or drug administration.

As mentioned in the previous section, a total lack of insulin can yield extremely high levels of ketone bodies in plasma secondary to increased hepatic production and decreased peripheral utilization. This pathological ketosis causes metabolic acidosis and leads to anorexia, decreased water intake, and depression. Especially when vomiting develops, the situation may deteriorate rapidly and when left untreated, death may ensue from hypovolemia and vascular collapse. Thus this is the dog with a history of polyuria and weight loss

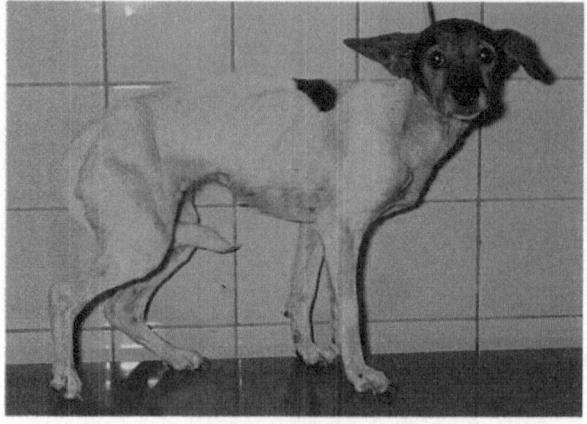

Fig. 5-6. A 7-year-old female mongrel dog that had developed diabetes mellitus during the luteal phase of the sexual cycle. At the time of presentation the dog had already lost several kg of body weight. The dog was ovariohysterectomized to prevent another progesterone (and thereby GH) exposure, which would have caused a drastic increase in the otherwise very stable insulin demand.

that not received insulin and that is presented as an emergency in a hypovolemic crisis.

On laboratory examination there is usually the paradox of the polyuric dog that does not have a low urine specific gravity, due to the high glucose content. In addition, there may ketonuria. Urine examination may also disclose bacterial cystitis. Occasionally gas forming bacteria (Escherichia coli, Aerobacter aerogenes, Clostridia) are involved, which may result in emphysematous cystitis (Fig 5–7). Plasma biochemistry will reveal hyperglycemia and hyperlipidemia. In case of an active pancreatitis the plasma concentrations of lipase and amylase will be elevated.

Differential diagnosis. For the differential diagnoses of polyuria and weight loss despite good appetite, the reader is referred to the algorithms in Chapter 15. Here the differential diagnosis will be confined to that of glycosuria. Although glycosuria reflects hyperglycemia in over 95% of patients, one category of nondiabetic glycosuria must be considered: renal glycosuria. Dysfunction of the proximal renal tubule, such as in Fanconi syndrome, may result in glycosuria despite a normal amount of glucose in the blood.[19]

Diagnosis. Fasting glucose levels that are on several occasions above 7.5 mmol/l establish the

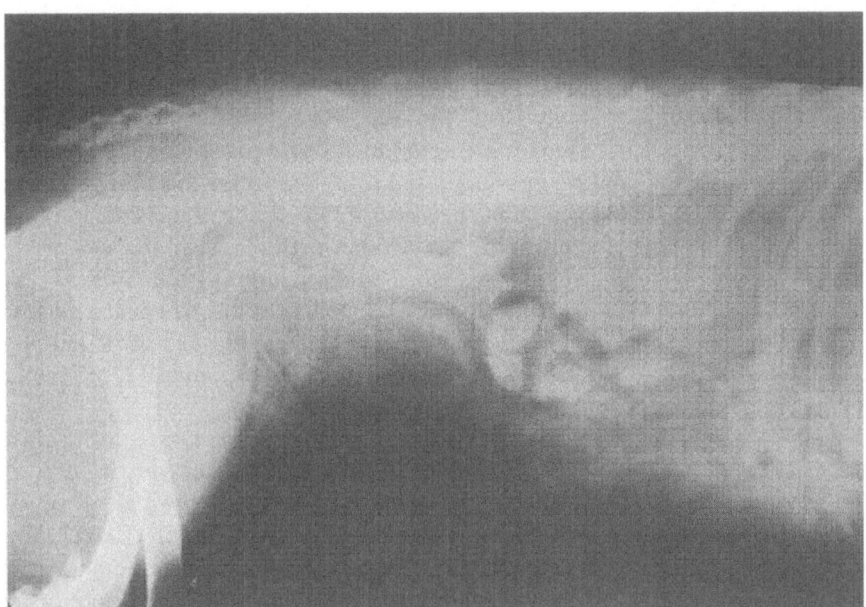

Fig. 5-7. Lateral radiograph of the abdomen of a 3-year-old Heidewachtel with diabetes mellitus, which reveals a diffuse gas pattern in the bladder wall caused by emphysematous cystitis.

diagnosis of diabetes mellitus in the dog. Occasionally circulating glucose concentrations are only transiently higher than 7.5 mmol/l. For example, dogs with acute pancreatitis initially may have hyperglycemia but only a small number develop permanent diabetes mellitus.

When the glucose concentrations are between the upper limit of the reference range (6.0 mmol/l) and 7.5 mmol/l or only occasionally clearly elevated or even normal but with suspicion of impaired glucose disposal, a glucose tolerance test may be performed. This is an assessment of the body's ability to dispose of a glucose load. The intravenous glucose tolerance test (Fig. 5–8) is preferred over the oral test because it is less subject to variation. The response to an oral load, although more similar to the physiologic response to food intake, also depends on gastrointestinal variables such as gastric emptying and carbohydrate intake on previous days. A protocol for an intravenous glucose-tolerance test is given in Chapter 13.

Treatment. In principle there are at least two main approaches in the treatment of diabetes mellitus: (1) to augment insulin release from the B-cells, and (2) insulin replacement therapy. For the former approach sulfonylurea compounds became available several decades ago. However, from the beginning of the introduction of these oral hypo-glycemic drugs it has been clear they are ineffective in dogs. Many diabetic dogs are presented in a stage of complete B-cell atrophy, thus in the absence of cells that can be stimulated. As explained earlier, in the secondary forms due to excessive exposure to counterregulatory hormones, the initially high insulin production causes the islets to atrophy, a process that will be promoted by further stimulation with these oral hypoglycemic drugs.

Therefore in dogs with diabetes mellitus, insulin replacement is the treatment of choice, with the support of dietary measures. However, it may not always be necessary to start immediately with insulin administration. If diabetes began during the luteal phase of the estrus cycle, rather than due to progestin injections or glucocorticoid excess, and clinical signs have been present for no more than three weeks, immediate *ovariohysterectomy* may result in complete reversal without insulin therapy. Trying to regulate the dog before surgery is usually counterproductive, as during the time needed to accomplish this, the damage to the islets may progress to complete atrophy, i.e., irreversible insulin-dependent diabetes mellitus.

If ovariohysterectomy is performed immediately, the dog will be hyperglycemic and will have an osmotic diuresis. Adequate intravenous administration of fluids during and following surgery is essential until the dog is able to drink. Plasma

104

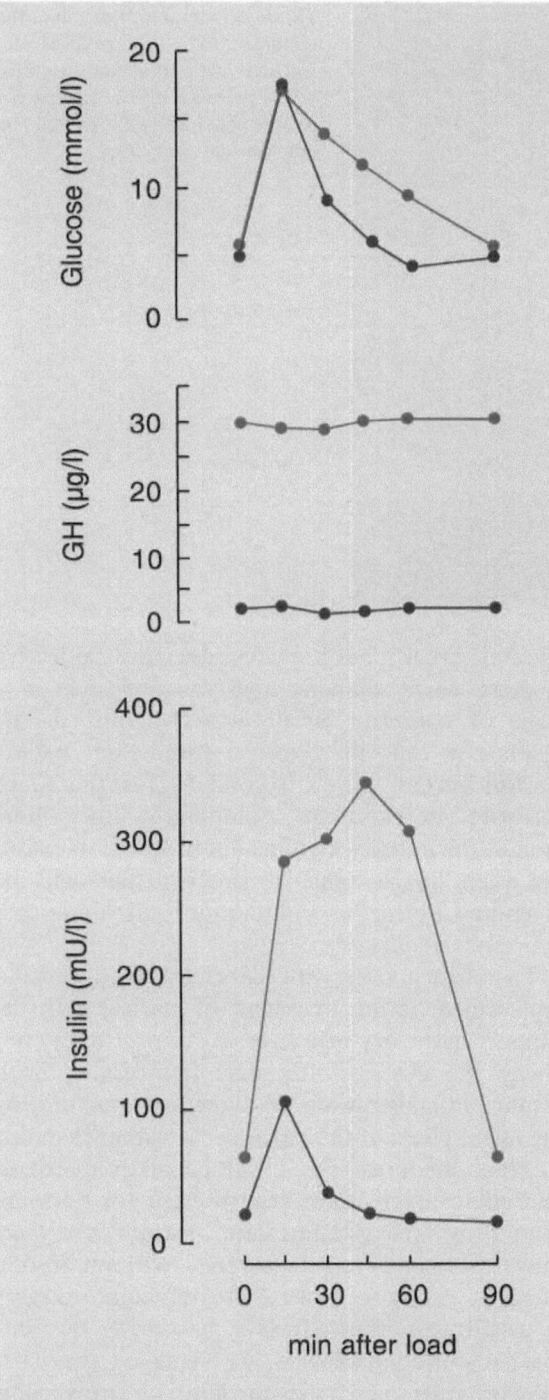

Fig. 5-8. Mean concentrations of glucose, GH and insulin during intravenous glucose tolerance tests in normal dogs (n = 6) (blue) as compared with the values of a dog with progestin-induced GH excess (red). Note that the progestin-induced GH excess was associated with strongly enhanced insulin secretion, but that nevertheless the glucose disposal was delayed.

glucose should be measured the following morning before food is given. If it is above 15 mmol/l, treatment with insulin should be started, but if it is only 10–12 mmol/l or lower, the dog should be fed one or two small meals and plasma glucose should be measured again on the following morning and the same decision made. Even if plasma glucose continues to decline without insulin therapy, it should be measured again within one week. During this period meals should be small and low in carbohydrate, e.g., meat and vegetables alone. If plasma glucose rises to 15 mmol/l or more, insulin therapy is started.

If ovariohysterectomy is delayed until after initial regulation, no food is given on the day of surgery and one-third of the normal dose of insulin is given at the usual time. If adequate regulation has not been achieved and the dog's insulin requirement is not yet certain, it may be safer to give no insulin on the day of surgery but to provide adequate fluid intake intravenously to avoid dehydration. Plasma glucose should be measured on the next morning before the dog is fed and if it is 15 mmol/l or higher, insulin should be continued. If it is 10–12 mmol/l or lower, insulin should not be given, two small meals should be fed and plasma glucose should be measured again on the following day. Sometimes, when good regulation has been achieved before ovariohysterectomy, the requirement for insulin stops almost immediately and if insulin is given without first checking plasma gluoce, severe hypoglycemia can result.

The aim of *insulin replacement* should be to reestablish a normal physiologic state as good as possible by administering insulin in such a manner as to provide a continuous low level of circulating insulin and to produce an 8- to 10-fold insulin rise with each meal. This aim is certainly not achieved with the traditionally recommended NPH (neutral protamine Hagedorn or isophane) insulin. The protraction of the action by the additions is insufficient (Fig. 5–9). Most dogs would need twice daily injections of this type of insulin to adequately control the diabetic state.[20,21] Although not 100% ideal, the above mentioned aim is much better met with an insulin preparation containing 30% amorphous zinc insulin and 70% crystalline zinc insulin. Amorphous zinc insulin is absorbed quickly from the subcutis and has a

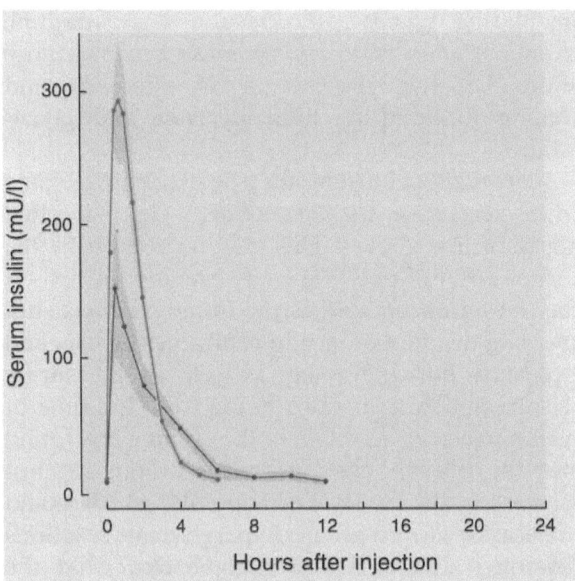

Fig. 5-9. Mean (± SEM) insulin concentrations in 7 dogs after subcutaneous administration of 0.5 U/kg body weight of regular insulin (beige) or NPH insulin (blue). The dispension as a suspension with protamine (derived from fish sperm) causes insufficient protracted action. (Adapted from Goeders et al., 1987.[20])

short duration of action. Crystalline zinc insulin has a later peak absorption and long duration of action (Fig. 5–10). Thus this mixed insulin zinc suspension of porcine origin (IZS-P)[a] delivers two peaks in plasma insulin concentration: one around 4 h and another around 11 h after injection.[22] Elevated plasma insulin concentrations persist for about 17 h (range 14–24 h). This indicates that in most dogs a once daily administration in combination with a 7.5 h feeding schedule (Fig. 5–10) satisfactorily substitutes for the levels of insulin, but that in some dogs this insulin preparation may be more beneficial if administered twice daily.

The treatment schedule described here is based upon the characteristics of this IZS-P preparation. The first meal is given with the insulin injection in the morning and the second meal is given 7 h later. A typical daily schedule is to give the insulin injection and first meal at 8.30 h and the second meal at 16.00 h. Plasma glucose measurements to adjust the dose of insulin are made within an hour before the second meal because then the lowest values are to be expected. Several owners of dia-

[a] Caninsulin®, Intervet, Boxmeer, NL (40 IU/ml)

betic animals have been taught to collect blood and to measure glucose themselves and do this without great difficulty.[23]

A safe starting dose is 1 unit per kg body weight. A small addition to the total dose can be made, namely 1 extra unit for dogs under 10 kg, 2–3 units for dogs of 10–20 kg, and 4 units for dogs over 20 kg. On the first day of treatment the owner feeds the dog and injects the insulin at the same time, e.g., 8.30 h. The uneaten food is removed after one 1 h, at both meals. The dose is increased by about 10% each day until the afternoon plasma glucose level is 6–8 mmol/l. If there has been a rather large decrease in one day (e.g., from 20 mmol/l or more to around 12 mmol/l), the same dose is continued for another day. When plasma glucose has been lowered to 6–8 mmol/l, it should be checked one more day and then about one week later, to be certain that regulation is stable.

In the beginning some dogs may not eat the morning meal immediately because their appetite is depressed by the hyperglycemia. Nevertheless the above schedule is pursued and the food is taken away. After a few days the dog will adapt to the schedule. After regulation is achieved, it is better to give the food first and then, as the dog is eating, to give the insulin injection. If the dog has vomited in the previous 24 h, it is advised to wait for 15–20 min before giving the insulin, to be

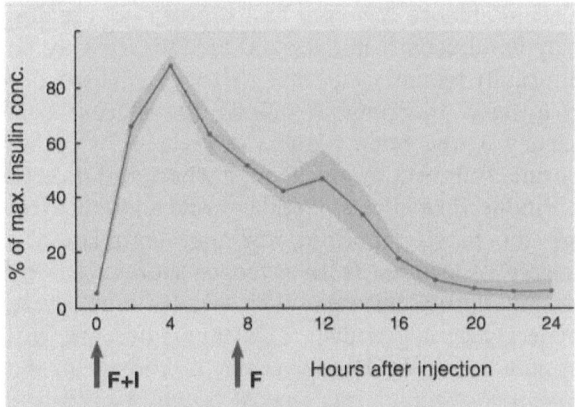

Fig. 5-10. Mean percentage (± SEM) of maximum plasma insulin concentrations of 10 diabetic dogs following subcutaneous injection of a two component insulin, containing 30% amorphous zinc insulin and 70% crystalline zinc insulin. The plasma insulin concentrations were transformed into percentages of the maximum plasma concentration reached in each dog. (Adapted from Graham et al., 1994.[22]) F + I = Feeding + insulin injection; F= Feeding.

certain the the meal is not vomited also. After regulation has been achieved, if the first meal is refused or only a small amount is eaten (often the first sign of an illness), or if food is being withheld because of surgery, diarrhea or vomiting, one-third of the dog's usual dose of insulin is given.

Satisfactory regulation can usually be achieved within 5–7 days and occasionally in only 2–3 days, but there may be some resistance to insulin during the beginning of treatment, so that several 10% increases have to be made. The resistance can decrease suddenly and afternoon plasma glucose may found to be as low as 2–3 mmol/l. When this occurs, the dog should be fed immediately and an extra meal should be given at 18.00 h. On the following day the dose should be decreased by 20% and plasma glucose should be measured again in the afternoon.[23]

If 3 or 4 increases of 10% in the dose have had little effect, increases in steps of 20% may be made. If this also has little effect after 3 or 4 times, even larger increases may be made. In hyperadreno-corticism, 2–4 units/kg may be required, but doses above 4 units/kg may be needed in insulin resistance caused by progestin injections.

When the dose of insulin is too high, signs of hypoglycemia may develop in the afternoon, usually between noon and the time of the afternoon meal. This can result in convulsions if not corrected. When the dose of insulin is too high but plasma glucose decreases at a slower rate, the dog may be unusually hungry and anxious, or may be unusually lethargic and dull. When plasma glucose is lowered to about 3 mmol/l, the glucose deficiency in the brain triggers the release of epinephrine, followed by glucagon, cortisol and growth hormone. The effects of epinephrine and glucagon are the most important, for they stimulate the release of glucose from glycogen stores, thereby raising plasma glucose rapidly. Moderate to severe hyperglycemia results. This hyperglycemic rebound following hypoglycemia is known as the *Somogyi effect*. Plasma glucose usually exceeds the renal threshold within two or three hours and can reach 20–30 mmol/l during the evening and night. Urine glucose is negative during the day but becomes increasingly positive during the evening, causing polyuria, and is strongly positive by the next morning. If not recognized and the insulin dose is based upon the urinary glucose rather than on plasma glucose, the insulin dose may be erroneously increased and the effect becomes more severe, i.e., hypoglycemia in the afternoon and evening followed by hyperglycemia and glycosuria.[23]

Short action of insulin may be observed in some dogs, according to the rather wide individual variation (see above). This may be noticed by the abrupt onset of polyuria every evening. Initially it may be misinterpreted as the Somogyi effect, but lowering the dose of insulin results in polyuria and glycosuria during the day as well. By measuring plasma glucose every two hours from the time of insulin injection until late in the evening it is found that the plasma glucose concentrations do not decrease below the level of 3 mmol/l, which would be necessary to trigger the hyperglycemic reactions (Somogyi effect). It will become clear that the duration of action of the insulin is only 12–14 h.

This problem is handled by twice daily administrations of insulin and further spreading of the meals over the day. The total daily amount of food is divided into three equal meals. The first meal and dose of insulin are given early in the morning and the second meal 5–5½ h later. The morning insulin dose is determined by measuring plasma glucose just before this meal. The third meal and the second dose of insulin (= one-half of the morning dose) are given 11–12 h after the first. If in doubt, the second dose of insulin can be assessed by measuring plasma glucose 3–4 h later. Another (4th) meal is usually not required, but the owner should be alert to the possibility of occasional signs of hypoglycemia late in the evening and then a snack or small meal can be given. For this reason it is best to start the daily program early, the three meals being given at for example 7.00, 12.30 and 18.30 h.[23]

Hypoglycemia can occur in any diabetic dog, during initial regulation or even after months of good regulation. It can be caused by overdosage of insulin, by failure to eat or by vomiting of food, by unusual excitement or physical activity, or it can occur without any obvious explanation. It is most likely to occur during the 3–4 h before the second meal, but can occur at any hour of the day or night.

Unexpected hunger and mild anxiety develop when plasma glucose is reduced to around 3 mmol/l. As glucose is decreased to 2 mmol/l or less, there is increasing anxiety, confusion and disorientation, with ataxia and stumbling or falling in the rear legs. Then muscle spasms begin, soon followed by grand mal convulsions with extreme excitabiltiy. Even if the dog is rescued from this severe degree of hypoglycemia by the administration of glucose, mild to moderately severe permanent brain damage can result. To avoid this risk, the owner must be instructed that hypoglycemia must be treated immediately, at home, and that time spent in telephoning or coming to the veterinarian may be fatal for the dog. Hence the owner must overcome panic and immediately administer glucose orally, continuing until the dog is able to take food. A 10-ml disposable plastic syringe and a box of powdered glucose to aid in giving glucose solution orally should be provided before the first dose of insulin is administered. When traveling or walking the owner should carry this glucose and a small portion of food.

The diet is as important as the administration of insulin in the succesful treatment of diabetes. It must be *constant in composition and amount from meal to meal and from day to day*. The most reliable way to be certain that the diet is constant and well-balanced, is to use a commercial food. To minimize fluctuations in postprandial blood glucose concentrations dry kibble foods or so-called dinners containing a predominance of digestibible complex carbohydrates should be fed. Semi-moist foods should be avoided because of the hyperglycemic effects of the disaccharides and propylene glycol, present in these foods.[24] There is evidence that foods with high fiber content improve the glycemic control.[25] They delay starch hydrolysis and glucose absorption, thereby slowing the increase and attenuating peak postprandial glucose concentration. However, there are disadvantages such as the the associated masses of faeces and the possibility that the low caloric density interferes with the desired weight gain or even may cause further weight loss.[7]

The following diet stands somewhere midway between these considerations. It consists of a commercial food, to which meat is added. Meat is not only added to the commercial food for reasons of palatability, but also to replace a portion of the carbohydrate by protein, allowing the generation of glucose via gluconeogenesis. In the twice-daily regimen the amount fed at each meal is 5 g of dry food per kg body weight, together with 5 g meat per kg body weight. After regulation is achieved, the total amount of food per meal may have to be decreased or increased, to maintain the dog at a satisfactory body weight, but the two meals should equal each other in amount and composition. When the amount of food is increased, the dose of insulin can then be increased following plasma glucose measurements, but when the amount of food is decreased, the dose of insulin should also be decreased on the same day, by about the same proportion, and plasma glucose should be checked that afternoon.

Insulin resistance (dosage $\geq$ 2 U/kg) may not only be caused by excess of counterregulatory hormones. It may also have trivial causes such as inactivated insulin by lack of refrigeration, too vigorous shaking of the bottle, and improper dilution. In addition, insulin resistance may be observed with seemingly unrelated conditions such as renal insufficiency and hypothyroidism. In uremia the resistance resides in peripheral tissues, primarily muscle.[26] When glomerular filtration rate further declines, renal clearance of insulin becomes markedly reduced and an improvement in glucose disposal may occur. Reducing the uremia by eliminating the prerenal component with fluid therapy will also enhance tissue sensitivity to insulin, but it will be clear that sometimes it may be difficult to predict what will happen to insulin requirements. In a recent report on insulin resistance in 3 hypothyroid dogs, it was suggested that the associated hyperlipemia had promoted down-regulation of insulin receptors.[27]

Alternative modes of regulation may include semiquantitative measurements of urine glucose concentrations. This usually results in insufficiently controlled diabetes mellitus, thereby increasing the risk of early appearance of complications such as lens cataract and urinary tract infection.

Then there is the possibility of measurements of glycated serum proteins, referred to as fructosamines. They are the result of non-enzymatic glysosylation of the amino group on the lysine residue. The reaction is irreversible and therefore fructosamine concentrations reflect glycemic control over the previous 2 to 3 weeks. This parameter appears to be a useful adjunct in long-term metabolic control.[28] Serum fructosamine measurements have also been proposed as a screening test for diabetes mellitus.[28a]

Treatment of ketoacidosis requires volume repletion with high priority. The deficit is usually about 10% of body weight. Infusion of Ringer's lactate should be started on arrival. Low doses of regular insulin[b] are administered intramuscularly at hourly intervals or as continuous intravenous infusion.[29] The total-body potassium deficit is usually masked by the acidosis that causes potassium to move extracellularly. Plasma potassium concentration may decrease rapidly due to both insulin treatment and correction of acidosis, which makes it necessary to begin replacement therapy after a few hours. The matter of bicarbonate therapy is controversial.[6] Rapid correction of acidosis may have detrimental effects on oxygen delivery to tissues. The hemoglobin-oxygen dissociation curve is normal in diabetic ketoacidosis because of the opposing effects of acidosis and deficiency of red blood cell 2,3-diphosphoglycerate (2,3-DPG). If the acidosis is reversed rapidly, the deficiency of 2,3-DPG becomes manifest, increasing the avidity with which hemoglobin binds oxygen and impairing the release of oxygen in peripheral tissues. In addition, with reversal of the acidosis, respiratory compensation will cease and as a result pCO_2 will rise. As CO_2 crosses the blood-brain barrier more rapidly than HCO_3^-, there is the possibility of paradoxical cerebral acidification. If bicarbonate is given at all, the infusion should be stopped when the pH reaches 7.2 to minimize possible side effects. It should be realized that with fluid therapy, insulin and potassium replacement, and intact kidney function, the acidosis usually disappears anyway.

Once insulin has restored glucose uptake by the insulin-requiring tissues and suppressed the hyperglucagonemia, hypoglycemia may follow unless exogenous glucose is provided. Because glucose levels always decrease before ketone levels, glucose infusions are begun when the plasma glucose concentrations reaches about 10 mmol/l. This allows continuation of the insulin administration needed to reverse the ketosis. In Chapter 14 a detailed protocol is presented.

[b] Purified regular pig insulin is no longer commercially available and therefore human preparations are used, such as Actrapid HM® (Novo) and Humuline Regular® (Lilly) with both 100 U/ml

Prognosis. All of the day-to-day therapy and many management decisions are in the hands of the owner. This requires a good understanding of the pathophysiology of diabetes, so that the owner becomes the dog's veterinarian for this disease. This should preferably include that he/she collects blood samples and measures plasma glucose. This allows meticulous control leading to low blood glucose levels and adequate energy supply. In this approach there are good chances for many happy years without hypoglycemic or hyperglycemic crises. In addition, with good control of the plasma glucose concentrations the development of complications such as lens cataract is postponed. Whereas in man the vascular changes in the retina are of major importance in contributing to blindness, in the dog they are reported to be much less severe.[30]

5.2.2 Diabetes mellitus in the cat

Several of the clinical manifestations and principles of therapy are similar for the dog and cat. Therefore in this section only those aspects of diabetes in cats are covered that are different from those of dogs.

Pathogenesis. Amyloid deposits in islets of Langerhans are a characteristic morphologic abnormality in cats with diabetes mellitus[31] (Fig. 5–11). The principal component of this amyloid is Islet Amyloid Polypeptide (IAPP or amylin). This is a 37-amino-acid-peptide that is produced in the B-cells and that is co-released with insulin (Fig. 5–12). There is evidence that under certain conditions IAPP can counter insulin action in peripheral tissue. Thus IAPP responds to the same physiologic stimuli as insulin, but has opposing biologic actions. In the pancreas IAPP inhibits insulin release possibly as an autocrine regulator.[32] The amino acid sequence of IAPP in both man and the cat predisposes to polymerization into large fibrillar deposits characteristic of amyloid. Factors leading to overproduction of IAPP may lead to deposition of IAPP and set in train a downward spiral of B-cell damage.[30] In this sequence of events there is a similarity between diabetes mellitus of cats and Type-II diabetes of man. It should be added that it is agreed that amyloid formation plays a role in the development

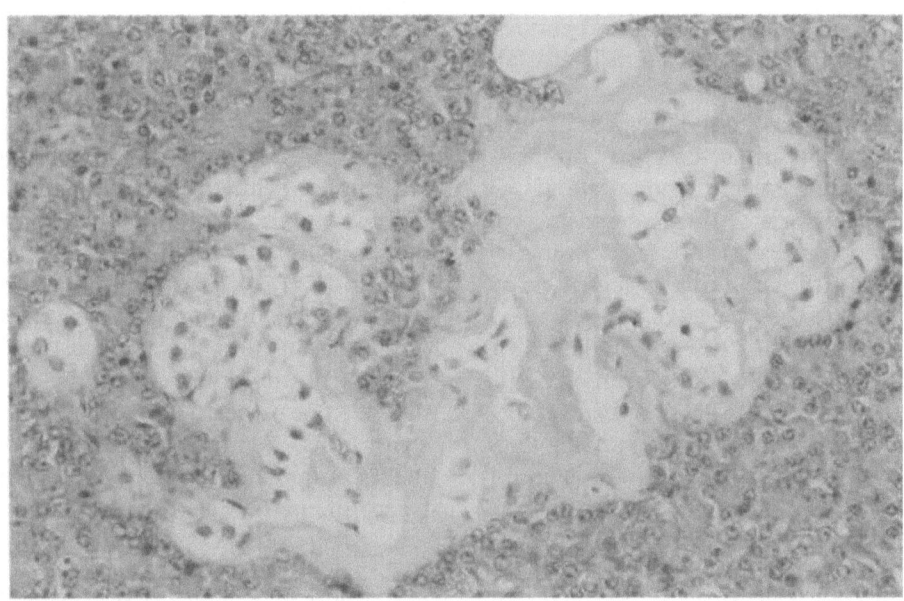

Fig. 5-11. Pancreatic islet of a cat with diabetes mellitus (H & E, 250×). There are massive amorphous deposits of amyloid (pink material), together with hydropic degeneration of islet cells.

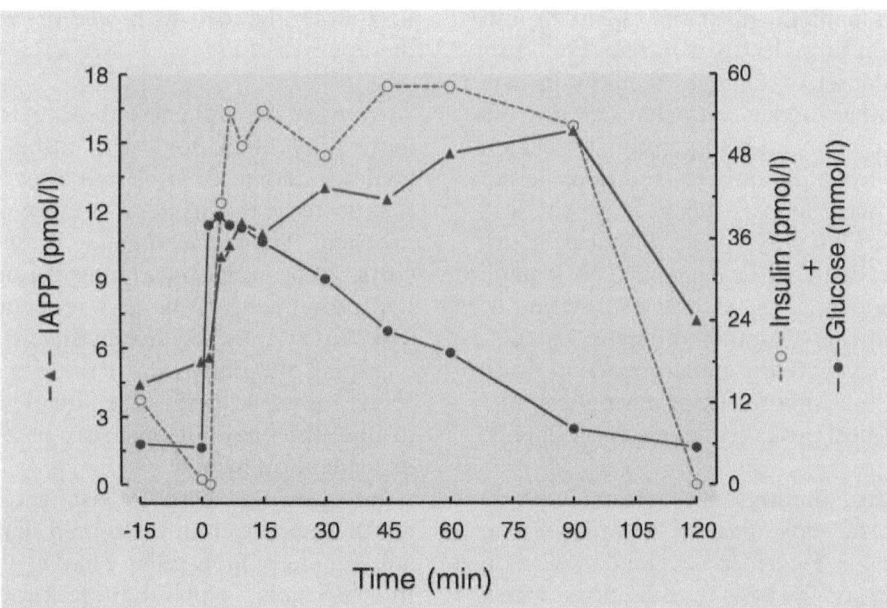

Fig. 5-12. Plasma concentrations of glucose, insulin and islet amyloid polypeptide (IAPP or amylin) during an intravenous glucose tolerance test (1 g glucose/kg body weight) in a cat, illustrating the co-release of the two peptides in response to the glucose stimulus (Courtesy of A.M.P. Nap.)

and progression of this type of diabetes mellitus, but it is probably just one factor in a multifactorial disease process.[33]

Possibly related to the just described pathogenetic events, cats more often than dogs are presented in a state of mild hyperglycemia and while still having an appropriate B-cell response to elevations of glucose concentrations in plasma.[34] In some of these cats the insulin requirement may vary initially and then after weeks or months they may no longer need insulin therapy. Other cats may become permanently insulin dependent. The progression of the loss of islet function seems to be somewhat slower than in dogs. This may explain why in cats more often than in dogs the elimination of excess of (endogenous or exogenous) counterregulatory hormones such as glucocorticoids results in permanent cure of the diabetes mellitus. For the background of the role of counterregulatory hormones the reader is referred to the previous section and Sections 2.2.3 and 4.3.

Clinical manifestations. Feline diabetes mellitus is seen most often in middle-aged and older cats and is more common in males than in females.[35] For the owner the onset of diabetes mellitus in cats usually has a rather sudden character. One day the cat develops polyuria and polydipsia, for which glycosuria and hyperglycemia are found to be the cause. If veterinary help is delayed, weight loss develops in spite of polyphagia. Physical examination may reveal hepatomegaly due to hepatic lipidosis. Unlike in dogs, cataract formation is rare in diabetic cats. Another difference is that, diabetic cats may develop a plantigrade posture with the hocks touching the floor during walking. This posture is most probably the result of diabetic neuropathy.

The laboratory findings may resemble those mentioned for the dog and are summarized in Tables 5–2 and 5–3. However, cats tend to develop more severe hepatic lipidosis than do dogs, which may even lead to hyperbilirubinemia. Of the electrolyte disturbances hypokalemia is relatively frequent. Hypophosphatemia has recently been reported as a cause of hemolytic anemia.[12]

Differential diagnosis. The clinical signs bear some resemblance to those of hyperthyroidism in cats (Section 3.4.1), but the accent is reversed: poly-phagia and weight loss usually predominate in hyperthyroidism while polyuria and polydipsia predominate in diabetes mellitus, at least initially.

Diagnosis. The diagnostic criteria for dogs and cats are similar, with the remark that cats are much more prone to stress-induced hyperglycemia. It is not uncommon to find plasma glucose concentrations up to 10 to 15 mmol/l in cats that are in stress caused by another disease. When there is doubt about the significance of the hyperglycemia found, it is advisable to send the cat home and to instruct the owner to monitor urine glucose concentrations. A more attractive approach includes the measurement of the plasma concentrations of fructosamine (see also 5.2.1); values < 350 µmol/l exclude persistent hyperglycemia.[28]

The presence of residual B-cell function can be established by measuring the insulin response to a glucose load or glucagon administration.[34] However, the differentiation between responsive and non-responsive B-cells is often made retrospectively, after the clinician has had several weeks to follow the cat with and/or without insulin therapy.[7]

Treatment. As explained above cats are presented more often than dogs with rather mild diabetes mellitus and residual B-cell function. Measures that decrease the insulin resistance may resolve the problem. These may include cessation of glucocorticoid or progestin administration, treatment of hyperadrenocorticism, and reduction of obesity. The latter may be achieved, for example, by confining the daily intake to 25 g of canned cat food.[23] Even in cases that already required some insulin, the final outcome may be a cat that is not dependent on insulin.

In principle there is also the possibility of another approach in these mild diabetic cats with still functioning B-cells. That is the use of oral hypoglycemic agents, that are known to augment insulin secretion and after some time also may improve the effectiveness of insulin at target cells. There is some experience with the sulfanylurea compound glipizide[c] in diabetic cats. When used in conjunction with correction of obesity, administration of 5 mg twice or three times a day has

---

[c] Glibinese®, Pfizer (5 mg glipizide/tablet)

been reported to be effective in some cats.[36] Initially the cats are examined weekly. Improvement in blood glucose concentration usually occurrs within 1 to 2 months of initiating glipizide therapy. Vomiting is the most frequent adverse reaction. The duration of the improvement is variable and may last from a few weeks to over a year. In many cases the final outcome is discontinuation of glipizide therapy and control of the disease with insulin therapy. The use of these drugs is certainly not as succesful as in man with Type-II diabetes mellitus.[37] It should be added that even in man there is considerably controversy about the safety of sulfonylurea agents in the therapy of diabetes.[38] Although not definitely demonstrated, it may very well be that the stimulated insulin secretion also leads to increased release of IAPP, which could promote the ongoing B-cell destruction by amyloid formation.

Insulin administration remains the main mode of treatment of feline diabetes melltius. The insulin preparation used in routine treatment of diabetes in cats is the same as that used in dogs (see 5.2.1). A constant diet that is equal from meal to meal is best achieved with canned or dry food or a combination. The total amount fed should be the same as the cat received before the onset of the diabetes. If the cat subsequently remains underweight, or becomes overweight, the amount of food can be changed accordingly and the dose of insulin can be adjusted as required at the same time. Cats which spend a large part of the day outside may obtain some food from other sources. They should be allowed to continue as before. If all other factors in treatment are handled correctly, usually this does not lead to serious problems.[23]

The daily schedule is exactly as described for the dog (see 5.2.1). Treatment and its explanation to the owner are less complex for the cat than for the dog. Ovariohysterectomy is not required (see 2.2.3, 7.2.2) and the incidence of hyperadrenocorticism is low. After regulation is achieved by measurements of plasma glucose, most owners of cats maintain quite good regulation by use of random measurements of urine glucose and clinical signs. The use of morning urine glucose measurements alone is as unreliable in the cat as in the dog, and failure to understand the Somogyi effect can lead to severe and potentially fatal insulin overdosage.

A safe starting dose of Caninsulin® is 1 U per kg body weight. The total dose can be increased in steps of ½ U, guided by plasma glucose measurements about one-half hour before the afternoon meal. If, during initial regulation, three or four successive increases of ½ U have had little or no effect, the dose may be increased in steps of 1 to 2 U. If this also has little effect after three or four increases, larger steps may be used.

In some cases initially the total dose of insulin may have to be increased to 10–15 U before plasma glucose is lowered. Although the resistance can then disappear suddenly, resulting in signs of hypoglycemia and requiring a rapid reduction in the dose, it usually disappears gradually over a few days. The correct maintenance dose may then be found to be around 5 U, for example. The cause of this temporary insulin resistance remains unknown.

A more persistant insulin resistance should alert one to the possiblity of hyperadrenocorticism (see 4.3) or a growth-hormone producing pituitary tumor (see 2.2.3). Especially in cases of growth-hormone excess, severe insulin resistance may be encountered. Doses of 60–80 U have been required to lower plasma glucose satisfactorily. Affected cats may have signs of acromegaly (see 2.2.3). Nevertheless some may live for many more months in spite of the GH excess, provided that the expensive control of the diabetes mellitus is acceptable to the owner.

The causes, clinical signs, and treatment of hypoglycemia are the same as in the dog and should be explained to the owner. A small bottle of 50% glucose can be kept in the refrigerator. Timely oral administration of 2 ml of this solution is adequate in most cats in the event of signs of hypoglycemia. A disposable 5-ml syringe should be provided for this purpose.

An alternative treatment schedule may be needed when the owner is not at home during the day. One solution has been to give the insulin injection and first meal at 23.30 h and the second meal at 7.00 h. For adequate control the owner must be taught to collect blood and to measure blood glucose. In most cats, blood can be collected with little difficulty from the jugular vein, using a 26-gauge needle. Plasma glucose concentration is measured just before the second meal. The period of highest risk of hypoglycemia in the event of

112

overdosage of insulin is in the 2–3 h before the second meal and so initially this treatment schedule requires that the cat spends the night in the bedroom of the owner so that the owner will be awakened and be able to respond quickly if the cat was having difficulty in the early hours of the morning.[23] We have also encountered owners who have solved the problem of absence during the day by giving food and insulin in the morning and giving access to the second meal via an electric device that opens the lid of the bowl at 7 h after the first meal. Adjustments of the insulin dose are only performed during the week-end.

Prognosis. Cats tend to be easier to regulate than dogs and have fewer hypoglycemic episodes and short-term changes of insulin dosage. Indeed, many diabetic cats remain on the same dose for many months without difficulty.

5.3 Hypoglycemia

Hypoglycemia is usually defined as a glucose concentration in plasma below the level at which symptoms are expected to occur, e.g., below 2.5 mmol/l. These concentrations may give rise to neurological signs because glucose is the primary energy substrate of the brain. In contrast to other tissues the brain cannot utilize free fatty acids as an energy source. Although the brain can use metabolites of free fatty acids, i.e., ketone bodies, this provides only for about half of the energy requirement. Moreover in (adult) dogs, fasting leads to an appreciable ketosis only after days to weeks.[39] Thus preservation of the function of the central nervous system in post-prandial or fasting states primarily requires an increase in the production of glucose.

Initially glucose is derived almost exclusively from hepatic glycogen (see also Fig. 5–4). However, glycogenolysis can only sustain the plasma glucose concentration for a short period of time; after about two days of fasting liver glycogen stores are completely depleted.[40] Secondly, glucose production in the liver is activated. The precursors for hepatic glucose synthesis are lactate/pyruvate and amino acids derived from muscle, as well as glycerol released from adipose tissue. In the adult dog the catabolic state of fasting is primarily the

result of the decrease in insulin release; the secretion of the counterregulatory hormones glucagon and growth hormone does not change significantly.[39]

Hypoglycemia can be expected in situations of (1) increased utilization (demand-side hypoglycemia), and (2) decreased availability of glucose (supply-side hypoglycemia). When the just mentioned adaptive mechanisms cannot compensate for increased peripheral utilization of glucose, the syndrome of hypoglycemia may develop. It can be the result of endogenous or exogenous insulin excess (see previous section). In principle, increased glucose utilization might also be associated with large tumor masses which metabolize glucose at high rates. However, in man there is increasing evidence that some of these tumors elaborate an incompletely processed insulin-like factor (pro-IGF-II).[41]

Supply-side hypoglycemia may result from impaired hepatic gluconeogenesis and glycogenolysis due to liver failure (cirrhosis, porto-systemic shunts). In addition, a deficiency of glucocorticoids may lead to insufficient gluconeogenesis (see Section 4.1) and consequently to hypoglycemia. Long-term lack of substrate, i.e., long-term starvation, may also lower circulating glucose concentration, to which especially young individuals are susceptible (see 5.3.2).

In dogs and cats with hypoadrenocorticism and liver insufficiency plasma glucose concentrations are usually only mildly decreased (> 2.6 mmol/l) and thus often an incidental finding. In this chapter the discussion will be confined to the two conditions that are well-known to be associated with severe hypoglycemia: islet cell tumor and juvenile hypoglycemia.

5.3.1 Hypoglycemia due to islet-cell tumor

B-cell tumors or insulinomas (Fig. 5–13) continue to produce insulin despite the provoked hypoglycemia. On immunohistochemical examination these B-cell tumors often appear not only to contain insulin but they also immunostain for somastatin, glucagon, and pancreatic polypeptide.[42,43] In addition, IAPP immunoreactivity and IAPP-derived amyloid deposits have been found in these tumors.[44]

Insulinomas are usually solitary but may be

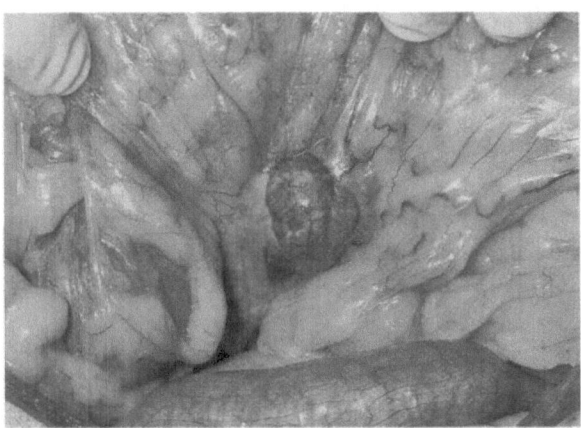

Fig. 5-13. Insulinoma of a 10-year-old male Malines Shepherd, exposed during surgery.

multiple. Especially in the dog these tumors are often malignant, with metastases occurring mostly in regional lymph nodes and surrounding tissues (mesentery and omentum). Distant metastases are usually confined to the liver.

Clinical manifestations. B-cell tumors occur most often in medium- to large-breed dogs without a pronounced breed or sex predisposition. At diagnosis the dogs' ages vary between 4 and 13 years, with an average of about 8 years.[45] Insulinomas are rare in cats; reports are confined to single cases.[46]

The most common signs are muscle tremors, episodic muscle weakness or ataxia, and collapse. Hypoglycemia due to increasing hyperinsulinism will eventually result in epileptiform convulsions in all cases, but a good history almost always reveals that there was weakness or ataxia or that there were other signs consistent with hypoglycemia, days or weeks before the onset of convulsions. In some cases it is helpful to ask whether the weakness and/or tremor were specifically seen in post-prandial (early morning) periods during exercise. Initially the convulsions are often self-limiting as they (further) stimulate the release of counterregulatory hormones (epinephrine, cortisol) that increase the blood glucose concentration, but with increasing severity of the insulin excess the animals may be presented in a state of permanent epilepsy and irreversible brain damage.

When the owners have satisfied the animal's increased hunger, there may be some weight gain. Apart from this occasional obesity on physical examination no abnormalities are found, except for the rare case that is complicated by peripheral neuropathy. The associated proprioception deficits and depressed spinal reflexes are the result of degenerative changes in radial and ischiadic nerves.[42] Apart from the hypoglycemia, also results of routine laboratory examination are usually unremarkable.

Differential diagnosis. As already mentioned above the other possible causes of hypoglycemia (hypoadrenocorticism and liver failure) are very rarely so severe that they give rise to signs of the hypogycemia syndrome. In these conditions the clinical features are dominated by those of the primary disease and the hypoglycemia is an associated finding without grave consequences.

Diagnosis. Against the background of the just described differential diagnosis, a presumptive diagnosis can be made in the majority of cases when a fasting plasma glucose concentration ≤ 3.0 mmol/l is found repeatedly. The hallmark of the diagnosis is of course the association of persistent hypoglycemia and inappropriately high plasma insulin concentrations. Thus when in doubt the animal can be fasted with close observation (!) and hourly glucose measurements until the plasma glucose concentration is below 3.5 mmol/l. Then plasma samples are obtained for measurements of insulin concentration. Low glucose concentrations with co-existing plasma insulin concentration > 10 mU/l are diagnostic.[47]

It should be added that there have been many reports on the calculation of [insulin]:[glucose] ratios and the use of tolerance tests employing glucose and glucagon. These tests are unreliable and may be associated with severe hypoglycemia. In addition, insulin-secreting tumors retain a degree of responsiveness to a glucose challenge and therefore this stimulation test cannot be used for the demonstration of autonomous hypersecretion. On the contrary, the insulin response to a glucose load tends to be high and may remain high at the lower end of the glucose tolerance curve.[47]

Abdominal ultrasonography and computed tomography can be used for the identification of a

114

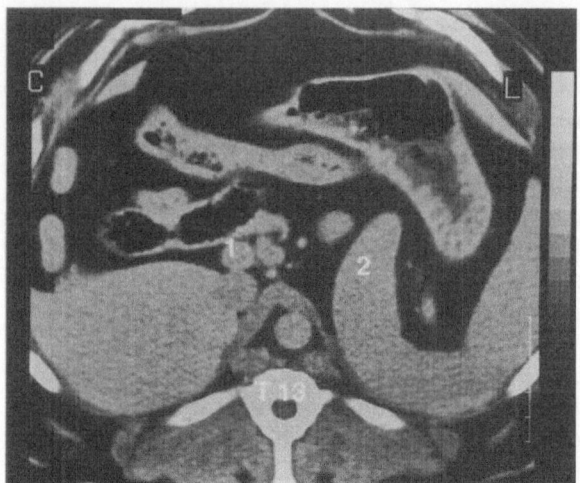

Fig. 5-14. Contrast-enhanced CT image of the abdomen at the level of the 13th thoracic vertebra (T13) of a 7-year-old Labrador Retriever with insulinoma. Between the portal vein (1) and the dorsal extremity of the spleen (2) two nodules are visualized in the region of the left pancreatic lobe.

pancreatic mass and for potential metastases in surrounding structures and the liver (Fig. 5–14), but they have a low detection rate for primary tumors. A recent development is the use of ^{111}In-labelled somatostatin analogue octreotide that binds with the usually abundant somatostatin receptors of the insulinoma (and metastases). The thus concentrated radionuclide can be visualized with regular scintigraphy and better with "single photon emission computed tomography" (SPECT)[48] (Fig. 5–15). These scans also have

predictive value for the effectiveness of treatment with octreotide (see below). Experiences with this approach in the dog are as yet very limited. During the scanning procedures the animals are not at great risk for a hypoglycemic crisis. The plasma glucose concentrations appear to be stabilized by the required anesthesia, whereby the use of α_2-agonists may be beneficial as they stimulate GH release, which antagonizes insulin action (see 5.1, 5.2).

Treatment. Pending the results of diagnostic procedures or surgery the risk of a hypoglycemic crisis should be reduced by limiting physical exercise and avoiding excitement. The administration of glucose, sucrose, and semi-moist commercial food has to be avoided. Instead, a low-carbohydrate diet (e.g., 3–4 parts meat or egg with 1 part dry food) should be given, divided into 4–5 small meals per day.[23] If signs of hypoglycemia persist in spite of these measures or if the animal has already been having frequent convulsions, glucocorticoids can be given. They interfere with the action of insulin and promote gluconeogenesis (see 4.3, 5.2.1). The initial daily dose of prednisolone is 0.5–1.0 mg/kg is divided in two doses. This often controls the signs of hypoglycemia. If not, the dose can be increased gradually. If these measures fail and convulsions are likely to occur, or the animal is presented with convulsions, the emergency protocol should be started (Chapter 14). This includes intravenous

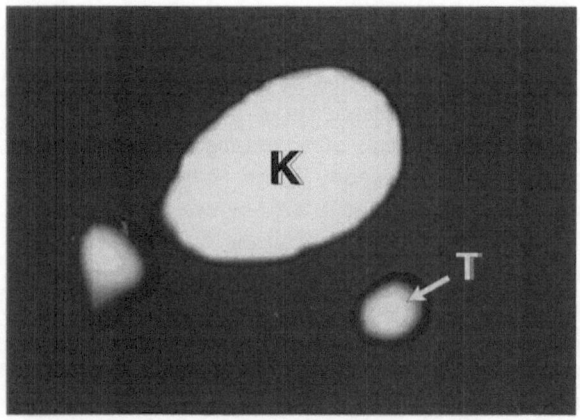
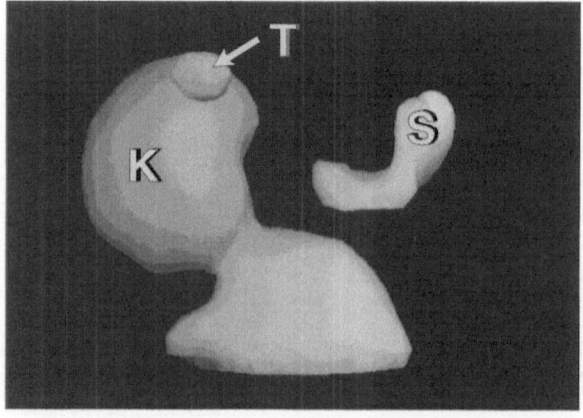

Fig. 5-15. Left: Sagittal image of an abdominal SPECT made 7 h after injection of [^{111}In-DTPA--Phe[1]]-octreotide in an 8-year-old male German Pointer with a solitary B-cell tumor in the pancreatic body close to the exocrine pancreatic ducts. K = right kidney; T = insulinoma. Right: Ventral image of a three-dimensional reconstruction of the same dog; lettering as in the picture on the left. S = spleen (Courtesy of J.H. Robben.)

glucose administration, but should be followed as soon as possible by measures to lower insulin release.

Surgery is not only started as an attempt to resect the insulin-producing tissue, but also for a complete inspection of the abdomen for metastases, which may reveal important prognostic information. Partial pancreatectomy is performed with a minimum of manipulation, as this may cause life-threatening pancreatitis.[49] Depending on the situation encountered during surgery, lymph node excision and partial hepatectomy may also be carried out. Intravenous infusion of 5% glucose solution during and after surgery usually prevents hypoglycemia, especially when done under guidance of hourly blood glucose measurements. Also in order to prevent the development of pancreatitis, intravenous fluids are continued for 48 h after surgery and nothing is given orally until the third day. The outcome immediately after surgery may be hypoglycemia, euglycemia, or hyperglycemia. Hypoglycemia is usually the result of incomplete removal of the tumor and/or metastases. Hyperglycemia is often transient and may last for days or weeks until the unaffected and suppressed islets have regained normal function. Rarely insulin therapy is needed to bridge this period.

Cases that cannot be cured by surgery may still be candidates for medical treatment. As mentioned above, there is the possibility of glucocorticoid administration, but especially when high doses are needed this therapy may give rise to unacceptable side-effects, i.e., iatrogenic hypercorticism. Therefore, when long-term treatment is foreseen one may start with diazoxide.[d] This is a benzothiadiazide diuretic that inhibits insulin secretion. In addition, it stimulates hepatic gluconeogenesis and glycogenolysis and inhibits peripheral use of glucose. The initial daily dose is 10 mg/kg body weight. By dividing the daily dose and by administration with food the adverse reactions (anorexia and vomiting) may be prevented. In some cases much higher doses (up to 50 mg/kg/day) are needed to controle the signs of hypoglycemia. Finally the diazoxide therapy may be combined with glucocorticoid therapy.

The somatostatin analogue octreotide[e] (see also

Fig. 2–22) inhibits the secretion of insulin by normal and neoplastic B-cells, provided that the tumor cells have expressed somatostatin receptors. In dose rates of 1 µg/kg tid subcutaneously, octreotide is probably effective, but there are no reports on long-term follow-up. In addition one should be aware of the possibility of tumors without somatostatin receptors. In these cases there will be no effect on the insulin secretion, whereas the release of the counterregulatory hormones glucagon and growth hormone will be inhibited and consequently the hypoglycemia may worsen. Also, the expenses involved may pose a problem, as well as the need for multiple injections per day.

Prognosis. At the time of surgery about 40% of cases have developed macroscopically visible metastases. Nevertheless some of these animals may do well for some time on medical treatment. About 10–20% may die from surgical complications, chiefly pancreatitis with local peritonitis and shock. For the 40% of the dogs that are helped by surgery, the mean survival time without symptoms or the need for medication is about 1 year and this can be extended to 1½ years total survival (range 6 months to 3 years or more) by resuming the dietary measures and medication with diazoxide or prednisolone or both. In dogs hypoglycemia due to B-cell tumor usually recurs, which suggests that most have metastasized before they are diagnosed and surgery is attempted.[23]

5.3.2 Juvenile hypoglycemia

In puppies of miniature breeds such as Yorkshire Terriers and Chihuahuas insufficient food supply of any cause (starvation, gastrointestinal disturbances, inactivity due to cold) may cause hypoglycemia.

Pathogenesis. Puppies have relatively high rates of glucose utilization, disproportionally large brains, and relatively limited stores of gluconeogenic substrate. During fasting the hepatic glycogen stores are rapidly depleted and the possibly still immature gluconeogenesis cannot supply the large amounts of glucose needed. Puppies of small breeds develop hypoglycemia within 24 h of fasting. This leads to hypoinsulinemia and hyper-

---

[d] Proglicem®, Schering-Plough, 100 mg diazoxide/capsule
[e] Sandostatin®, Sandoz, 50, 100 or 200 µg octreotide/ml)

glucagonemia, i.e., a ketogenic endocrine setting[50] (see also Fig. 5–4). Impaired liver function such as in porto-systemic shunting may contribute to the precipitation of the condition; these animals are especially at risk in the peri-operative fasting period.

Clinical manifestations. The signs and symptoms of juvenile hypoglycemia are not dissimilar to those of other forms of hypoglycemia, although probably in part due to the ketosis, the animals are more commonly presented with lethargy or in coma. In addition there may be muscular weakness, muscle twitching and generalized convulsions. On admission they are mostly in a good nutritional state and without remarkable abnormalities on physical examination.[51]

Diagnosis. The blood glucose concentration may be extremely low, usually less than 1.5 mmol/l.

Treatment. Intravenous administration of a 20 or 50% glucose solution (0.8 and 0.2 ml/100 g body weight, respectively) is indicated if neurological signs, even mild muscle spasm, are present.[51] When the pup can take the glucose solution orally, it is administered at regular intervals until the appetite has returned. Then small amounts of food are given. If needed, (oral) rehydration is started with guidance of blood electrolyte measurements.

Prognosis. If the hypoglycemia is corrected before brain damage has occurred, the prognosis is good. With increasing age and body weight the chances for developing the syndrome of hypoglycemia decrease.[50]

5.4 Gastrinoma; Zollinger-Ellison Syndrome

The term gastrin comprises three biologically active peptides, ranging in size from 14 to 34 amino acids. The normal pancreas does not contain appreciable amounts of gastrin. It is secreted by G cells located in the gastric and duodenal mucosa. Nevertheless most gastrin-secreting tumors, called gastrinomas, occur in the pancreatic islets. In 1955 Zollinger and Ellison first described in man the syndrome of increased gastric acid secretion due to hypersecretion of

gastrin by pancreatic tumors. The syndrome occurs in middle-aged and old dogs and cats as an uncommon disease and the gastrinomas are usually malignant.[52,53]

Clinical manfestations can be traced back to the main biologic actions of gastrin, i.e., stimulation of the hydrochoric acid secretion by gastric parietal cells and trophic effects on the gastric mucosa. The acid hypersecretion and hypertrophic gastritis resulting from gastrin hypersecretion lead to anorexia, vomiting, weight loss, and diarrhea. The development of erosive esophagitis and duodenal ulcers may be associated with hematemesis and melena. In addition, there may be polyuria and polydipsia.

On physical examination the animals are usually lethargic and in a bad nutritional state. Laboratory examination may reveal regenerative anemia, leucocytosis, (mild) hyperglycemia, and hypoproteinemia.

Diagnosis. Suspicion may arise when on endoscopic examination the combination of esophagitis, hypertrophic gastritis, and gastric and/or duodenal ulceration is found. When accessible, measurements of plasma concentrations of gastrin may provide a definitive diagnosis. In the reported cases plasma gastrin concentrations were 3–100 times normal.[53] However, in principle elevated gastrin concentrations may also be found in other conditions such as renal failure and chronic gastritis. Cases with borderline gastrin values may be further studied with a secretin provocative test, but reference values still have to be established.[53]

Treatment. The ideal treatment of gastrinoma is surgical resection, but this measure is rarely curative because of unresectable metastases. As for B-cell tumors (see 5.3.1), somatostatin may be effective to inhibit gastrin release from these non-B-cell tumors.[53]

Symptomatic measures concentrate on inhibition of gastric acid secretion. Gastric parietal cells not only have receptors for gastrin but also for histamine and acetylcholine. Gastric acid secretion is regulated by a concerted action of these three secretagogues and therapeutic control can be achieved by use of specific antagonists such as histamine blockers and anticholinergics. The histamine H_2-receptor antagonist cimetidine[f] (5–10 mg/kg every 6 h) may be effective in the short term but with time progressively higher doses are required. C....ombination with an anticholinergic drug may contribute to the temporary relief. The effectiveness of an inhibitor of the parietal cell Na/K-ATPase such as omeprazole[g] has not yet been reported in dogs with gastrinoma.[53]

Prognosis. The high grade of malignancy of gastrinomas makes the long-term prognosis poor.

---

[f] Tagamet®, SmithKline Beecham, 200 mg cimetidine/tablet.

[g] Losec®, Atra, 20 and 40 mg omeprazole/tablet

6. Testes

6.1 Introduction

In the dog the testes are positioned obliquely within the scrotum, with their long axis directed caudodorsally. Attached to the testis is the epididymis, which is relatively large in dogs. It lies along the dorsolateral border of the testis and is made up of the head, the body and the tail. The head communicates with the testis cranially and is the thicker part. The body is the middle part and is slightly smaller than the head. The tail is attached to the caudal extremity of the testis and is continuous with the ductus deferens. In the cat the testes are located closer to the anus and the long axis is directed caudoventrally.

Tubules with seminiferous epithelium make up about 80% of the testis. They are composed of supporting cells and spermatogenic cells (Fig. 6–1). Seminiferous tubules are the site of spermatogenesis, i.e., where spermatogonia develop into spermatozoa. This process consists of four distinct phases: the mitotic phase, in which immature, undifferentiated spermatogonia undergo rapid cell proliferation; the meiotic phase, in which spermatocytes develop; the spermiogenic phase, in which spermatids differentiate; and the spermiation phase, in which spermatids are released into the tubular lumen. With increasing age there is increased degeneration of seminiferous tubules[1] and a decrease in the relative number of germ cells.[2]

Sertoli cells provide support for the seminiferous tubules and are involved in the release of spermatozoa (spermiation). They contain receptors for follicle stimulating hormone (FSH) and androgen receptors and are thought to regulate the development of the germ cells via the synthesis and secretion of molecules which act upon the surrounding germ cells. They also contain the aromatase enzyme complex that converts testosterone into estradiol.[3]

In the basal region of the seminiferous epithelium the plasma membranes of adjacent Sertoli cells form specialized junctional complexes which form the structural basis of the Sertoli cell barrier. The primary function of this Sertoli cell barrier, previously known as the blood-testis barrier, is probably to ensure that proper conditions for germ cell development are maintained in the tubules. Some molecules enter the tubules nearly instantaneously, while others are almost completely excluded. For example, testosterone and glucose appear to have accelerated entry rates, while peptide hormones (including the gonadotropins) are generally excluded. Peptide hormones produced or secreted into the tubular lumina are retained there by the barrier and probably do not function as endocrine factors outside the testis.[4]

Between the seminiferous tubules lie groups of interstitial or Leydig cells. They are the main constituent of the endocrine portion of the testis and produce the androgens that drive the spermatogenic process.[5]

Hormone synthesis and secretion. The main hormones that are secreted by the testes are androgens and estrogen. Androgens are produced by the interstitial or Leydig cells, which are stimulated by LH. The primary androgen is testosterone. Like other steroid hormones it is produced from cholesterol, which is converted intramitochondrially to pregnenolone. Pregnenolone is further metabolized extramitochondrially to several other steroids via various pathways (see also Fig. 4–3). Apart from direct interaction of testosterone with the androgen receptor many effects are exerted after conversion to the higher affinity androgen receptor ligand dihydrotestosterone by an NADPH-

119

A. Rijnberk (ed.), Clinical Endocrinology of Dogs and Cats, 119–130.
© 1996 *Kluwer Academic Publishers.*

120

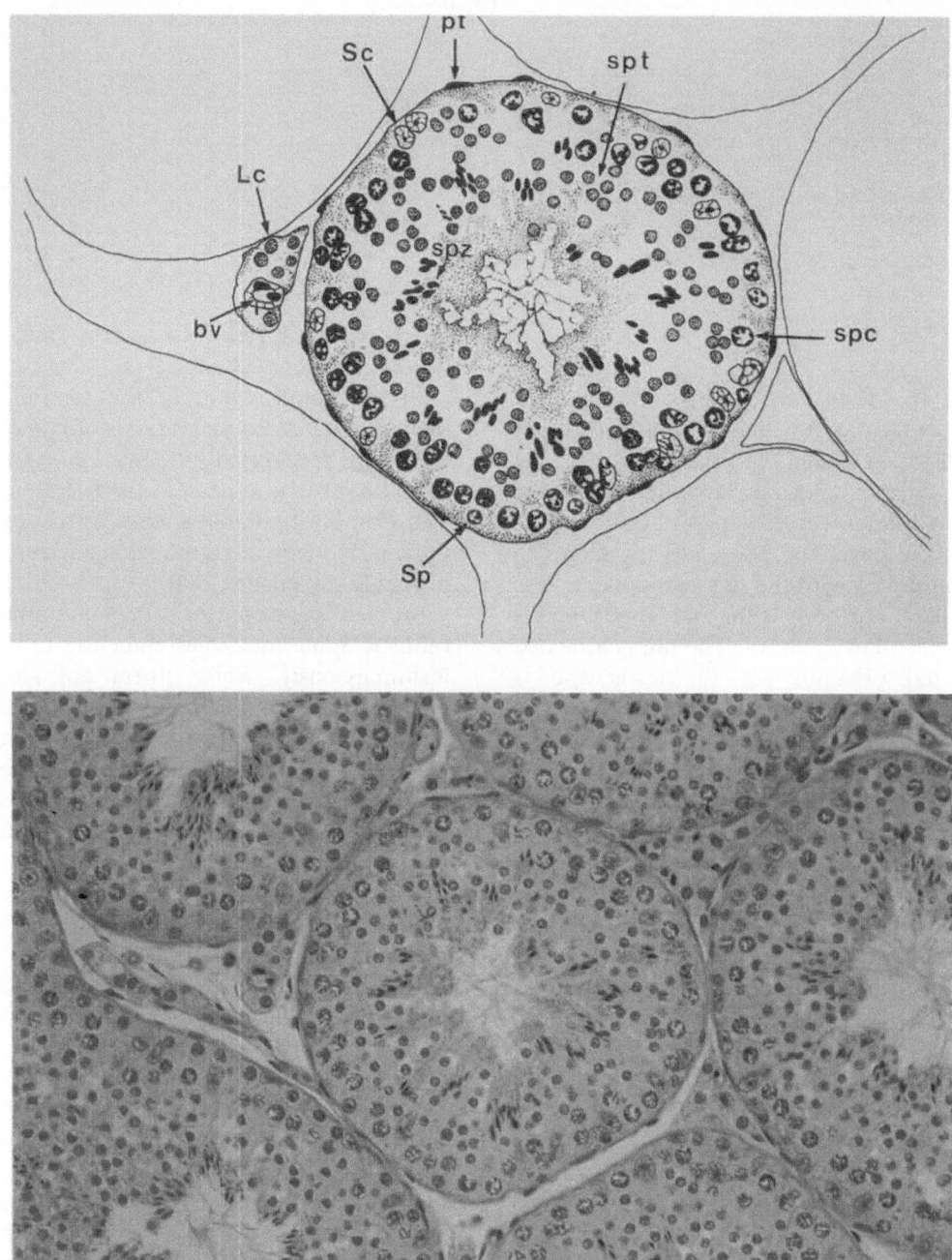

Fig. 6-1. Cross section of a seminiferous tubule of a dog. PAS-hematoxylin, ×475. Sc = Sertoli cells, spc = spermatocytes, spt = spermatids, spz = spermatozoa, sp = spermatogonia, pt = peritubular cells, Lc = Leydig cells, bv = blood vessels. (Courtesy Dr. K.J. Teerds, Department of Functional Morphology, Faculty of Veterinary Medicine, Utrecht University, The Netherlands. Drawing: H. Halsema.)

dependent 5α-reductase. Testosterone can also be converted to other hormones such as estradiol.[6]

Estrogens are produced by the Leydig cells as well as by the Sertoli cells. However, the testicular contribution to the total estradiol production appears to be small (in the order of 20–25%) as compared to the peripheral aromatization of androgens to estradiol.

Testicular steroids are secreted by diffusion into blood, lymph, and tubular fluid. Blood is quantitatively the most important effluent system because the flow rate is 20 times that of lymph or tubular fluid.

Another hormone secreted by the testis is inhibin, a glycoprotein hormone that is primarily produced by the Sertoli cells. It consists of two dissimilar, disulphide-linked subunits termed α and either β_A or β_B. The β subunit of inhibin shares a sequence homology with members of the transforming growth factor β family such as TGFβ, activin and anti-Müllerian hormone (AMH).

Regulation of testis function. Testicular function is controlled by gonadotropins. Androgen secretion is regulated by luteinizing hormone (LH), whereas spermatogenesis is controlled by FSH and locally produced androgens (Fig. 6–2).

LH is secreted by the hypophysis in a pulsatile pattern with a frequency of approximately 4.5 pulses every 6 h. LH pulses are usually followed by a testosterone pulse within 60 min.[7] Diurnal rhythmicity has been described with lowest levels in the morning and peak levels in the afternoon (LH) or evening (testosterone).[8] LH secretion is under negative feedback control by testosterone.

Like LH, FSH is secreted in pulses, but the pulse frequency is different. LH and FSH synthesis and secretion are differentially regulated by the frequency of GnRH pulses from the hypothalamus.[9] FSH secretion is under negative feedback control by inhibin as well as by testosterone, but the relative role of these hormones is unclear. Neither FSH nor testosterone are able to exert full control, and the system as a whole is slowly reacting.

Within the testis, androgens act as paracrine agonists rather than as hormones. Together with other locally produced factors such as endogenous opioids and proteins produced by the peritubular

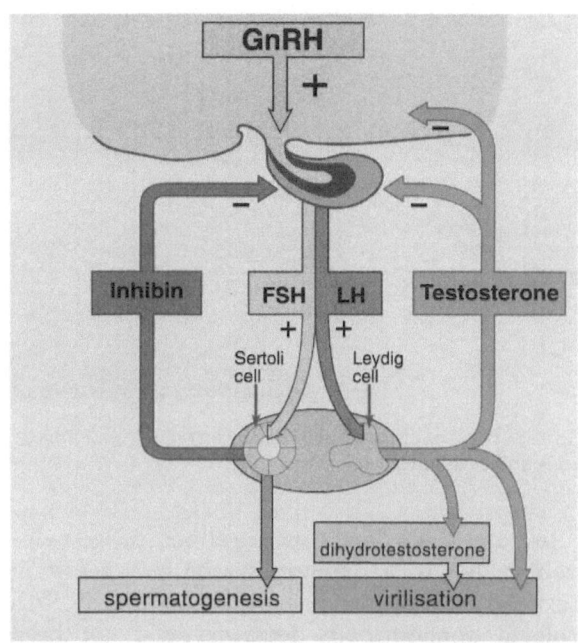

Fig. 6-2. Hormonal control of testis function. Androgen secretion is regulated by LH, with feedback from testosterone. Spermatogenesis is controlled by FSH, with feedback control from inhibin. Testosterone is converted to dihydrotestosterone in several target tissues. (Modified from: Belchetz, 1987.[61])

cells (P-Mod-S), they regulate Sertoli cell function and thereby indirectly the process of spermatogenesis.[3,10]

6.2 Hypogonadism

The term male hypogonadism delineates all forms of endocrine and secretory hypofunction of the testes. The term hypogenitalism is used to indicate underdeveloped external genitals. Hypogonadism is generally distinguished into two forms: (1) primary or hypergonadotrophic hypogonadism, and (2) secondary or hypogonadotrophic hypogonadism. Atrophy of the testes in the presence of normal or increased plasma concentrations of gonadotropins may result from many diseases, such as orchitis of either infectious (Brucella canis) or autoimmune nature, trauma and testicular torsion. In rare cases it may be due to a chromosomal defect. An example of this are male tricolor cats with a 39/XXY karyotype[11] (see Chapter 8). The ultimate form of primary hypogonadism is found in the castrated male dog or tomcat.

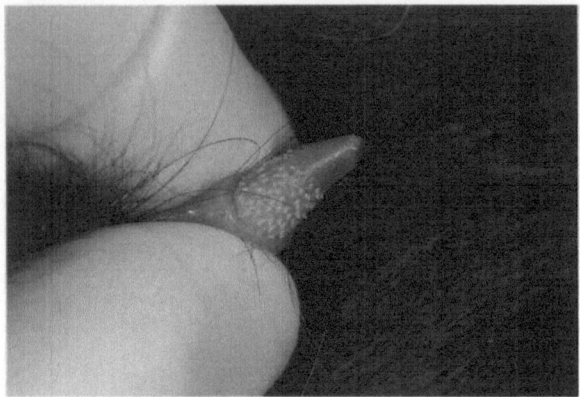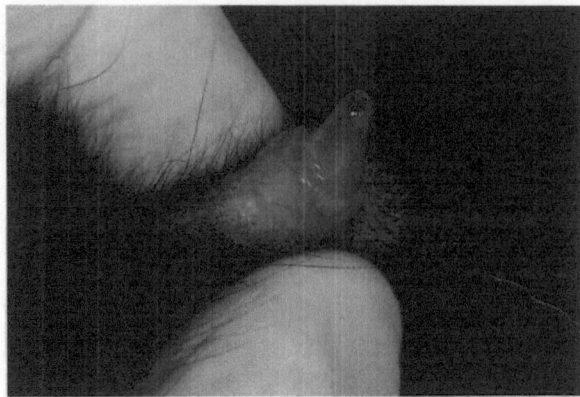

Fig. 6-3. Penis of an intact (left) and a castrated (right) tomcat. The penis of the intact male has typical barbs; these are absent on the penis of the castrated cat.

In rare cases low concentrations of gonado-tropins due to a pituitary tumor may result in secondary hypogonadism (Section 2.2.5). An isolated gonadotropin deficiency has not been described for dogs or cats so far. Anti-androgens such as cyproterone-acetate may act as proges-tagens and their therapeutic use may result in inhibition of the secretion of gonadotropins. This may result in reversible secondary hypogonadism. The same holds true for corticosteroids. Both endogenous and exogenous corticosteroids reduce plasma concentrations of LH.[12]

Clinical manifestations. Testicular atrophy is characterized by small and soft testes. The atrophy does not affect the epididymis, which is relatively large and firm when compared with the adjacent testis. If the condition occurred at a young age the shortage of androgens may result in underdevelop-ment of secondary sexual characteristics, i.e., hypogenitalism. Tomcats will not exhibit the typical feline masculine appearance and the pre-puce, and penis remain underdeveloped. The penis lacks the barbs that are typical of male felidae (Fig. 6–3). Hypogonadism also affects certain aspects of behavior. There is a decreased tendency to marking and roaming, and usually less aggressive behavior toward other cats.[13]

Differential diagnosis. Hypogonadism (including possible previous castration) should be dif-ferentiated from cryptorchidism. Recognition of ectopic testes by palpation is difficult in obese animals and in abdominal cryptorchids. In

tomcats the presence of barbs on the penis may indicate secretion of androgens by cryptorchid testicles (Fig. 6–3). The presence of a functional testis can be demonstrated unequivocally by a GnRH-stimulation test (Chapter 13).

Diagnosis. The consistency of the testes is deter-mined by palpation. The size can be measured with calipers (Fig. 6–4) or estimated with Prader's orchidometer (Fig. 6–5). In the dog the dimensions of the testes depend on the body mass.[14] They range from 1.5 × 1.5 × 2 cm in toy breeds to 3 × 3 × 5 cm in large breeds. In the cat the testes have a diameter of approximately 1 cm.

Treatment. Most cases of hypogonadism are due to castration. This condition is usually desired by the owner and is no reason for treatment. In the rare cases in which treatment of hypogonadism is requested replacement therapy with androgens

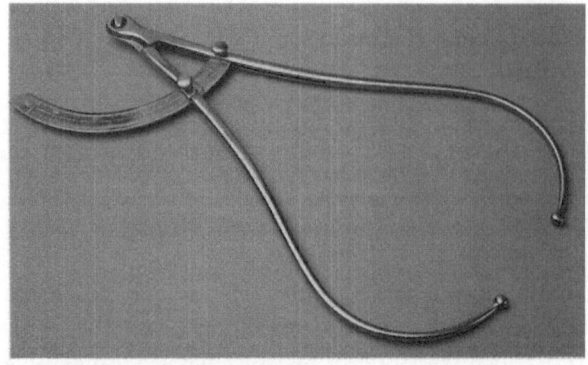

Fig. 6-4. Calipers used for measuring testicular size.

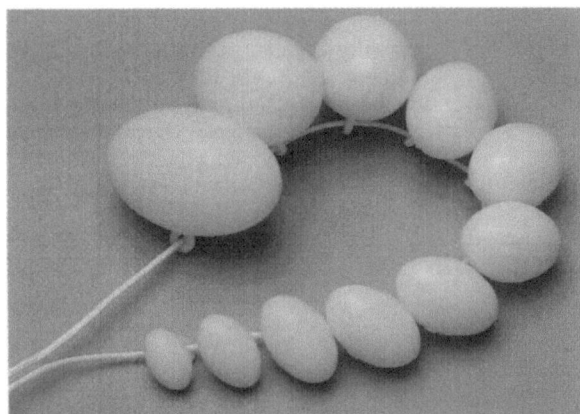

Fig. 6-5. Prader's orchidometer. The volume of the testis is estimated by comparison with the ellipsoids. The size is indicated in ml. The epididymis should not be included in the assessment of testicular volume.

may be given. Daily oral administration of 1 mg testosterone[a]/kg body weight or 0.1 mg fluoxy-mesterone[b]/kg, or weekly injections of a long-acting testosterone formulation[c] may be used. After the starting dose of 1 or 0.1 mg/kg the dose is adjusted to effect for maintenance.

Prognosis. Primary hypogonadism is usually incurable, but the testosterone deficiency may be substituted lifelong with replacement therapy. In secondary hypogonadism the prognosis depends on the course of the primary disease (see Section 2.2.5).

6.3 Cryptorchidism

Cryptorchidism is a developmental defect in which complete descent of one or both testes into the scrotum does not occur. The reported incidence in dogs varies from 1.2%[15] to 9.7%, depending on the population studied. It is a congenital disease and is considered to be a sex-limited inherited trait in dogs.[17] Cryptorchidism occurs more often in purebred dogs than in crossbreds, and bilateral cryptorchid dogs are reported to be more inbred than unilateral cryptorchids. Although a single

[a] Andriol®, Organon (40 mg testosterone-undecanoate per capsule)
[b] Halotestin®, Upjohn (5mg fluoxymesteron per tablet)
[c] Sustanon®, Organon (Three testosterone-esters)

autosomal recessive gene has been cited as a probable cause, transmission of the defect is probably due to more than one gene. Cryptorchid dogs are considered to be homozygous for the defect; their removal from the breeding line generally causes a decrease in frequency of the defect. Because cryptorchidism is a sex-limited trait that can only be detected in males, the genotype of the (carrier) female can only be assessed by progeny testing. This requires large numbers of puppies and makes the condition difficult to eliminate from a canine population. Cryptorchidism has been found in at least 68 canine breeds.[17] A retrospective study of 2,912 dogs identified 14 breeds with a significantly increased risk:[18] Toy Poodle, Pomeranian, Yorkshire Terrier, Miniature Dachshund, Cairn Terrier, Chihuahua, Maltese, Boxer, Pekingese, English Bulldog, Old English Sheepdog, Miniature Poodle, Miniature Schnauzer, and Shetland Sheepdog. The incidence of cryptorchidism in the cat has been reported to vary from 1.7%[19] to 3.8%.[20] Persian cats were overrepresented in both studies.

Normal testicular descent can be divided into three phases: intra-abdominal, intra-inguinal and extra-inguinal migration. The process of descent is controlled by the gubernaculum testis (Fig. 6–6). This is a mesenchymal cord that extends from the caudal pole of the testis to the inguinal canal. During the process of descent, the gubernaculum increases in size just distal to the external opening of the inguinal canal. This enlargement or outgrowth exerts traction upon the intra-abdominal part of the gubernaculum and this pulls the testis and epididymis distally through the abdomen toward the inguinal area and then through the inguinal canal. These are the intra-abdominal and intra-inguinal phase of descent. After completion of the outgrowth the gubernaculum regresses and pulls the testis further caudally. This is the extra-inguinal migration that moves the testis into the scrotum. Complete absence of the outgrowth reaction has not been observed, but substantial underdevelopment does occur with low frequency. In these cases there is a partial migration of the testis from its original position just caudal to the kidney to the vicinity of the internal inguinal opening. The final result in such cases is either permanent low abdominal cryptorchidism or

124

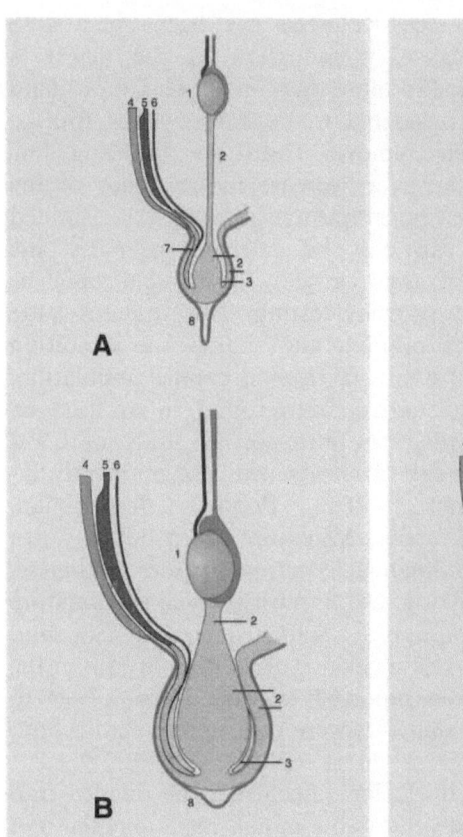
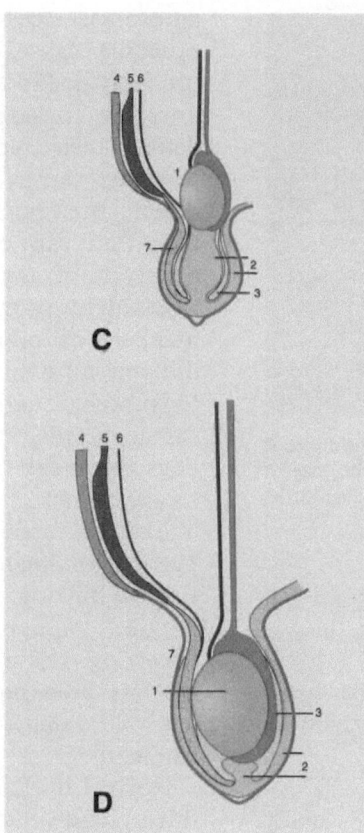

Fig. 6-6. Schematic representation of four successive stages (A→D) of normal descent of the testis. (1) Testis, (2) gubernaculum, (3) vaginal process, (4) external oblique abdominal muscle, (5) internal oblique abdominal muscle, (6) peritoneum, (7) cremaster muscle, and (8) external spermatic fascia. (Modified from: Wensing CJG, 1980.[62])

delayed testicular descent. Abnormal location of the gubernaculum can take three forms (Fig. 6–7): (A) the extra-abdominal part of the gubernaculum does not expand beyond the inguinal canal but, instead, thrusts back into the abdominal cavity (reversed outgrowth). The traction normally developed by the outgrowth is absent, and the testis fails to leave its original position caudal to the kidney. This results in high abdominal cryptorchidism. (B) The outgrowth takes place partly in the inguinal canal and is partly intraabdominal. Only slight displacement of the testis in the direction of the internal inguinal opening will then occur. (C) The outgrowth reaction is partly extra-abdominal. If this occurs, descent will progress further, and the testis may even reach the internal inguinal opening. The final outcome is difficult to predict, but low abdominal or inguinal cryptorchidism is the most likely result.

The hormonal control of testicular descent is poorly understood. There are no indications that gonadotropins play a role. In dogs, the initial outgrowth of the gubernaculum requires the presence of androgens, and testosterone induces gubernacular regression during the final phase of testicular descent, but additional testicular factors are necessary for complete descent.[21–23]

Clinical manifestations. The most striking abnormality is the absence of one or both testes from the scrotum. Bilateral cryptorchid dogs are considered to be infertile. Unilaterally cryptorchid dogs generally are regarded as potentially fertile, but their fertility is probably lower than that of normal dogs[17]. Plasma concentrations of testosterone and estradiol do not differ among unilateral inguinal cryptorchid, unilateral abdominal cryptorchid, and normal dogs.[24] Unilateral cryptorchid cats display behavior characteristic of intact males.[20]

Cryptorchidism is associated with an increased risk for testicular neoplasia in the cryptorchid testis. Certain types of testicular neoplasia may cause feminization and blood dyscrasias (See section 6.4).

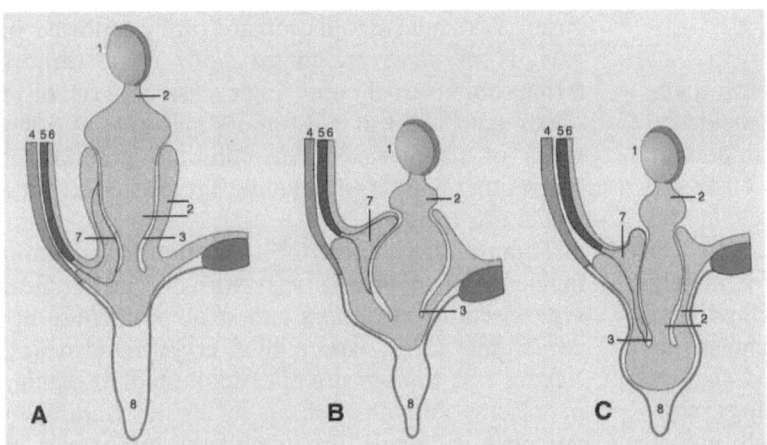

Fig. 6-7. Schematic representation of three forms of abnormal descent of the testis. A Reversed outgrowth of the gubernaculum. B. Outgrowth of the gubernaculum partly in the abdomen. C. Outgrowth of the gubernaculum partly outside the abdomen. The figures refer to the same structures as in Fig. 6–6. (Modified from: Wensing CJG, 1980.[62])

Differential diagnosis. Unilateral cryptorchidism should be differentiated from monorchism, in which there is no testicular tissue present. Monorchism has been described in two cats.[20]

Diagnosis. Cryptorchidism is diagnosed by inspection and palpation. Cryptorchid testes may be found in the abdomen, at the inguinal ring, or in the inguinal canal. Abdominal testicles cannot be palpated. Testicles in the inguinal area can sometimes be palpated, but in young animals it is difficult to determine the position of the testes reliably because of their small size during the first weeks of life. In addition, the cremaster muscle may hold immature testicles in the inguinal canal or retract them from the scrotum when the animal is exposed to stress during physical examination. Cats have large inguinal fat pads which make inguinal testicles extremely difficult to palpate. Bilateral cryptorchidism in cats can be suspected by the presence of barbs on the penis (Fig. 6–3).

There is disagreement in the literature about the time of testicular descent in the dog and cat. Detailed data have been published only for beagle and mongrel puppies.[25] In these breeds the testicles reach their final position in the scrotum at 35 and 40 days postpartum. Based on these findings, puppies should be examined at between 6 and 12 weeks of age. If the testes have not descended by 8 weeks of age cryptorchidism may be tentatively diagnosed. However, testicular descent has been reported to be complete as late as 6 months of age in some dogs.[26,27] For this reason a periodic re-examinations should be scheduled until 6 months of age.

Treatment. Human chorionic gonadotropin (hCG) and gonadotropin releasing hormone (GnRH) have been tried and reported anecdotically to be effective.[28,29] The scientific basis for this form of treatment is not clear, since there is no evidence that testicular descent is controlled by gonadotropins. As the inguinal canal is usually closed in abdominal cryptorchids, success can only be expected in inguinal cryptorchidism. Testosterone has been tried as a therapy for cryptorchidism with little or no success.[30] Surgical placement of the retained testicle in the scrotum (orchidopexy) has been shown to improve testicular function and may even result in normal fertility.[31,32] However, it is generally considered unethical because it conceals a congenital abnormality and promotes spread of the defect within the population. Surgical removal of the retained testis or castration are frequently advised because this eliminates the risk of developing testicular neoplasia and prevents spread of the defect within the population. Although cryptorchid testes have a higher risk of developing Sertoli cell tumor and seminoma than scrotal testes, the risk of fatal complications such as pancytopenia or metastasis is still very low. A decision analysis has shown that the risk of tumor-related mortality and morbidity is of the same order of magnitude as the risk of mortality and morbidity due to anesthesiological or surgical complications.[33] Based on these findings there is no strong reason to advise castration in cryptorchid dogs.

126

6.4 Testicular neoplasia

Testicular tumors are relatively common neoplasms in dogs. They have an estimated incidence of 67.8 per 100,000 male dogs[34] and represent 5–15% of all neoplasms in this species.[35] There are three major types of testicular neoplasia in the dog: Sertoli cell tumor, seminoma, and Leydig cell tumor. These tumors occur with approximately equal frequency. Cryptorchidism is an important risk factor. In cryptorchid dogs, the incidence of Sertoli cell tumor is 23 times higher and that of seminoma 16 times higher than in dogs with scrotal testes. The incidence of Leydig cell tumors in cryptorchid and scrotal testes is similar.[35-39] Other tumors (gonadoblastoma, leiomyoma of the tunica vaginalis, schwannoma, and undifferentiated sarcoma/carcinoma) have been described in individual dogs,[40-42] but these are exceptional

cases. Testicular neoplasms are rarely reported in cats. None were present in 1,567 feline tumors (from both sexes), but single case reports have documented Sertoli cell tumors and several other types of neoplasia.[43] The common practice of castrating male cats at a young age may contribute to the low incidence.

Tumor size, secretion of hormones, and incidence of metastasis vary with the histological type. Sertoli cell tumors and seminomas may become quite large, especially in cryptorchid testes. Leydig cell tumors are the smallest of testicular neoplasms and may be an incidental finding at necropsy. Bilateral tumors and the occurrence of different tumor types in a single dog are not exceptional.[36,44-46] Approximately 8–39% of the Sertoli tumors in dogs are associated with a feminization syndrome.[16,46,47] Feminization has also been reported in a dog with a seminoma and in a limited number of dogs with Leydig cell tumors, but these are exceptional cases. Feminization in dogs with testicular tumor may be associated with blood dyscrasias.[47-52] Feminization and blood dyscrasias have been attributed to increased secretion of estrogens by the tumor, but this has been investigated in only a small number of dogs.[50,53,54] In one study elevated plasma levels of estradiol were found in only 3 of 10 dogs.[50] In another study there was no significant difference between plasma estradiol levels in tumor bearing and healthy control dogs,[53] but recent experiments using a different estradiol radioimmunoassay showed elevated plasma concentrations of estradiol before and after stimulation with the GnRH-analogue Buserelin[a] in 5 dogs with feminizing testicular tumors compared to 5 healthy control dogs (Fig. 6–8). These findings indicate that feminization in dogs with testicular tumors is probably caused by an increased secretion of estrogens by the tumor. It was also found that Sertoli cell tumors secrete increased amounts of bioactive inhibin,[53] but the significance of this finding is unclear at present.

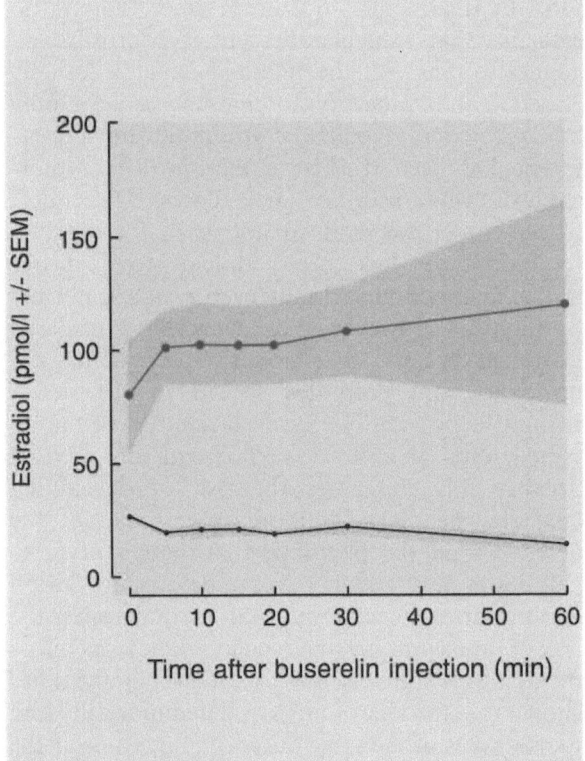

Fig. 6-8. Plasma concentrations of estradiol in 5 male control dogs (blue) and 5 dogs with Sertoli cell tumors (beige) at various times after i.v. administration of 0.5 µg buserelin/kg body weight. (Van Sluijs F.J., De Jong F.H., unpublished results.)

Clinical manifestations. Testicular tumors cause noticeable testicular enlargement. In cryptorchid dogs this may result in a palpable abdominal mass. Dogs with testicular neoplasia may have bilater-

[a] Receptal, Hoechst, Frankfurt, FRG

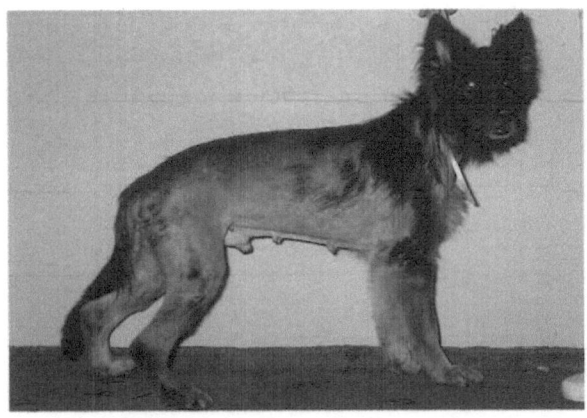
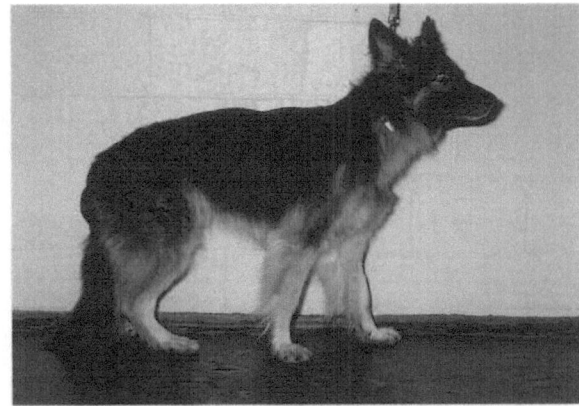

Fig. 6-9. - Bilaterally symmetrical alopecia in an 8-year-old German Shepherd dog with a Sertoli cell tumor in an abdominal testis (left). Complete regrowth of the hair coat had occurred 6 months after surgical removal of the tumor (right).

ally symmetrical alopecia (Fig. 6–9), atrophy and pigmentation of the skin and signs of feminization such as gynecomastia (Fig. 6–10), a pendulous prepuce (Fig. 6–11), atrophy of the penile sheath, and atrophy of the contralateral testis, and they may be attractive to other male dogs. There may be blood dyscrasias varying from thrombocytopenia to pancytopenia. In severe cases this may lead to hemorrhagic diathesis and anemia (Fig. 6–12).

Differential diagnosis. Testicular enlargement due to tumor should be differentiated from orchitis and testicular torsion. The skin disorders may mimic other endocrine diseases such as hypothyroidism (see Section 3.3), hyperadrenocorticism (see Section 4.3) and possibly growth hormone deficiency (see Section 2.2). Blood dyscrasias may

also be caused by a variety of other conditions such as idiopathic or immune-mediated thrombocytopenia, myeloproliferative disorders, and aplastic anemia.

Diagnosis. Testicular neoplasia in dogs and cats is diagnosed by palpation of a testicular mass in a scrotal or ectopic testis. The consistency is usually firm and the tumors are rarely painful on palpation. In dogs with testicular enlargement due to orchitis or testicular torsion the swelling is mostly soft and painful. In cryptorchid dogs, testicular tumors may not be noticed unless skin disorders or signs of feminization develop. Survey radiography and ultrasonography may help to define the presence of an enlarged ectopic testis. Ultrasonography may also be used to detect small neoplasms in the contralateral testis that may be missed by palpation.

Treatment. Testicular tumors are treated by orchidectomy. Removal of the tumor is usually simple, but blood transfusions may be necessary in patients with severe blood dyscrasias. In cases of bilateral testicular involvement orchidectomy should be bilateral. In cases of unilateral testis tumor the contralateral scrotal testis, which may be atrophic due to suppression of GnRH secretion by feedback of the autonomously hypersecreting tumor, can be left in place. Ectopic contralateral testes are best removed because of the high incidence of Sertoli cell tumors in non-scrotal testes.

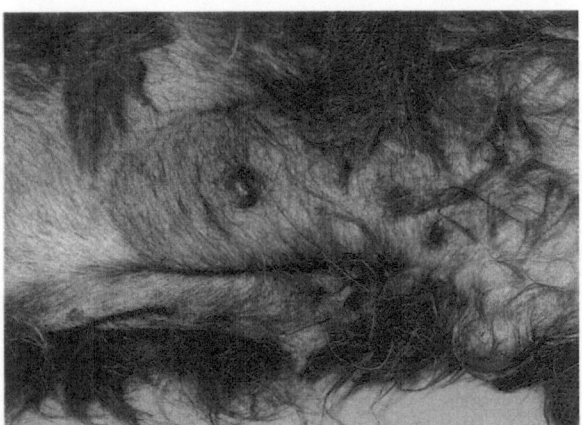

Fig. 6-10. Gynecomastia in a 7-year old Bouvier with an abdominal Sertoli cell tumor.

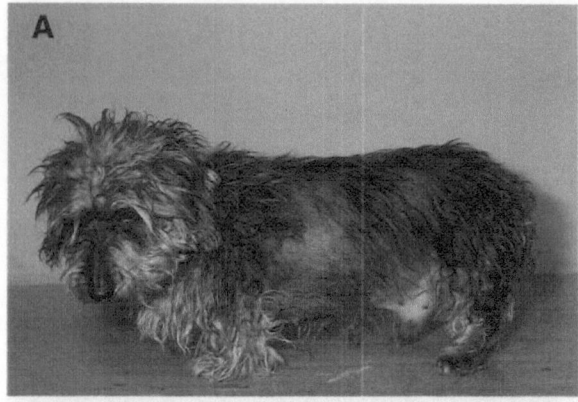

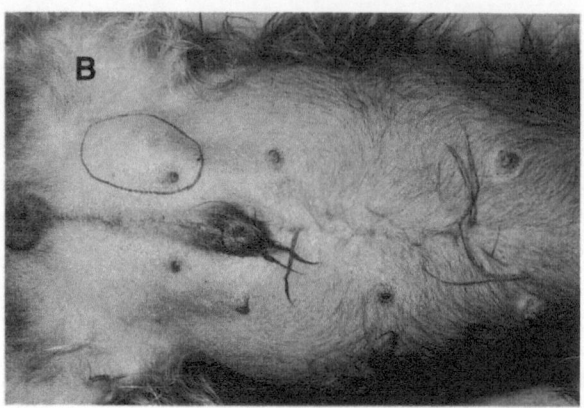

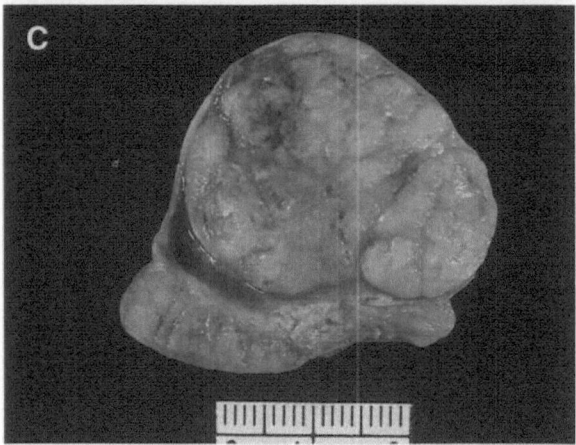

Fig. 6-11. A 10-year old Dachshund with pendulous prepuce and bilaterally symmetrical alopecia (A). These signs were caused by a mixed Sertoli cell tumor/seminoma in an ectopic testis in the inguinal area (B and C) and resolved after removal of the tumor.

Prognosis. The prognosis after surgical removal of the affected testis depends on the type of tumor but is usually good. Associated skin disorders and signs of feminization are reversible (Fig. 6–8), but more severe forms of blood dyscrasia are not amenable to treatment and may result in fatal

complications. Metastases are uncommon but may occur with all types of testicular tumors. The reported incidence is 1 to 10% in Sertoli cell tumors, 3% in seminomas, and 2 to 3% in Leydig cell tumors.[16,37–39,46]

6.5 Male infertility

Infertility in the male dog (or cat) may be congenital (no offspring) or acquired (sired offspring). Possible causes of congenital infertility include an abnormal hypothalamic-pituitary-gonadal axis, chromosomal and/or sexual differentiation abnormalities (see Chapter 8), segmental aplasia of the ducts, cryptorchidism (see Section 6.3), and defects in spermatogenesis. Acquired fertility disorders may be caused by testicular hyperthermia due to inflammation or environmental factors, testicular neoplasia (see Section 6.4), infections of the reproductive tract, endocrine disorders,

Fig. 6-12. Petechia on the penis of a dog with thrombocytopenia, which can occur as a result of estrogen-induced bone marrow depression. (Courtesy of R.J. Slappendel.)

exposure to toxins, or medication, or may be idiopathic. The latter is the most common cause of infertility in men (ca. 75%), and a similar high incidence is suspected in the dog.[55,56] Endocrine disorders that are associated with infertility are hypothyroidism and hyperadrenocorticism. Hypothyroidism caused by lymphocytic thyroiditis has been shown to be related in incidence to lymphocytic orchitis and reduced fertility in a colony of Beagles[57] (see also Section 3.3.1). In hyperadrenocorticism the increased production of cortisol exerts a negative feedback on the secretion of LH by the pituitary, resulting in a decreased secretion of testosterone by the Leydig cells.[12]

Clinical manifestations. Male infertility may vary from complete absence of libido to the inability to sire offspring in spite of normal mating. Depending on the cause there may be other signs that are characteristic of the underlying condition.

Diagnosis. Diagnosis of male infertility is based on a complete physical examination, serological testing for Brucella canis, semen analysis, and testicular biopsy. Particular attention should be paid to endocrine diseases such as hypothyroidism (see Section 3.3) and hyperadrenocorticism (see Section 4.3).

Possible findings of semen analysis include oligozoospermia (< 200 million sperm in the entire

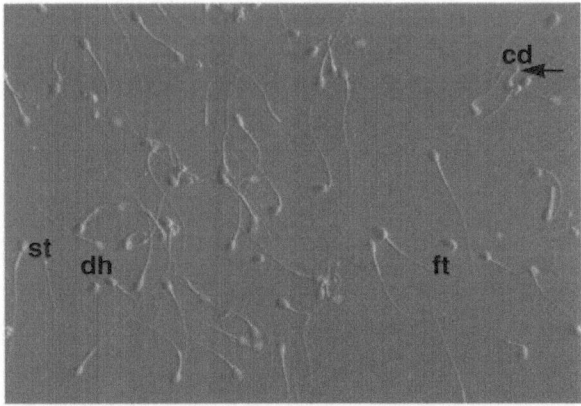

Fig. 6-13. Differential interference contrast photograph (× 300) of semen from a healthy dog with 85% normal spermatozoa. Abnormalities include detached head (dh), sperm tail without head (st), cytoplasmic droplet (cd), and folded tail (ft). (Courtesy Prof. Dr. B. Colenbrander, Department of Herd Health and Reproduction, Faculty of Veterinary Medicine, Utrecht University, The Netherlands.)

semen-rich fraction of the ejaculate); teratozoospermia (< 70% of sperm cells with normal morphology); asthenozoospermia (< 50% progressively forward motility); leukozoospermia (> 2,000 WBC per microliter in the ejaculate); azoospermia (no sperm observed in the ejaculate); and hemozoospermia (blood seen grossly or on cytology). More than one abnormality may be present in a single sample (Fig. 6–13).

Testicular biopsy is indicated in dogs which are persistently azoospermic or severely oligospermic.[55] A wedge biopsy is preferred over a percutaneous needle biopsy because specimens obtained with needle biopsies contain insufficient tubules in circular cross section to allow detailed histomorphometric analysis of spermatogenesis.[58] Testicular biopsy is not entirely harmless and should be undertaken with care. Hemorrhage and necrosis with subsequent fibrosis at the biopsy site and testicular atrophy have been described after percutaneous needle biopsy,[58] and similar lesions of greater severity were found after Trucut and incisional biopsies.[59]

Leukozoospermia indicates prostatitis with or without benign prostatic hyperplasia, orchitis, epididymitis, and/or urinary tract disease. Orchitis and epididymitis are diagnosed by ultrasonography and fine needle biopsy. The latter method should be used with care. Epididymal aspiration may cause hematoma, fibrosis or sperm granuloma, which could cause obstruction.[55] Infections of the reproductive organs require bacteriological culture of the ejaculate. Mycoplasma and E. coli are the organisms most frequently cultured from infections of the reproductive tract.[56,57]

Teratozoospermia may be associated with insufficient testosterone production, past hyperthermic events, reproductive tract infection, and genetic or familial disorders. It is often observed in combination with leukozoospermia and infection. Asthenozoospermia may be caused by ciliary dyskinesia, anti-sperm antibodies, benign prostatic hyperplasia, reproductive tract infection, or by improper collection or handling of the sample. Oligozoospermia may be caused by toxin exposure, medication (sex steroids, anabolic steroids, glucocorticoids, ketaconazole, cimetidine, and chemotherapeutic agents), reproductive tract infection, reproduction tract blockage, and benign prostatic hyperplasia. It may also be due to an incomplete ejaculate.

Azoospermia may be the result of a congenital defect or epididymal blockage. As in oligozoospermia it can be due to an incomplete ejaculate. The semen of azoospermic animals should therefore be collected several times under different circumstances to ensure that a full ejaculate is obtained. Collection should be made at least three times at 2-month intervals before more invasive diagnostic procedures are attempted. Low concentrations of alkaline phosphatase (< 10,000 IU/l) in several ejaculates indicate ductal blockage due to bilateral sperm granuloma rather than incomplete ejaculation. In these cases fine needle aspirates may be taken from the epididymides, but this may cause sperm granuloma and induce antisperm antibodies. A search for chromosomal abnormalities should be started in dogs with a lifelong history of hypoplastic testes and no sperm. Testicular biopsy is warranted in dogs with azoospermia but may induce production of antisperm antibodies and formation of a fibrotic scar in the testis.

Treatment. Treatment of male infertility depends on the underlying cause. Infections of the reproductive tract are treated with long-term (4–6 weeks) appropriate antibiotic therapy. Antibiotics that penetrate and maintain therapeutic levels in the male reproductive tract are trimethoprim-sulfa and fluorinated quinolones. Acute orchitis and/or epididymitis require rapid diagnosis and treatment. Unilateral orchidectomy is successful in preserving a normal spermogram from the remaining testis in more than 75% of the cases. Aggressive antibiotic therapy may also be successful, but sperm granulomas often form, leading to epididymal blockage. Blockage of the reproductive tract can be treated surgically, but the chances of success are small. Owners of treated animals should be made aware of the fact that the spermatic cycle in the dog requires approximately 62 days, and that an additional 15 days are needed for sperm transport through the epididymis. Response to treatment may require several cycles of spermatogenesis and, therefore, several months may be needed for regeneration and improvement.

Prognosis. Leukozoospermia due to infections of the reproductive tract has a guarded prognosis because there is a considerable risk of epididymal blockage by scar tissue. Teratozoospermia has a guarded prognosis, but exceptionally well-planned matings may be successful. Abnormal morphology of sperm cells does not correlate with birth defects in the offspring; however, some defects in sperm maturation seem to be hereditary. There are reports of offspring from a dog with only 8% normal morphology when a total of 250 million sperm cells were used for vaginal artificial insemination over several days.[60] Asthenozoospermia has a guarded prognosis, but in some cases sperm motility can be improved considerably by extending the semen with an extender. Oligozoospermia and azoospermia generally have a poor prognosis, but semen quality may improve if primary conditions are present that can be treated successfully.

7. Ovaries

7.1 Introduction

The ovaries are situated immediately caudal to the kidneys and thus lie at the level of the third or fourth lumbar vertebrae. They are attached to the dorsolateral wall of the abdominal cavity by the broad ligaments and to the middle and ventral thirds of the last one or two ribs (dog) or to the diaphragm (cat) by suspensory ligaments. The ovaries are connected to the cranial ends of the uterine horns by the proper ligaments of the ovary (Fig. 7–1). The ovaries are in the dog completely and in the cat partially enclosed in a peritoneal pouch, the ovarian bursa. The ovarian bursa contains the uterine tubes and is usually opaque in the dog due to its fat content (Fig. 7–2). The surfaces of the ovaries, which are free of serosa, are covered by germinal epithelium. Germ cells from the germinal epithelium of the cortex grow inward and follicles, many of which degenerate and become atretic, develop. During the follicular phase tertiary follicles grow and can be seen macroscopically at the surface as follicular fluid increases. Lateral to the ovaries, the infundibula are opened to collect ovulated ova. In the dog the fimbriated extremities lie mainly in the ovarian bursae, but generally a portion protrudes through the slit-like opening of the bursa.

7.2 Estrous cycle, pregnancy, and parturition

7.2.1 Dog

In the healthy bitch the onset of puberty is between 6–18 months of age. Following each estrous cycle, which has a length of about 3 months, an anestrus with a variable duration follows. The mean interval from one estrous cycle to the next is

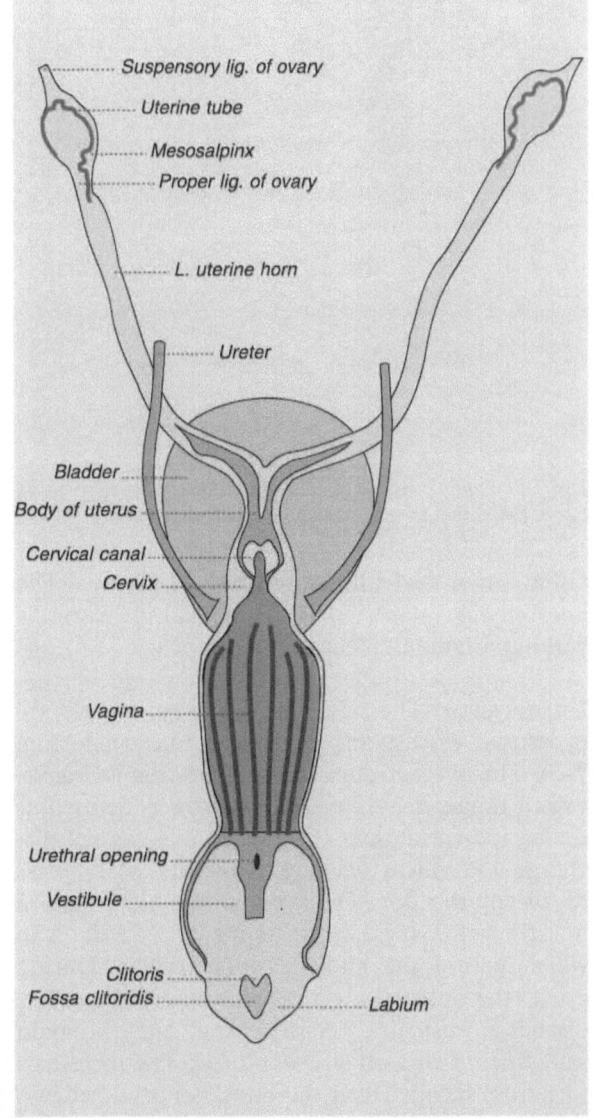

Fig. 7-1. Dorsal view of genitalia of the bitch. The vestibule, vagina, cervix, and body of the uterus are opened on the midline. The first parts of the uterine horns have also been opened. (Modified from Evans and Christensen, 1993.[1])

131

A. Rijnberk (ed.), Clinical Endocrinology of Dogs and Cats, 131–156.
© *1996 Kluwer Academic Publishers.*

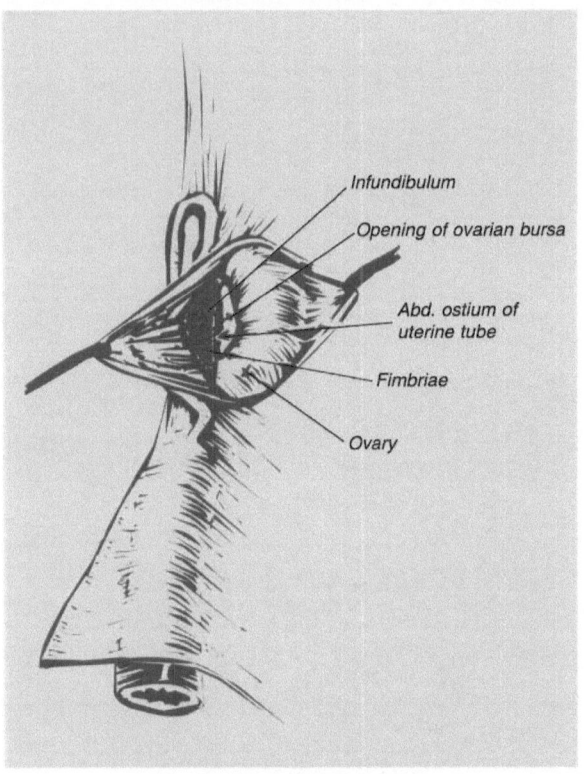

Fig. 7-2. Lateral aspect of left ovary with opened ovarian bursa. (Modified from Evans and Christensen, 1993.[1])

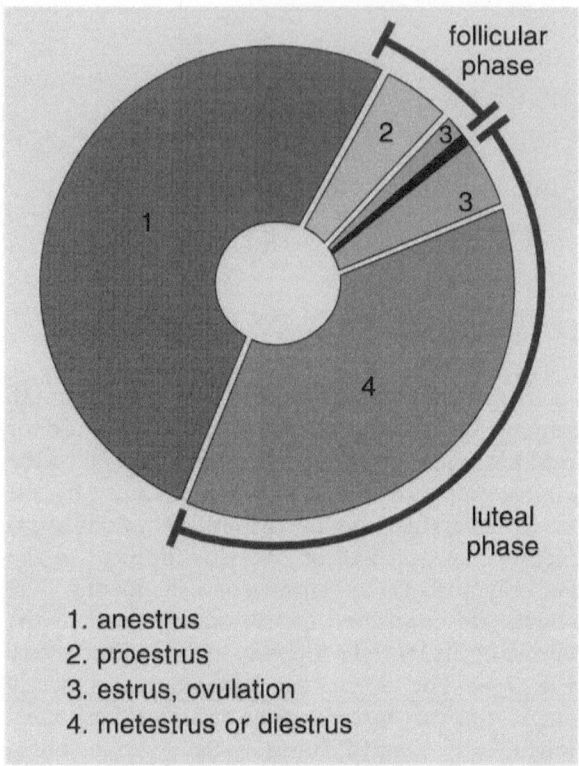

1. anestrus
2. proestrus
3. estrus, ovulation
4. metestrus or diestrus

Fig. 7-3. Diagram of the estrous cycle and anestrus in the dog.

about 7 months with a range of 4–12 months. The interestrous interval may be regular or variable within individual bitches.

Estrous cycle. The stages of the estrous cycle are proestrus, estrus, and metestrus (diestrus) (Fig. 7–3). The average duration of proestrus is 9 days, with a range of 3–17 days. Proestrus is defined as the period from onset of sanguineous vaginal discharge and vulvar swelling to the first willingness to accept the dog. On average the estrus has a duration of 9 days, with a range of 3–21 days, in which period the bitch accepts mating. During estrus the vulva starts to shrink and soften. The discharge usually persists, and may remain sanguineous or turn straw-colored. The metestrus (diestrus) begins when the bitch is no longer willing to accept the dog. It has an average duration of about 70 days if we assume that it ends when the progesterone concentration declines (for the first time) to a level of ≤ 3 nmol/l.

In addition to this behavior-oriented classification of the cycle, it is also possible to classify

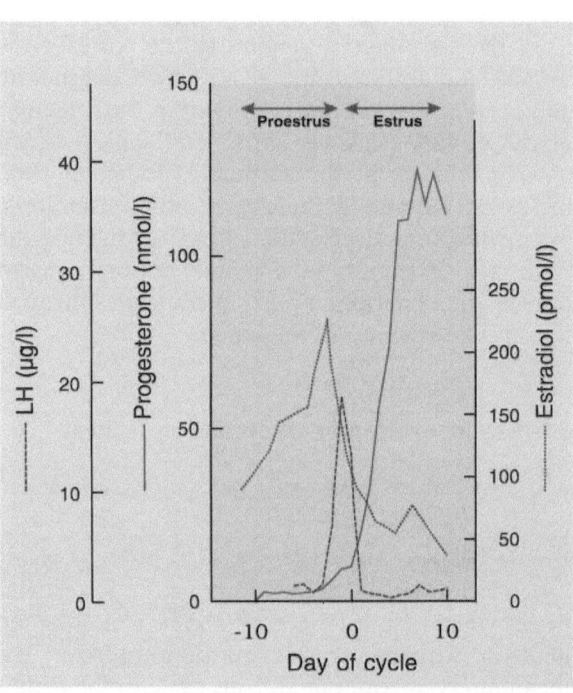

Fig. 7-4. Concentrations of estradiol, LH, and progesterone in plasma in relation to estrus behavior of the bitch.

according to ovarian function and to distinguish the follicular phase, the phase of preovulatory luteinization and ovulation, and the luteal phase (Fig. 7–3).

Follicular phase. As tertiary follicles develop in the ovaries they produce estradiol, leading to peak levels in plasma of 180–370 pmol/l in late proestrus, about 1–2 days before the preovulatory LH surge (Fig. 7–4). During laparoscopic examination follicle development is not readily apparent on the ovary because of the ovarian bursa and because the follicles remain below the ovarian surface until just prior to ovulation. The external signs of proestrus, such as hyperemia and edema of the vulva and bloody vaginal discharge, are caused by the high level of estradiol (Fig. 7–5). This also causes lengthening and hyperemia of the uterine horns, enlargement of the cervix, and thickening of the vaginal wall. The percentage of superficial cells in the vaginal smear increases and the percentage of parabasal and small intermediate cells decreases (Fig. 7–6). Superficial cells dominate as the follicular phase progresses (Fig. 7–7). However, it should be realized that although vaginal cytology gives an indication of the stage of the cycle it is not a trusted indicator of the preovulatory LH surge or of ovulation. Vaginoscopy reveals that the vaginal mucosal folds are swollen, very pale, and have smoothly rounded surfaces (balloons) (Fig. 7–8). At the end of the follicular phase, i.e., during the decline in estradiol and the rise in progesterone concentrations in plasma, shrinkage begins in response to reduced estradiol-dependent water retention. These cyclic changes are most marked in the dorsal median fold and

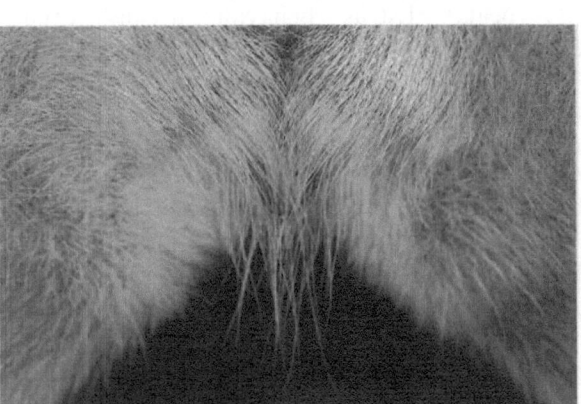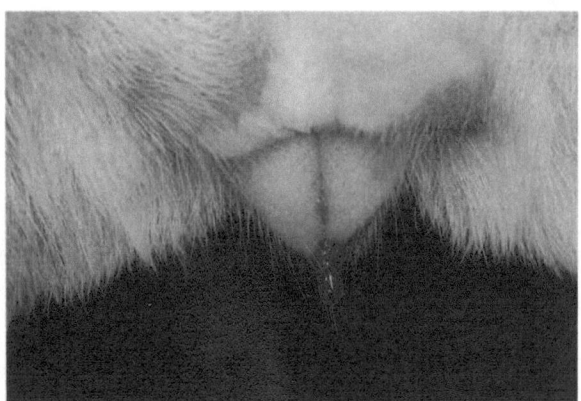

Fig. 7-5. The vulva of a beagle bitch during (left) anestrus, and during (right) proestrus/estrus.

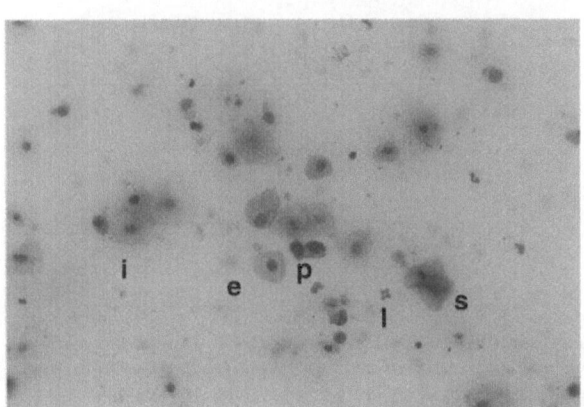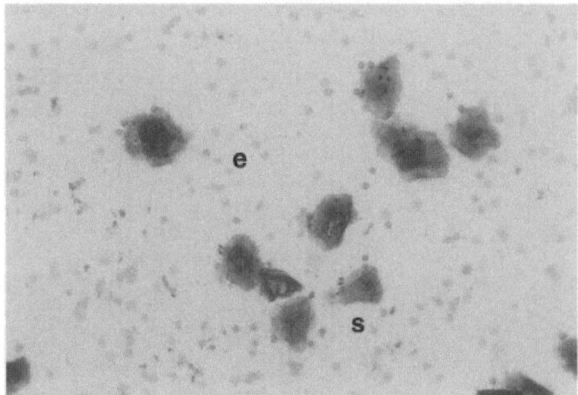

Fig. 7-6. Vaginal cytology in the bitch at the onset of the follicular phase, showing primarily intermediate (i) cells, some superficial (s) and parabasal (p) cells, erythrocytes (e), and leukocytes (l). (200×, May Grünwald Giemsa.)

Fig. 7-7. Vaginal cytology in the bitch during the second half of the follicular phase, at ovulation and the onset of the luteal phase. This smear shows superficial cells (s) and erythrocytes (e). (200×, May Grünwald Gremsa.)

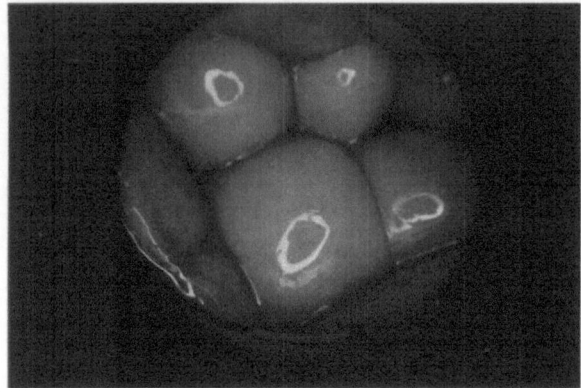

Fig. 7-8. Vaginoscopy in the bitch at the onset of the follicular phase. Note the swollen, pale mucosal folds with smooth rounded surfaces (balloons) and the bloody secretion between the folds.

precede those of the mid vaginal mucosa (Fig. 7–9).

Both LH and FSH concentrations in plasma are low during the follicular phase. Progesterone levels remain low but fluctuate. This fluctuation may become more pronounced during the second part of the follicular phase, possibly as a result of partial luteinization.

Preovulatory luteinization and ovulation. The preovulatory surge of LH lasts 24–72 h. It usually starts 1–2 days after the estradiol peak and coincides with declining estradiol and rising progesterone concentrations in plasma (Fig. 7–4). Rapid and extensive luteinization takes place during the preovulatory LH surge. Ruptured follicles therefore have many of the characteristics of rapidly developing corpora lutea (Fig. 7–10). Most ova in the dog are released in an immature state as primary oocytes. The first meiotic division and the extrusion of the first polar body are not completed until at least 48 h after ovulation. Progesterone levels are around 6–13 nmol/l at the time of the LH peak, and 15–25 nmol/l at the time of ovulation, 36–48 h later. Concurrent with the LH peak, a preovulatory surge in FSH occurs and peak concentrations are reached 1–2 days after the LH peak.[2] Estrus behavior usually occurs synchronously with the preovulatory LH peak (Fig. 7–4), but some bitches demonstrate estrus behavior days before the LH peak and others not until days thereafter or never. Shrinkage of the vaginal mucosa starts about midway in the follicular phase and continues through the phase

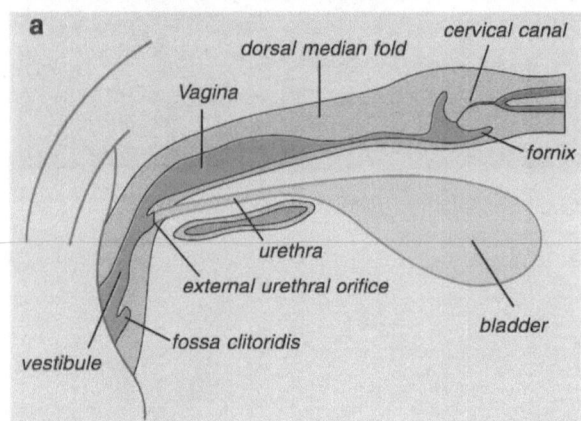

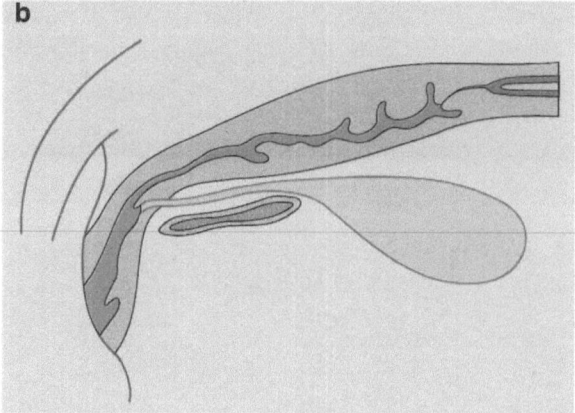

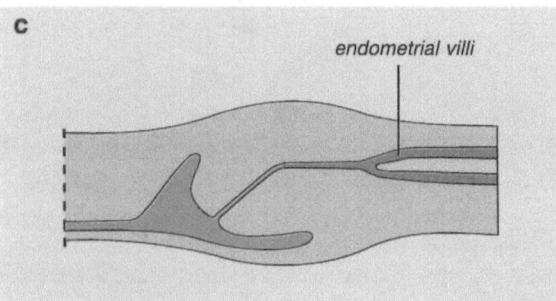

Fig. 7-9. Illustration of a sagittal section through the vestibule, vagina, and cervix of a bitch during (a) anestrus and (b) the proestrus/estrus period. In this stage the vaginal wall is extremely folded. (c) A close up of the cranial part of the vagina and the cervix during the anestrus period. Note the very short craniodorsally directed cervical canal; its apparent horizontal extension is in fact the caudal part of the uterus, which is covered with endometrial villi.

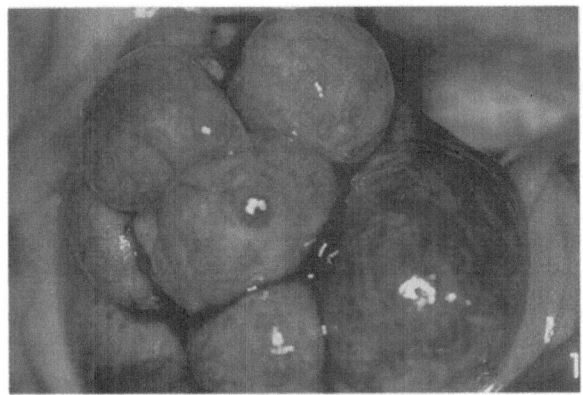

Fig. 7-10. Ovary of the bitch at the time of ovulation. The bursa which normally encloses the ovary has been removed.

of preovulatory luteinization and ovulation, whereby many longitudinal folds can be observed (Fig. 7–11).

Luteal phase. Concentrations of progesterone originating from the corpora lutea increase in the peripheral blood during the remainder of estrus and during the onset of metestrus (diestrus). Thus, in the bitch, estrus behavior is seen in the period of rising progesterone concentrations. A plateau in the progesterone level occurs 10–30 days after the LH peak. Thereafter, in non-pregnant bitches, progesterone concentration declines slowly and reaches a basal level of 3 nmol/l for the first time about 75 days after the start of the luteal phase (Fig. 7–12). The factors which are responsible for

initiating the regression of the corpora lutea in the dog are still unknown. Prostaglandin $F_{2\alpha}$ originating from the endometrium is not the causative factor as it is in the cow and sheep. This is demonstrated by the fact that hysterectomy does not influence the length of the luteal phase.[3] The secretion of prolactin fluctuates but average levels in the follicular and luteal phases are not significantly different (Fig. 7–12). However, in bitches with overt pseudopregnancy symptoms, a significant increase in prolactin secretion can be observed (see Section 2.2.4). Prolactin acts as a luteotropic factor in the second half of the luteal phase[4]. During the first half of the luteal phase the canine corpus luteum functions independently of pituitary support.[5] Thereafter experimentally induced inhibition of prolactin secretion causes a sharp decrease in progesterone secretion (Fig. 7–13). Whether or not LH has luteotropic properties in the bitch is still unclear. LH levels change little during the luteal phase, with the exception of a slight increase in the second half of the luteal phase (Fig. 7–12).

During the initial part of the luteal phase the transition from estrus to metestrus (diestrus) takes place. In this period of time the cytology of the vaginal mucosa changes from chiefly superficial cells to chiefly intermediate and parabasal cells and leukocytes (Fig. 7–14). This is an indication that the fertile period is over. At the time of the maturation of the oocytes the shrinkage of the vaginal mucosa continues and increasing numbers

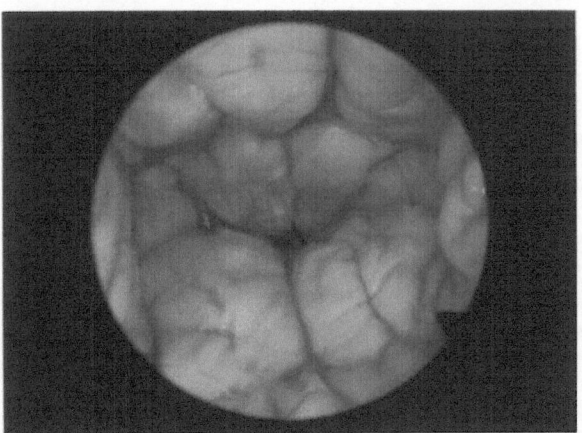
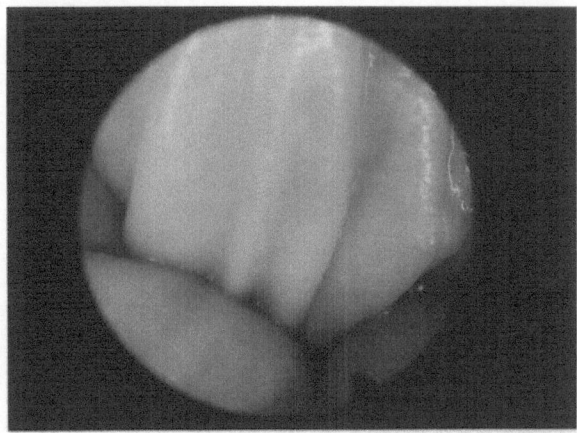

Fig. 7-11. Vaginoscopy at the time of ovulation. The plasma progesterone concentration in this bitch was 22 nmol/l. Left: The mucosal shrinkage leads to longitudinal folds. Right: Close-up of the shrinkage of the longitudinal folds of the dorsal median fold of the cranial vagina.

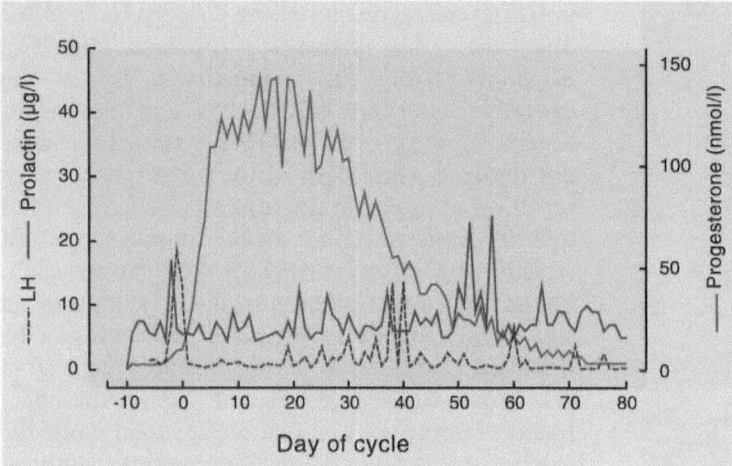

Fig. 7-12. Mean LH, progesterone, and pro-lactin levels in plasma of three dogs during the follicular and luteal phase. The data have been synchronized on day 1, the day after the onset of the follicular phase, on which the progesterone concentration in the peripheral blood had reached 16 nmol/l. (Modified from Okkens et al., 1990.[4])

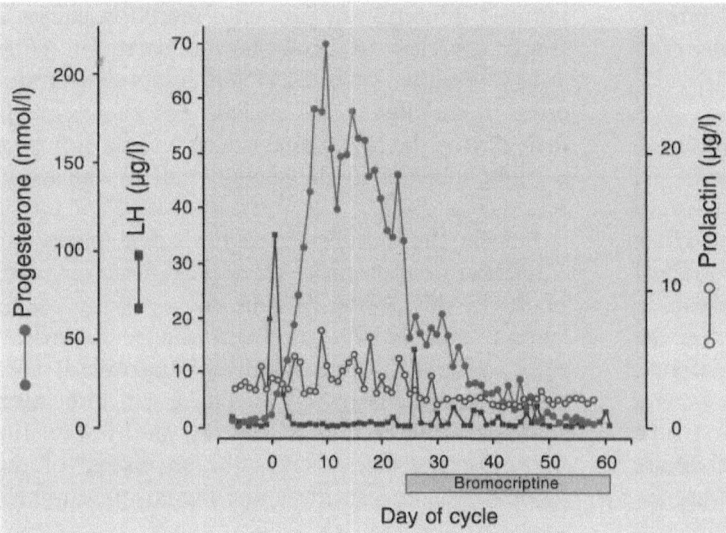

Fig. 7-13. Mean progesterone, prolactin, and LH levels in the plasma of four dogs, treated with bromocriptine, 20 µg/kg body-weight, twice daily, orally from day 20–24 after the onset of the luteal phase until the end of the luteal period (bar). The data have been synchronized on day 1, the day after the onset of the follicular phase, on which the progesterone concentration in the peripheral blood had reached 16 nmol/l. (Modified from Okkens et al., 1990.[4]) Note the shortened luteal phase due to bromocriptine-induced lowering of circulating prolactin concentrations.

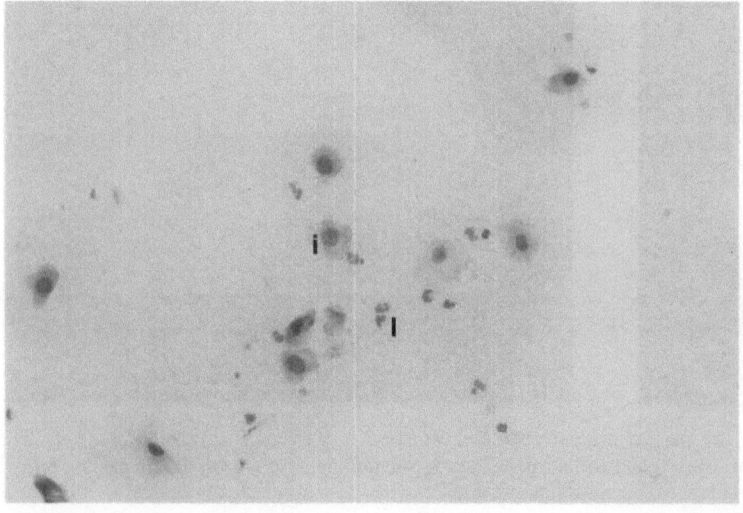

Fig. 7-14. Vaginal cytology during metestrus, which starts 6–10 days after the preovulatory LH peak. This smear shows intermediate cells (i), and leucocytes (l).

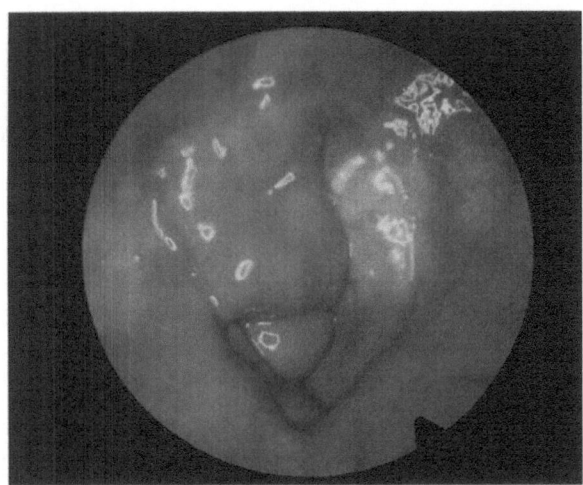

Fig. 7-15. Vaginoscopy during metestrus. Note the rounded profiles and the patchwork of red and white areas.

of sharp edged summit profiles appear. In the transition period from estrus to metestrus the mucosa thins and profiles become round. In the start of metestrus a patchwork of red and white areas can be seen (Fig. 7–15).

Anestrus. The time of the onset of anestrus depends on which criterion is being used to define the end of the luteal phase: e.g., after 2–3 months when mammary development subsides, the first time that the progesterone concentration reaches a level of 3 nmol/l, or the time at which the influence of progesterone on the endometrium is no longer evident. In any case, the transition from the luteal phase to anestrus is gradual and varies considerably among bitches. Although sporadic elevations are observed, estradiol concentrations are usually low and do not begin to rise until late anestrus. FSH concentrations are generally higher than during proestrus.[2] Mean LH concentrations are low, although there is an indication of a short period of an increased number of pulses at the end of anestrus. In advanced anestrus the sensitivity of LH responses to various doses of GnRH increases.[6] The estrous cycle can start at any time throughout the year and there appears to be little, if any, seasonal influence. Breed differences and strains within breeds can form the basis of variation in mean interestrous intervals. In the Collie, for example, this interval is 36 weeks, and in the German Shepherd about 20–22 weeks. Some breeds such as the Basenji and Tibetan Mastiff, however, have a single annual estrous cycle which is possibly influenced by a photoperiod. Environmental factors can also affect the interestrous interval: placing an anestrous bitch in close proximity to a bitch in estrus may cause the onset of proestrus to be advanced by several weeks. In addition, bitches housed together often have synchronous cycles.

It is still not clear which factors influence the transition from anestrus to proestrus. Endogenous opioids may modulate GnRH and LH release by reducing pulsatile secretion. There is some evidence that factors which decrease opiodergic activity promote LH release and the termination of anestrus.[7] Anestrus can be shortened considerably by administration of the dopamine-agonist bromocriptine, which suppresses prolactin secretion (see also Section 7.5).[8] However, it is still unclear whether this decrease in prolactin secretion causes the onset of follicular growth or whether (more probably) the main factor is the dopamine agonistic effect of bromocriptine. So far there is no evidence for a spontaneous decrease in circulating prolactin concentrations during late anestrus.[2]

Pregnancy and parturition. The length of gestation in dogs varies greatly. Naaktgeboren,[9] using data obtained from dogs of various breeds, reported a mean gestation of 62.0 days (n = 184), with a variation of 24 days (54–77). The length of gestation and litter size were negatively correlated. In a Beagle colony the mean gestational period was to be 65.3 days (n = 290), with a variation of 16 days (57–72).[10] The variation was, however, reduced to 3 days (64–66) (n = 54) when gestation was calculated as the interval from the preovulatory LH peak to birth. In another study the length of gestation was calculated in bitches of various breeds (n = 77) which were mated at a fixed time after ovulation. The optimal time for mating was based on the rapid increase in plasma progesterone concentration at the time of ovulation, which is strongly correlated with the preovulatory LH peak. The gestational period was 62.1 days, with a variation of 11 days (58–68).[11] It was negatively correlated with litter size when litters contained seven or fewer pups. Litter size appears to be an important determinant of the

138

length of gestation. In addition, it is possible that there is a relation between the breed of the bitch and the length of gestation. For instance, the gestation of German Shepherds (60 days) is shorter than the average (62 days).[11]

During pregnancy the hormone patterns in plasma are very similar to those described for the estrous cycle, with the exception of the hormonal changes during the last days of pregnancy and during parturition. In the bitch the duration of pregnancy is equal to or somewhat shorter than the luteal phase. Progesterone and estradiol concentrations follow a similar pattern during pregnancy and the luteal phase, but the total quantity of secreted hormones is probably higher during pregnancy. This may be due to an increased plasma volume. Progesterone is the hormone responsible for the maintenance of pregnancy in the dog. It is secreted by the corpora lutea but the concentration is not overtly influenced by the number of corpora lutea. Ovariectomy during pregnancy results in either resorption of the fetuses or abortion. Progesterone promotes endometrial gland growth, stimulates uterine secretions, promotes placental integrity, and inhibits uterine motility. Progesterone concentrations in plasma fluctuate in a manner similar to that during an estrous cycle until they decline to a level of 16 to 48 nmol/l, which is maintained for 1–2 weeks until the rapid fall to 3–6 nmol/l just before parturition.

The decrease in the progesterone concentration is essential for the onset of parturition and is negatively correlated with a progressive qualitative change in the pattern of uterine activity (Fig. 7–16).[12] During prepartum luteolysis and parturition there are elevated plasma concentrations of 13,14-dihydro-15-keto prostaglandinF$_{2\alpha}$, (PGFM), a fairly stable metabolite of prostaglandin F$_{2\alpha}$ (PGF$_{2\alpha}$), originating from the feto-placental unit (Fig. 7–17).[13] It is possible that PGF$_{2\alpha}$ is the factor which causes prepartum luteolysis. However, it is often necessary to give several injections of PGF$_{2\alpha}$ in order to induce parturition.

Maternal plasma cortisol levels are variable but are within the normal range during the last week of gestation (40 to 70 nmol/l) and, in most bitches, they are clearly elevated (110 to 220 nmol/l) on the day prior to parturition and are then low (28 to 70

nmol/l) during parturition (Fig. 7–18).[14] This cortisol increase, which perhaps causes an elevation of PGF$_{2\alpha}$, is possibly the trigger for the onset of parturition and the result of an increase in fetal cortisol secretion due to the maturation of the fetal pituitary-adrenocortical axis.

Prolactin levels in plasma rise during the second half of pregnancy. During the rapid decrease in

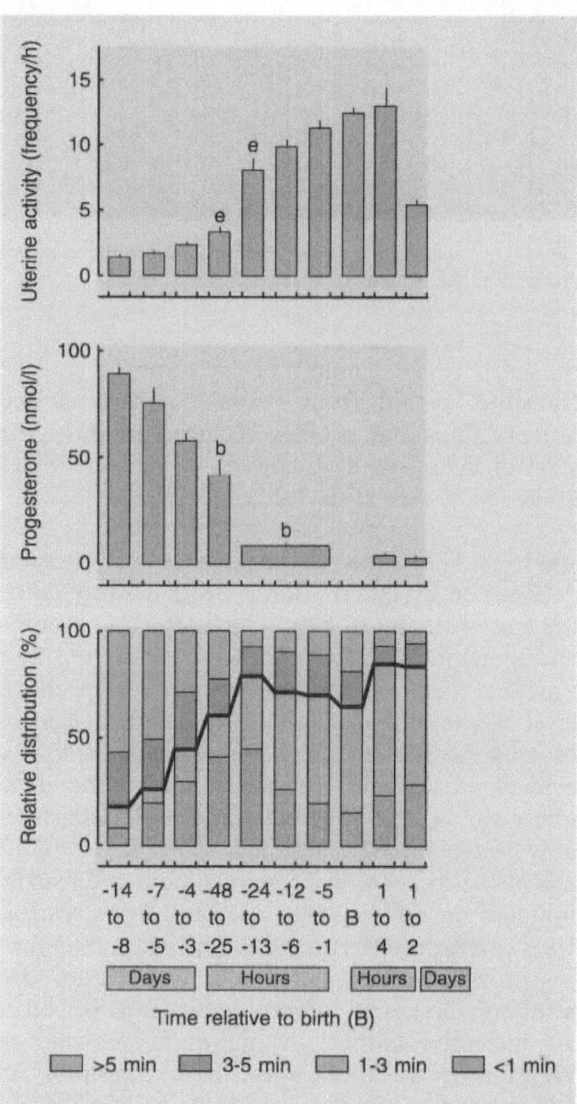

Fig. 7-16. Mean values of uterine activity (burst frequency/h, plasma progesterone concentration, and the relative distribution (%) of the individual duration of bursts of EMG activity for various periods around spontaneous parturition in 5 dogs. Differences between columns with a similar superscript were significant (P < 0.001). Birth (B) = period between birth of first pup and birth of last pup. (Modified from Van Der Weyden et al., 1989.[12])

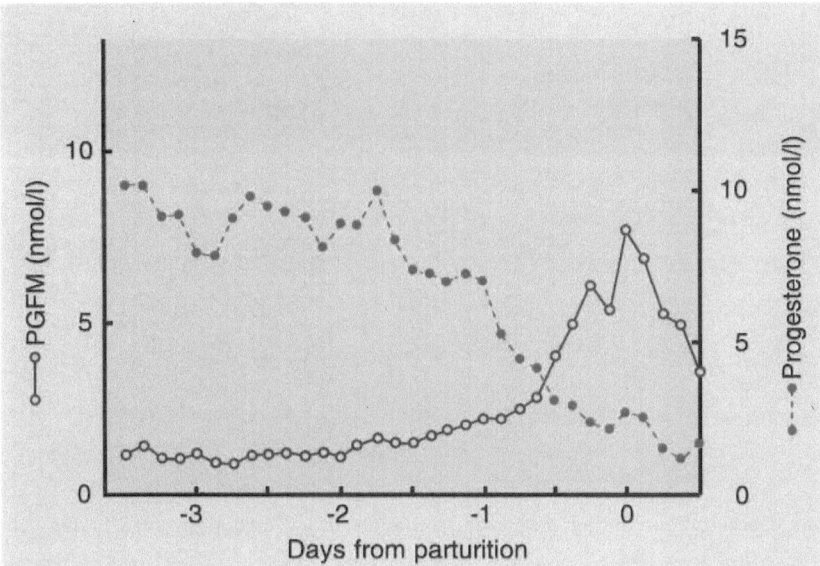

Fig. 7-17. Mean concentrations of progesterone and of 13,14-dihydro-15-keto-prostaglandin $F_{2\alpha}$ (PGFM) in plasma of 6 pregnant bitches around the time of parturition. All values were aligned to a common Day 65 of parturition for the sample obtained at or immediately after the birth of the first pup, which occurred in individual bitches at 64–66 days after the preovulatory LH surge. (Modified from Concannon et al., 1988.[13])

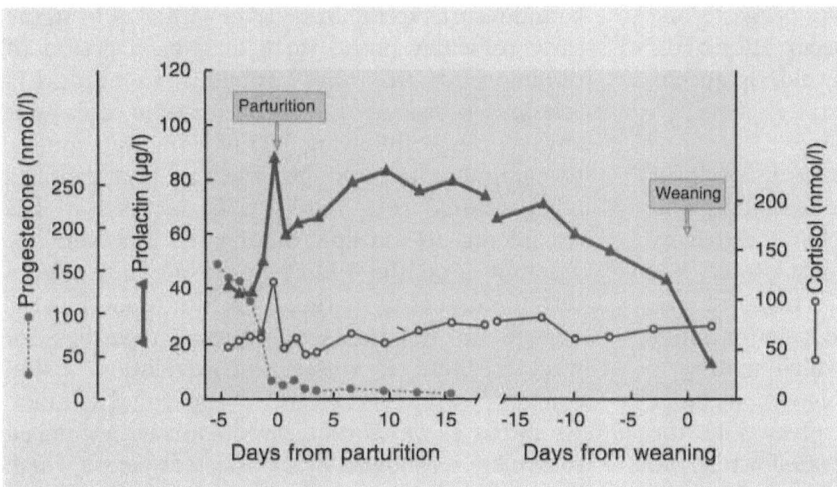

Fig. 7-18. Mean serum concentrations of progesterone, cortisol, and prolactin during the peri-partum period and lactation in a group of 6 beagle bitches. (Modified from Concannon et al., 1978.[14])

circulating progesterone concentrations prior to parturition a transient, large surge of prolactin occurs (Fig. 7–18).[14] Prolactin is, as in the estrous cycle, a luteotropic factor. Suppression of prolactin secretion by bromocriptine and cabergoline causes abortion in the second half of the pregnancy.

7.2.2 Cat

Puberty in the queen occurs at 4–18 months of age and the onset is influenced by the season of the year. It frequently occurs when the hours of daylight are increasing. Physical condition is also

an important factor: cats usually do not reach puberty until a weight of about 2.5 kg is reached. Short-haired breeds may reach puberty sooner than long-haired breeds.

Queens can go through several periods of estrus per season (seasonally polyestrus). Cats kept in a common household, however, can become non-seasonal breeders as a result of night-time illumination.

Queens are induced ovulators. Copulation, vaginal stimulation, or administration of gonadotropin or gonadotropin releasing hormones induce ovulation within 24–48 h. It is likely that ovulation can also be induced by external stimuli such as

140

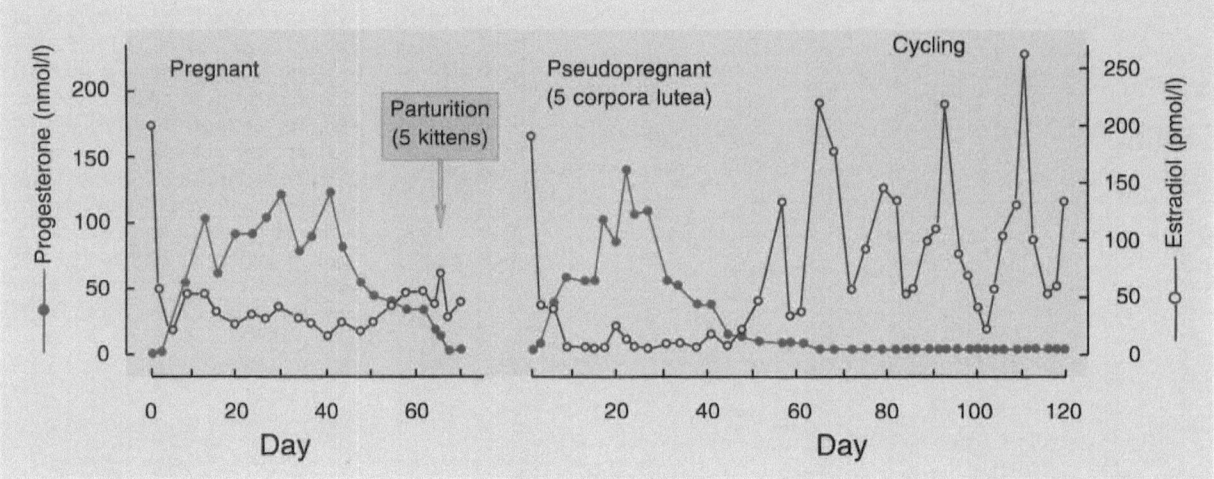

Fig. 7-19. Plasma estradiol and progesterone concentrations during pregnancy, pseudopregnancy, and poly-estrus in the cat. (Modified from Verhage et al., 1976.[15])

stroking the cat. Increases in plasma progesterone concentrations, which normally occur after ovulation, have been observed in mostly elderly queens which had not been mated.

Estrous cycle. The stages of the estrous cycle of the queen include proestrus, estrus, postestrus, and metestrus (diestrus). Proestrus is characterized by rubbing of the head and neck against objects but not permitting breeding by the male. It is observed in only a minority of the cycles and lasts for about 1–2 days. Estrus, the phase in which mating is allowed, lasts 7–9 days. Estrus behavior includes crouching with the forequarters pressed to the ground and the pelvic region elevated while the hind legs are stamped rhythmically, frequent vocalizing and restlessness. Estrus occurs during maximal follicular activity and estradiol secretion; estradiol concentration rises to 180–260 pmol/l and then decreases within 5–7 days after copulation (Fig. 7–19).[15] There are no notable changes in size and appearance of external genitalia. The absence of cellular debris in the vaginal smear is the earliest sign of follicular activity. There is a distinct increase in anuclear cells and a slight increase in partially cornified superficial cells. Intermediate cells decrease during the follicular phase and parabasal cells are absent in the second half of the follicular phase.

If breeding is permitted, LH release begins within minutes after copulation, peaks within 2–4

h, and returns to the basal level within 24 h. In the early follicular phase there may be a period of refractoriness to this copulation-induced LH release. A rise in LH concentration does not always occur following a single mating and is higher and more prolonged when multiple matings are permitted (Fig.7–20).[16] This increase in LH release due to multiple matings is, however, not indefinite and the LH response declines after a certain number of matings. The duration of estrus appears to be similiar in queens regardless of whether there is coitus with ovulation, coital contact without ovulation, or no coital contact. An estrus in which a queen has not been induced to ovulate is followed by a postestrus period which has an average duration of 8–10 days, after which the next estrus begins. Plasma progesterone concentrations are at the basal level during the postestrus period.

Ovulation usually occurs 24–48 h after copulation and the appearance of the LH peak, but it may take up to 90 h. After ovulation, pregnancy, or a luteal phase without pregnancy, which is called "pseudopregnancy" follows.

Pseudopregnancy in the queen does not give rise to signs and symptoms and is thus not comparable to pseudopregnancy in the bitch (see Section 2.2.4). In both pregnancy and pseudopregnancy, plasma progesterone concentration begins to rise 24–48 h after ovulation along with the development of luteal tissue. This luteal tissue is initially

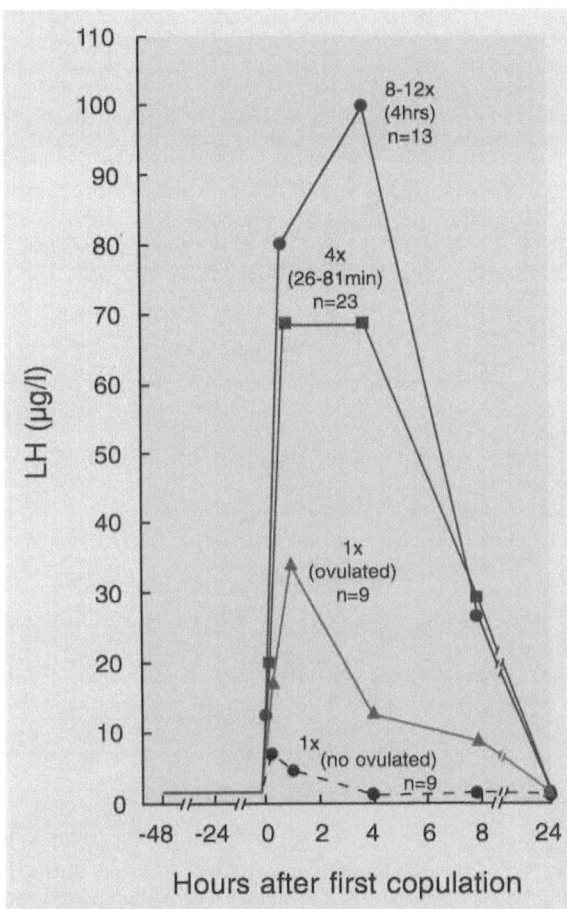

Fig. 7-20. Mean serum LH levels in cats confirmed to have ovulated following a single copulation (red), 4 copulations within a 26–81 min period (green), or 8–12 copulations during a 4 h period (blue), and in cats which did not ovulate following a single copulation (black). All copulations were on the third day of estrus. (Modified from Concannon et al., 1980.[16])

red and sometimes referred to as corpora rubra. It subsequently develops into yellow corpora lutea (Fig. 7–21). The progesterone-dominated phase lasts about 38 days in the pseudopregnant queen and approximately 60 days in the pregnant queen. Plasma progesterone concentrations in pseudopregnancy and pregnancy are similar until day 21. Thereafter the progesterone concentration decreases more rapidly in pseudopregnant cats than in pregnant cats (Fig. 7–19). The interestrous interval for a pseudopregnant queen is approximately 7 weeks. During the progesterone-dominated phase, particularly at the end of this phase, there can be follicle growth and regression which causes elevations in plasma estradiol concentrations.

Anestrus is a period without cycle activity. Estradiol and progesterone concentrations in the peripheral blood are at baseline levels. This phase occurs during late autumn and the onset of winter (October, November, December) in queens exposed to natural daylight in the northern hemisphere.

Photoperiod influences. Photoperiods influence the reproductive processes via the pineal gland and its main hormone, melatonin, which affects the hypothalamus-pituitary-gonadal axis. Melatonin and prolactin concentrations change congruently with photoperiod changes. Plasma concentrations of both hormones are highest during a period of darkness (Fig. 7–22).[17] Leyva et al. (1989)[18] found that folliculogenesis and estradiol secretion are stimulated during days with 14 h of light, with an

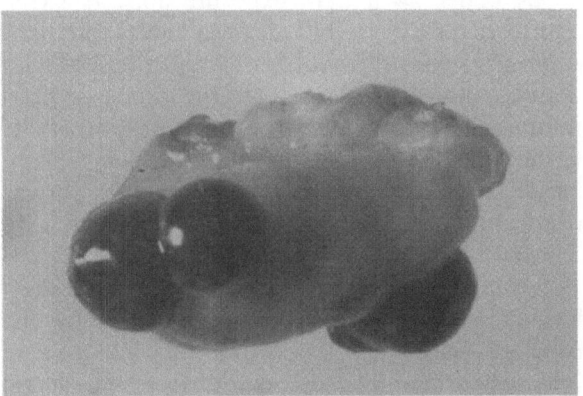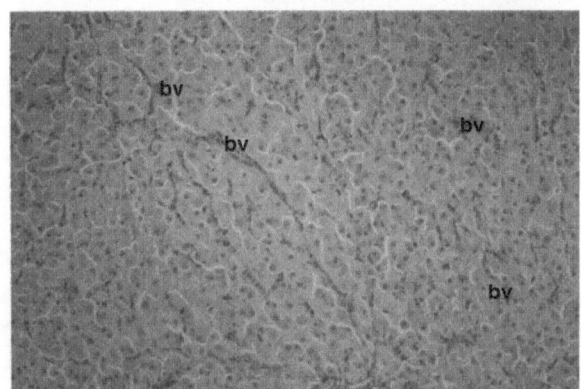

Fig. 7-21. Left: The ovary of a queen mated 6 days before, showing luteal tissue sometimes called corpora rubra because of its red color. Right: Microscopic section of a corpus luteum of a queen mated 21 days before. The corpus luteum mainly consists of large luteal cells and blood vessels (bv). (475×, H & E.)

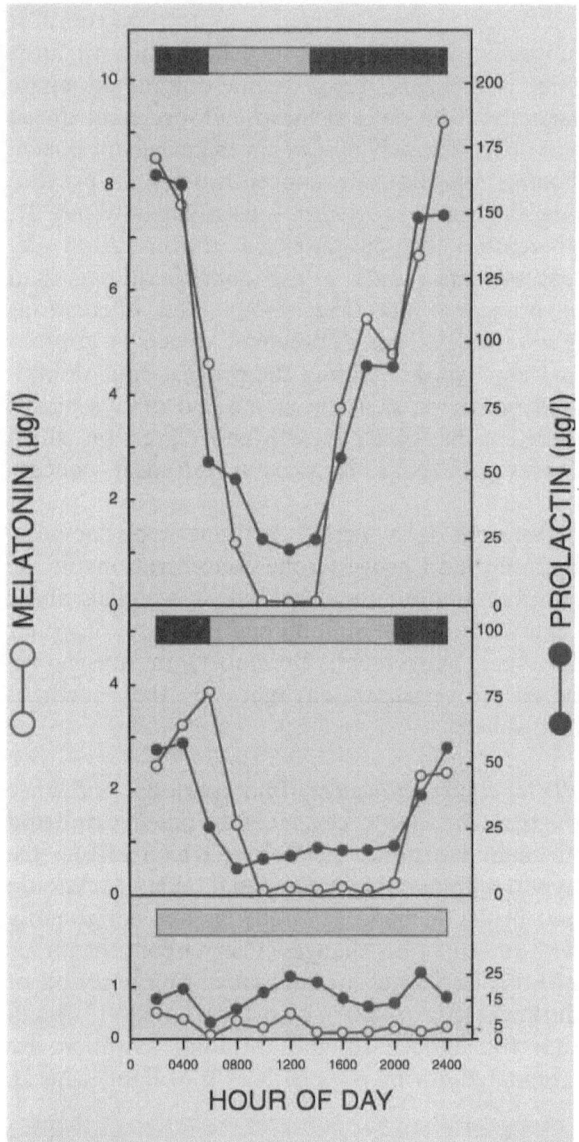

Fig. 7-22. The effects of three different photoperiods on mean plasma concentrations of melatonin and prolactin in 4 cats, determined at 2 h intervals. Horizontal bars indicate the timing of the particular lighting regimen; lower panel: 24 h light, middle panel 14 h light and 10 h darkness, upper panel 8 h light and 16 h darkness. (Modified from Leyva et al., 1984.[17])

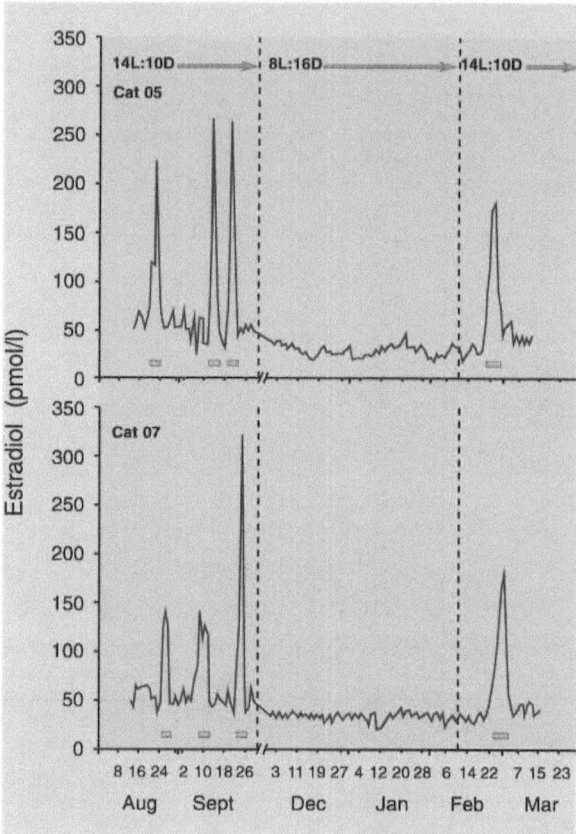

Fig. 7-23. Plasma estradiol concentrations in 2 cats during a photoperiod regimen of 14 h light, an 8 h light photoperiod and a subsequent return to 14 h light. Horizontal bars indicate periods of sexual receptivity. (Modified from Leyva et al., 1989.[18])

estrous cycle frequency of 2 per month. Estrous activity immediately ceases after a change from 14 h to 8 h of light and estradiol concentrations decrease rapidly (Fig. 7–23). Gonadotropin secretion is possibly decreased during a short light period. Continuous exposure to light, however, also does not appear to be optimal. Cycle fre-

quency decreases to 1 per month with 24 h exposure to light. The estradiol secretion during estrus under 24 h light exposure appears to be approximately twice that observed under 14 h light exposure, while the number of large antral follicles doubles about 45 days after the onset of continuous light. This may cause a depletion of the tertiary follicle population, after which a long period of time is necessary for tertiary follicle restoration.[18]

Pregnancy and parturition. In the cat, progesterone, produced throughout pregnancy by the corpora lutea, is responsible for maintaining pregnancy. The placenta either does not secrete progesterone or secretes it in amounts insufficient to maintain pregnancy. Progesterone levels in plasma increase continuously through day 25–30,

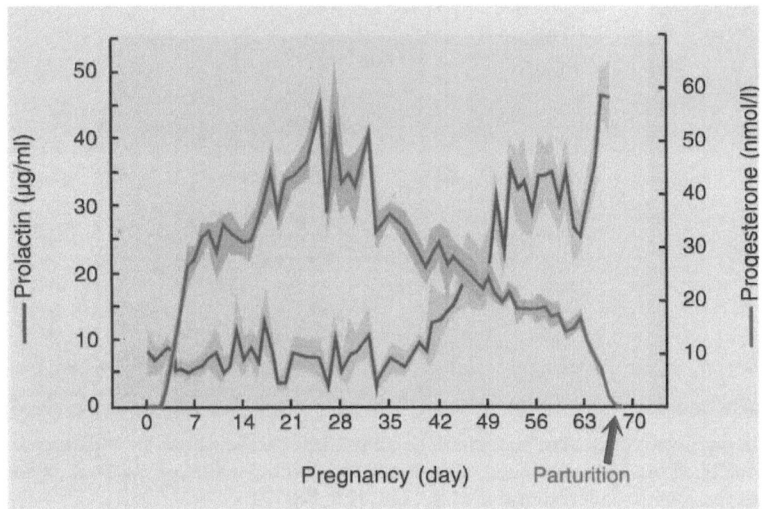

Fig. 7-24. Mean ± sem concentrations of prolactin (brown) and progesterone (red) in the plasma of eight queens during gestation. Day 0 is the day of copulation. (Modified from Banks et al., 1983.[20])

after which they slowly decline during the second half of pregnancy. Ovariectomy during any stage of the pregnancy results in a decline in progesterone concentration in the peripheral blood to < 3 nmol/l within 48 h after surgery, and abortion follows.[19]

It is not yet clear what causes the difference in pseudopregnant and pregnant corpora lutea. Pregnancy appears to involve a pregnancy-specific secretion of luteotropic hormones from placental or pituitary origin. Among these, prolactin appears to be an important factor. Prolactin secretion in the pregnant queen begins to increase around day 35, reaches a plateau at about day 50, and increases just before delivery (Fig. 7–24).[20] If it is suppressed by treatment with the dopamine agonist cabergoline, progesterone secretion decreases and abortion may follow. In the pseudopregnant queen no increase in prolactin secretion occurs. This may be the cause of the early regression of the corpora lutea.

There is an indication that $PGF_{2\alpha}$ is produced after about day 30. This production probably increases just before parturition and subsequently falls in the days thereafter.

Superfetation which has been suggested to occur in the queen may be related to estrus behavior during pregnancy. Superfetation has, however, never been proven. Another possible explanation for the presence of fetuses of different age could be an arrested development.

The first estrus after parturition can be expected within 1–21 weeks. Little is known about fertility

during the first estrus after parturition. If this estrus occurs during lactation, which is not uncommon, fertility may be lower than normal.

7.3 Cystic endometrial hyperplasia-endometritis

Pathogenesis and pathology. Cystic endometrial hyperplasia (CEH) is a disorder of the uterus of the bitch and the queen which can develop either as a consequence of repeated endogenous progesterone influence during successive luteal phases or as a consequence of exogenous progesterone. Therefore, it is a common disorder in older bitches, which have completed many luteal phases. It is not the result of "retained" corpora lutea. If the endometrial hyperplasia is accompanied by inflammation the condition is called CEH-endometritis.

In the queen it is also a disease of the older animal, unless it is induced by exogenous progesterone. As mentioned previously, queens do not always require coital contact to induce ovulation (see Section 7.2.2). A mild stimulus such as stroking is, in older animals, probably sufficient to induce ovulation. Queens with CEH-endometritis often have corpora lutea without an history of mating.[21] This probably means that several unnoticed ovulations have occurred and that as a consequence the animals have been repeatedly under progesterone influence. CEH-endometritis has also been observed in ovariectomized queens that have been treated with progestagens.

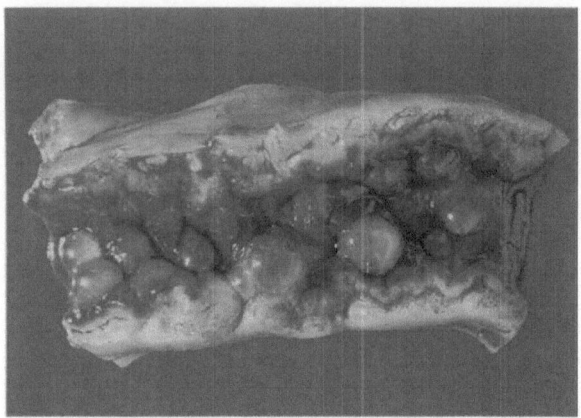 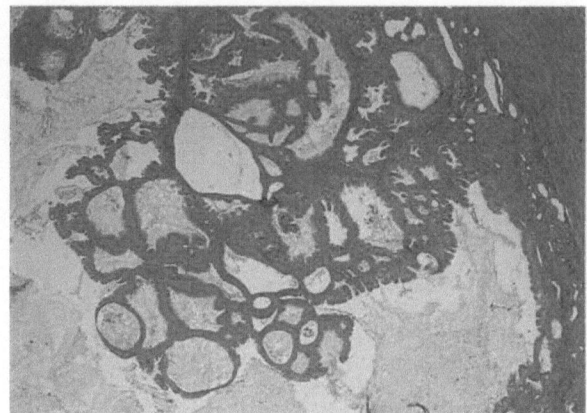

Fig. 7-25. Left: Cystic endometrial hyperplasia in an 8-year-old bitch. The endometrial wall is filled with congeries of bulging cysts. Right: Multiple cystic endometrial proliferation in the bitch due to cystic endometrial hyperplasia with papillary overgrowth of the endometrium, which is mainly composed of epithilial tissue with scant connective tissue. (4×, H & E.)

The glands which are closest to the uterine lumen change first (Fig. 7–25). Hypertrophic and hyperplastic glands however, can also be present in the myometrium (adenomyosis) or even in the serosa (endometriosis). CEH is usually diffuse, but it can be limited to parts of the uterus. If the cervix is closed, which is often the case under progesterone influence, a mucometra develops (Fig. 7–26). In CEH without infection, there are no inflammatory cells. If there is infection neutrophils and plasma cells are present.

Clinical manifestations. Bitches and queens with uncomplicated CEH do not exhibit signs of systemic disease. Infertility due to failure of im-plantation or to fetal resorption can, however, be observed. If infection is also present the signs and symptoms are often dependent upon cervical patency. When the cervix is open the systemic disease is usually milder than when it is closed. Massive quantities of pus may be found in the lumen of the uterus, especially if the cervix is closed (pyometra). In this situation the animals are lethargic and may be anorectic. With an open cervix vaginal discharge may vary in color from yellow to chocolate or red, depending on the presence or absence of blood. The enlarged uterus may cause abdominal distention. The bacterial infection may cause deposition of immune complexes in the glomerular capillary walls. This

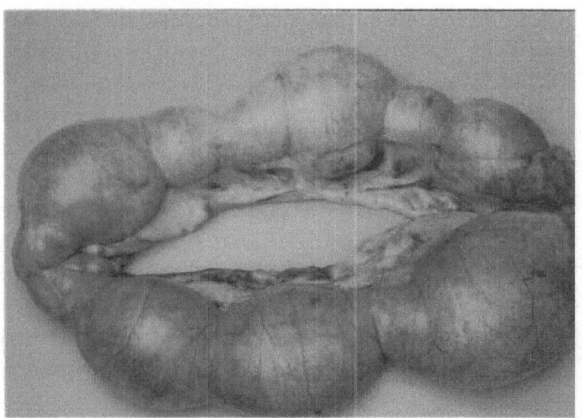 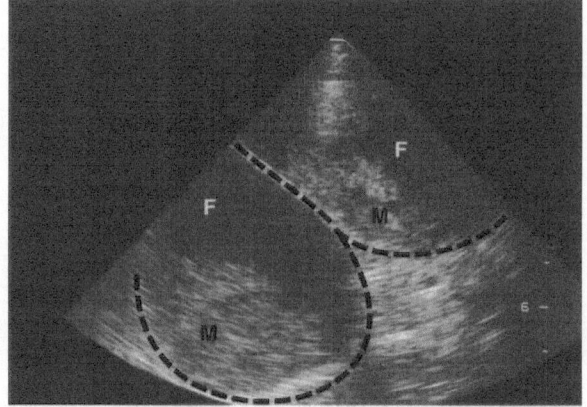

Fig. 7-26. Left: A mucometra with a thin uterine wall in a 7-year-old Bouvier des Flandres. The bitch was treated for several years with high doses of progestagens. Right: Transverse ultrasonogram of the abdomen of the same bitch. The uterus is severely dilated (delineated by interrupted line) and filled with fluid (F). Inspissated mucus (M) causes amorphous echogenicity in the dependent part of the uterine horns.

will cause proteinuria, but it usually does not give rise to permanent renal failure. The elevated concentrations of urea and creatinine in plasma are generally of prerenal origin, i.e., due to the hypovolemia. In this situation vomiting may be an aggravating factor, which can be ascribed to this uremia syndrome. One must also be alert to the possibility of peritonitis due to a perforated uterus.

In addition, the bacterial infection and more specifically E. coli antigens may cause loss of renal medullary hypertonicity.[22] This leads to a decreased ability to concentrate urine. The associated polyuria and polydipsia are common in dogs with CEH-endometritis, but rare in cats.

Anemia is present in about 40% of the bitches with CEH-endometrits. This may be the result of blood loss in the uterus, but the disease may also lead to decreased erythropoietin production.

Diagnosis. CEH-endometritis is a disease of the middle-aged or elderly bitch and queen. It occurs during the luteal phase of the estrous cycle or under influence of exogenous progestagens. The enlarged uterus can be palpated or visualized with radiography (Fig. 7–27) or, preferably, ultrasonography (Fig. 7–28). If, however, CEH is present without accumulation of fluid, it may be difficult or impossible to visualize the uterus. Laparoscopy or laparotomy with biopsies of the uterus for histological and bacteriological examinations are indicated if CEH is suspected, e.g., as a cause of infertility. In cases of endo-

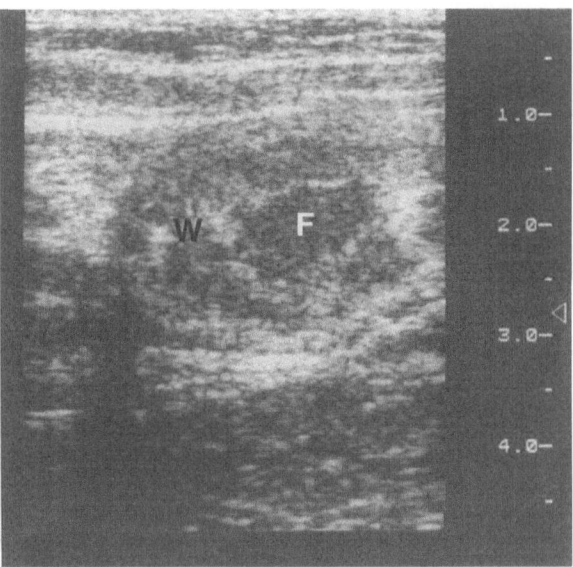

Fig. 7-28. Longitudinal ultrasonogram of the abdomen of a 9-month-old Doberman with endometritis. The uterus is moderately dilated, fluid filled (F), and has an irregularly thickened wall (W). The bitch was treated at the onset of the first proestrus with megestrolacetate, 1st and 2nd day 10 mg, the next 16 days 5 mg daily; she developed endometritis within one month after the start of the treatment.

metritis with an open cervix the discharge can be observed during vaginoscopy. Culture of the discharge usually reveals E. coli, and sporadically other bacteria. Neutrophilia, anemia, and hyperproteinemia are often found by routine laboratory examinations.

Differential diagnosis. Several of the various symptoms of CEH-endometritis can also be associated with pregnancy, tumors causing discharge, and vaginitis. For other causes of polyuria/polydipsia such as progestagen-induced growth hormone excess, diabetes mellitus, hyperthyroidism, and hyperadrenocorticism, the reader is referred to the relevant chapters, including Chapter 15.

Treatment. Ovario-hysterectomy is the therapy of choice for CEH-endometritis. If the affected bitch or queen is young and the owner wishes to breed the animal, medical therapy can be started but only if there is no systemic disease. Treatment may consist of an antibacterial agent administered for at least 2 weeks, selected on the basis of the results of the bacteriological culture and antibiogram. In

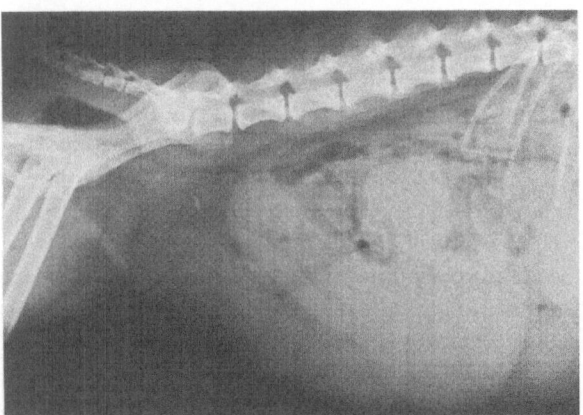

Fig. 7-27. Lateral radiograph of the abdomen of a 7-year-old mixed breed dog with pyometra. The dilated, fluid filled uterus causes displacement of the other visceral organs.

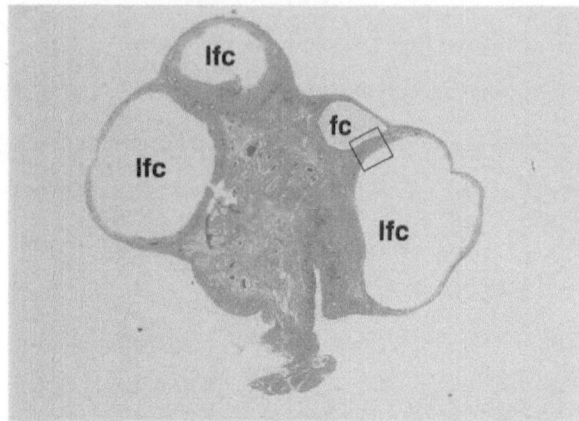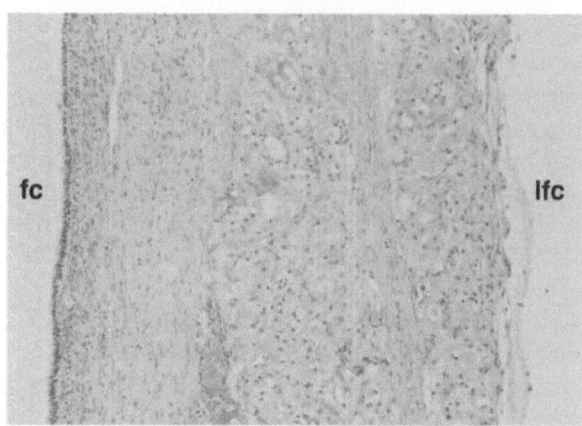

Fig. 7-29. Left: Follicular cyst (fc) and luteinized follicular cysts (lfc) in a 4-year-old bitch with shortened interestrous intervals and persistent estrus symptoms. During these estrus periods the progesterone concentrations in the peripheral blood were elevated but did not reach concentrations which normally occur at the time of ovulation. Right (Close- up of inset in the figure on the left): The wall of the follicular cyst (fc) and the wall of a luteinized follicular cyst (lfc). Note the luteinized cells bordering the luteinized follicular cyst. (H & E.)

addition, dinoprost,[a] a salt of $PGF_{2\alpha}$, may be administered at a dose rate of 100–250 µg/kg twice or thrice daily for 4 days. This causes premature regression of the corpora lutea if it is administered repeatedly in the second half of the luteal phase. Uterine contractions, cervical dilatation, and evacuation of the uterine contents can be expected. Side effects, observed mainly at the onset of therapy, may consist of salivation, vomiting, diarrhea, hyperpnea, ataxia, restlessness, and pupillary dilatation, starting within minutes after administration. Walking the dog during this time diminishes the side effects, as does a lower dosage administered more frequently. There is an increased risk of uterine perforation during this therapy and the risk is greater if the cervix is closed.

In the queen, it is sometimes possible to pass the cervix with a tom catheter and to introduce a water-soluble antibiotic, such as 100 mg ampicillin in 5 ml water, into the uterus. In the cat, estrus generally follows soon after completion of the therapy.

Prognosis. Endometritis in the dog after a mismating treatment with estrogens appears to have a fairly good prognosis, as opposed to the medically treated elderly bitch with severe CEH. In the latter animal ovariohysterectomy should be performed

[a] Dinolytic®, Upjohn

without delay. The prognosis for the cat is generally much better than for the dog. Many cats later conceive and deliver normal litters.

7.4 Persistent estrus

The bitch is considered to have a persistent estrus if ovulation has not occurred after about 25 days from the onset of proestrus, and estrus symptoms such as sanguinous discharge, estrus behavior and/or the presence of superficial cells in the vaginal smear. A continuous or persistent estrus can also occur in the queen.

Pathogenesis. Ovarian cysts and ovarian tumors can cause persistent estrus in dogs and cats. Cystic follicles and luteinized follicular cysts may synthesize and secrete estrogens or progesterone depending on the degree of luteinization (Fig. 7–29). Follicles normally undergo preovulatory luteinization, after which ovulation occurs and corpora lutea are formed. Luteinized follicular cysts fail to ovulate. There is probably a difference in the pathogenesis of cystic follicles in young dogs during their first and second cycles and in older dogs. In the young dog, persistent estrus is not uncommon.[23] In general, young dogs react well to treatment and a normal follicular phase and ovulation can be expected during their next cycle. In contrast, the problem is often recurrent in older

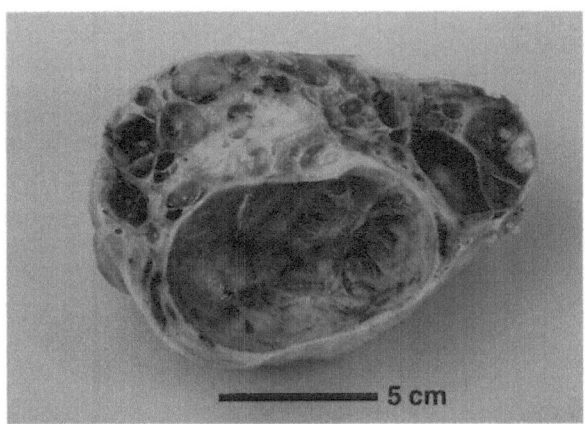

Fig. 7-30. Granulosa cell tumor of a 9-year-old Belgian Shepherd which had estrus behavior for 4 months. The progesterone and estradiol 17-β concentrations in the peripheral blood were 7 nmol/l and 270 pmol/l, respectively. The estradiol-17β concentration in the cyst fluid was 1195 pmol/l.

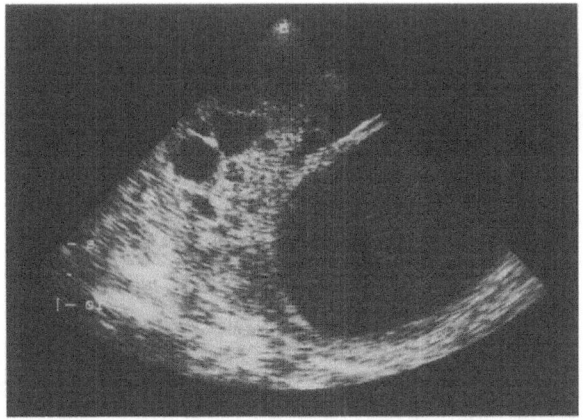

Fig. 7-31. Longitudinal ultrasonogram of the abdomen of the bitch of Fig. 7–30, revealing small and large cysts in the tumor.

dogs. In addition, cysts and symptoms of persistent estrus are observed regularly in bitches that have undergone an incomplete ovariectomy. Ovarian follicular cysts producing estrogens are also common in queens. They may arise from mature or atretic follicles and their occurrence may increase with age.

Hormone-producing ovarian tumors, which frequently originate from sex cord stroma, are the other important cause of persistent estrus (Fig. 7–30). They occur mainly in the older dog and cat, but are sometimes observed in young bitches or in bitches with ovarian tissue left in situ after an ovariectomy. The tumor is usually a granulosa cell tumor.

In addition, estrogens administered, for example, to terminate an unwanted pregnancy can occasionally cause a persistent estrus, possibly by inducing ovarian cysts. Liver disease has also been mentioned as a cause of persistent estrus, supposedly related to defective hepatic metabolization of reproductive hormones.[23]

Diagnosis. The diagnosis is based on the persistence of sanguinous discharge, vaginal cornification, estrus behavior, vaginoscopal findings and on concentrations of hormones such as progesterone and estradiol in the peripheral blood. The progesterone concentration is lower than 16 nmol/l but the estradiol concentration is not consistently elevated. A history of incomplete

ovariectomy or hormone therapy can contribute to the diagnosis. Abdominal palpation can be helpful in ruling out a tumor, although the size and consistency of these tumors vary considerably. Ultrasonography is very valuable in diagnosing cysts and cystic tumors (Fig. 7–31), although it is sometimes difficult to distinguish between normal structures such as preovulatory follicles and antra in young developing corpora lutea on the one hand and ovarian cysts on the other. Computed tomography provides better spatial resolution than ultrasonography and it is easier to perform and to interpret (Fig. 7–32).

Differential diagnosis. A split heat is a heat which stops before ovulation and starts again after an interval that varies from days to weeks. A split heat may be difficult to distinguish from persistent estrus if the interval is very short.

Therapy. Cysts can be treated with GnRH,[b] 10 µg/kg, once or repeatedly, but this does not always resolve the problem. If luteinization of cystic follicles or further luteinization of luteinized cysts takes place the estrus will stop, progesterone concentration will increase, and the vaginal smear will have intermediate and parabasal cells and leukocytes. If the problem persists estrus can be stopped by oral administration of low doses of

[b] Fertagyl®, Intervet

148

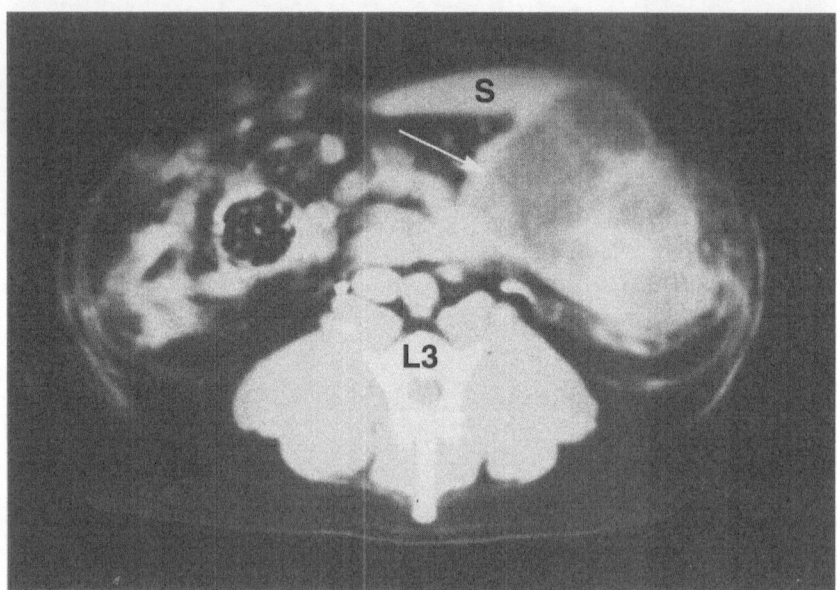

Fig. *7-32.* Contrast-enhanced CT image of the abdomen at the level of the third lumbar vertebra (L3) of a 4-year-old Collie with persistent estrus symptoms. Originating from the left ovary there is a large, cystic, space-occupying lesion (arrow) in close contact with the ventral extremity of the spleen (s).

megestrol acetate[c] (once daily, first week: 0.1 mg/kg; second week: 0.05 mg/kg). Tumors should be removed.

7.5 Infertility in the bitch

In the bitch fertility problems may arise during any stage of the reproductive cycle. They may result in a failure to mate, a missed conception, or premature termination of a pregnancy. Many of the observed fertility problems are, however, the result of inappropriate management of the bitch and can be solved if a correct breeding program is introduced.

7.5.1 Breeding management

Knowledge of reproductive physiology is indispensable for good breeding management. As mentioned in Section 7.2.1, the length of proestrus is usually 9 days, but it can last from as few as 3 to as many as 17 days. The length of estrus is usually 9 days but has a range of 3–21 days. The onset of estrus is usually synchronous with the pre-ovulatory LH surge, but occasionally it is as early as 2–3 days before or as late as 4–5 days after the LH peak. It should also be borne in mind that

[c] Ovarid®, Pitman Moore

some bitches never show estrus behavior. After ovulation, which can last for 24 h, the oocytes mature for the next 2–3 days, after which fertilization can occur. Sperm needs a capacitation period of at least 7 h.

Considering the above it is clear that breeding a bitch on a standard day in the cycle will usually give poor results. Breeding according to estrus behavior will give better results, although some bitches wil be bred too early and others too late. Determination of the ovulation period is therefore of the utmost importance. Several methods have been described to determine the ovulation period and the proper time for mating. The primary methods are measurement of the progesterone concentration in peripheral blood and vaginoscopy.

The ovulation period can be well defined through thrice-weekly measurements of the progesterone concentration in peripheral blood. The concentration increases slightly at the time of the preovulatory LH peak and rapidly at the onset of ovulation. At this time the progesterone concentration exceeds 16 nmol/l. The onset of the optimal period for mating is 24 h later and is based on the time needed for maturation of the oocytes and capacitation of the sperm (Fig. 7–33).[24] With determination of the time for mating using a rapid radioimmunoassay for measuring plasma progesterone concentration, it was found that 105 of

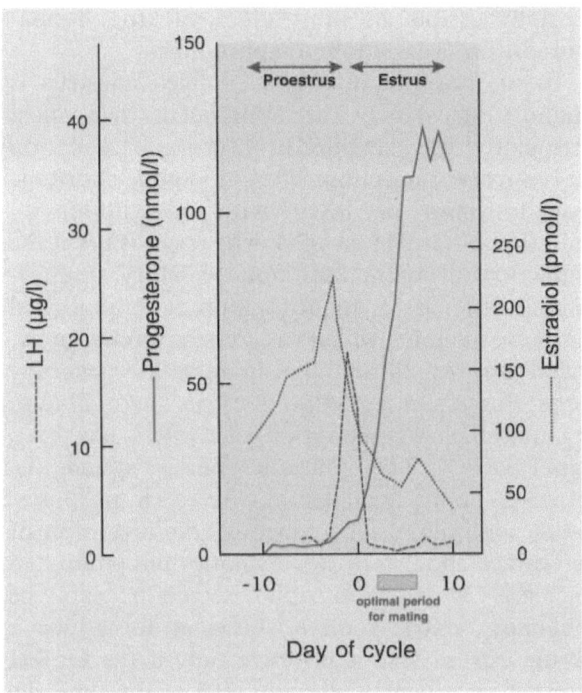

Fig. 7-33. The optimal mating time in relation to the concentration of estradiol, LH, and progesterone in plasma.

112 (94%) bitches with normal fertility became pregnant and 81 of 104 bitches (78%) with suboptimal fertility became pregnant.[24] In the latter group only 23% of previous matings had been successful.

Determination of the preovulatory LH peak would also provide an excellent parameter for the estimation of the ovulation time, but a rapid radioimmunoassay for the determination of LH concentrations in dog plasma is not yet available. Furthermore, more frequent blood sampling is required than for progesterone because of the risk of missing the preovulatory LH peak.

Vaginoscopy can also be used to try to establish the ovulation period (see 7.2.1). The mucosal changes are, however, a response to hormone-controlled alterations and are therefore secondary changes. Interpretation of the changes is also subjective. Vaginoscopy is thus a less reliable method for the estimation of the ovulation period. For the experienced veterinarian it is a useful tool for monitoring the stage of the cycle, but mating advice based on vaginoscopy should include the recommendation to mate at least twice, with an interval of 48 h.

Vaginal cytology is very useful in diagnosing early proestrus, progressing proestrus-estrus or metestrus (see Section 7.2.1). There are, however, no reliable changes in the smear indicative of the preovulatory LH surge or of ovulation. During the transition from estrus to metestrus the percentage of round cells increases rapidly and leukocytes reappear. However, an early metestrus smear can easily be confused with an early proestrus smear. Therefore the use of vaginal cytology is not a suitable method for determining the appropriate mating period for the bitch.

In spite of correctly timed breeding, some bitches will refuse the dog or other mating problems may arise. Some breeds, such as the English and French Bulldogs and the Newfoundland dog, are especially prone to having mating problems. The cause of the mating problem can be related to the dog (abnormal anatomy, inexperience, behavioral problems), the bitch (behavioral problems, vaginal abnormalities), or the owner (inexperience). With due regard for possible hereditary consequences artificial insemination may be performed.

7.5.2 Fertility disorders due to hormonal disturbances

Prolonged anestrus. The bitch which has not been in estrus by 18 months of age is considered to have primary anestrus. One of the major causes of primary anestrus is probably true hermaphroditism or pseudohermaphroditism (see also Chapter 8). If a bitch has been in estrus, an interval of more than 12 months or an interval which is double the usual interestrous interval for that individual bitch is considered to be a prolonged interestrous interval. One reason for a prolonged anestrus can be hypothyroidism. It should be pointed out, however, that hypothyroidism may initially lead to prolonged or abbreviated proestrus or mild estrus symptoms. Anestrus may also be induced with drugs such as progestagens or glucocorticosteroids. In the latter case and in spontaneous hyperadrenocorticism anestrus is probably the result of a decreased level of circulating gonadotropic hormones.[25] With ageing, the duration and frequency of cycles become more irregular and the interestrous interval increases after eight years of age. An apparent prolonged anestrus can be the result of a silent estrus or the owner's failure to observe estrus.

A general physical examination and a gynecological examination[26] should be performed and the following tests may be useful:

- Determination of the plasma progesterone concentration. If this is > 3 nmol/l, the bitch was probably in estrus and either the owner did not observe it or the bitch had a silent estrus period.
- Determination of plasma thyroxine concentration. If the result supports the suspicion, this may be followed by thyroid scintigraphy and/or a TSH-stimulation test (see Chapter 13).
- Determination of plasma LH and FSH concentrations. High levels of FSH and LH are an indication of absence (aplasia, ovariectomy) or failure of the gonads. Although not needed diagnostically it is interesting to note that these high values of LH and FSH can be further stimulated with GnRH.
- Stimulation of testosterone secretion. This test, using human chorionic gonadotrophin (hCG) or preferably GnRH, can be used to diagnose male pseudohermaphroditism or true hermaphroditism in phenotypically female dogs (see Chapter 13).
- Determination of the karyotype. Abnormalities in sexual differentiation may result in primary anestrus in phenotypically female dogs. The abnormalities may include the presence of abnormal complements of sex chromosomes as well as sex chromosomes that do not match the animal's phenotype[27] (see also Chapter 8).
- Laparoscopy or laparotomy. The genital tract can be examined macroscopically and tissue can be collected for microscopic examination. Pseudohermaphroditism and true hermaphroditism can be diagnosed.

Treatment is dependent on the pathogenesis of the prolonged anestrus. Hypothyroidism, for example, can be treated with a thyroxine supplementation (see Section 3.3). If the animal has silent heats, estrus can be detected by cytological examinations at regular intervals and close visual examination of the vulva, and the optimal mating period can be determined by progesterone measurement. Treatment, however, is not possible in most cases of true hermaphroditism or pseudohermaphroditism.

If no specific cause of prolonged anestrus is found, estrus may be stimulated. The most frequently used methods of estrus stimulation have involved injections of eCG (equine chorionic gonadotropin) or FSH, with or without an injection of GnRH or hCG. The result is often the induction of premature non-ovulatory luteinization of follicles or the formation of an abnormal corpus luteum which regresses prematurely. Therefore results of these methods are generally poor. Successful induction of estrus and ovulation by pulsatile administration of GnRH has been reported.[28,29] The pulsatile pump system is, however, only available for research purposes. With continuous subcutaneous administration of a GnRH agonist by an osmotic minipump, an increase in gonadotropin secretion can be obtained which is often sufficient to induce a fertile estrus. This is effective only if the GnRH agonist treatment is discontinued at the time the luteal phase starts, i.e., plasma progesterone concentration starts to rise. Continuing treatment results in receptor desensitization and thus LH secretion is suppressed.[7]

A completely different and often successful approach to induce a fertile estrus is the long-term oral administration of a dopamine agonist such as cabergolin (5 µg/kg per day[30]), or bromocriptine[d] (at least 20 µg/kg twice daily). It is still unclear whether the results are due to suppression of prolactin secretion which may inhibit gonadotropin release or whether there is a direct influence of the dopamine agonist. Both of the dopamine agonists give essentially the same results. When bromocriptine is administered during the luteal phase, the interestrous interval can be shortened from 245 days to 100 days (Fig. 7–34)[8,31] and when started during anestrus – 100 days after the ovulation – the next proestrus can be expected after about 45 days. The fertility of an estrus initiated by bromocriptine treatment appears to be normal.[30,32]

Persistent estrus. See Section 7.4.

[d] Lactafal®, Eurovet B.V., The Netherlands (Bromocriptine, Sandoz A.G., Switzerland)

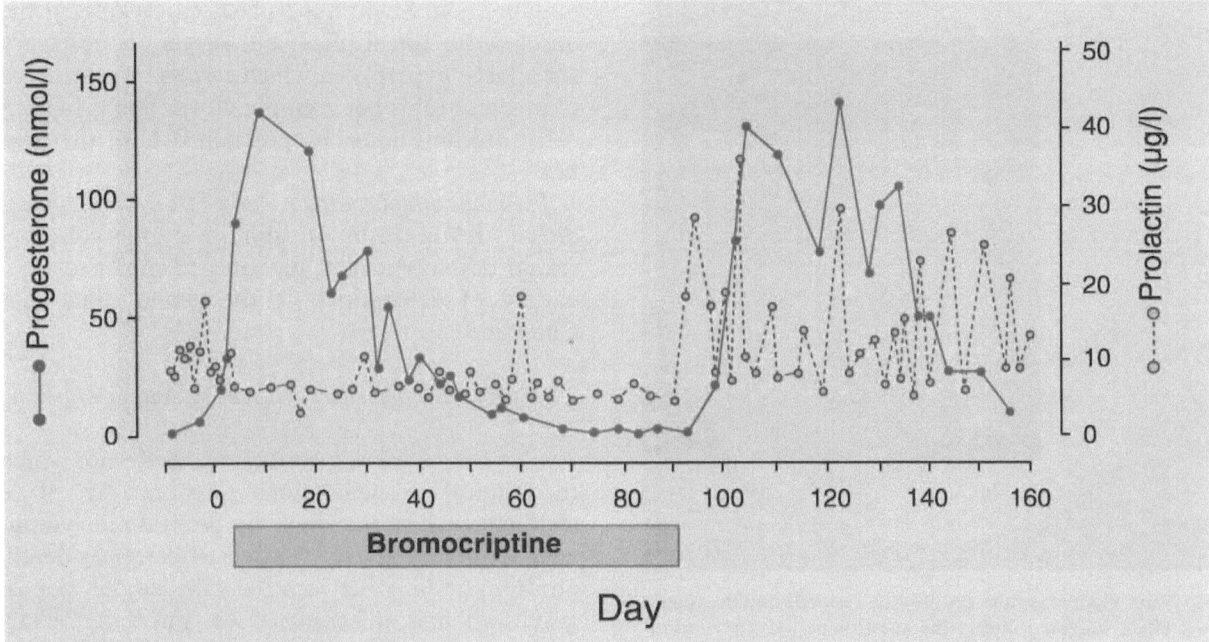

Fig. 7-34. Progesterone and prolactin levels in the peripheral blood of a dog treated with bromocriptine (bar) from the time of ovulation in the first cycle until the onset of the next follicular phase. The luteal phase and especially anestrus are considerably shortened. (Modified from Okkens et al., 1985.[8])

Cystic endometrial hyperplasia (CEH)-mucometra. See Section 7.3.

Split heat. A split heat is a heat which stops before ovulation and starts again after a few days or weeks. The vaginal discharge changes from red to brown, the smear contains intermediate cells, parabasal cells, and leukocytes, and the swelling of the vaginal mucosal folds diminishes. It is observed fairly often in both young and older bitches. It is probably caused by prematurely regressing follicles. Ovulation will generally occur if proestrus returns. Treatment is usually not necessary but close monitoring of the cycle is essential to determine the appropriate mating period.

Hypoluteoidism. Progesterone, secreted by the corpora lutea, is necessary for maintenance of pregnancy. Sterility may be caused by hypoluteoidism, but this appears to be extremely rare and may even be non-existent. It is questioned whether a condition that may be called luteal phase deficiency exists in man.[33] Because of the serious side effects of progesterone, such as CEH-

pyometra, bitches should not be treated with progesterone or progestagens after ovulation unless primary hypoluteoidism has been proven in previous cycles.

Lymphocytic oophoritis, which may be immune mediated, has been reported to cause primary anestrus.[27] However, Nickel et al. (1991)[34] described a case of oophoritis which was possibly immune mediated, in a bitch which had cycles with very short luteal phases and short interestrous intervals.

7.5.3 Fertility disorders due to anatomic abnormalities

Strictures and septa are common in bitches (Fig. 7–35). They can be congenital or acquired as a consequence of local treatment of vaginitis with irritating drugs. If the adhesions are extensive, there may be complete vaginal obstruction so that no sanguineous discharge is observed during proestrus or estrus. Congenital strictures and septa are usually located at the transition between the vestibule and the vagina; occasionally a stricture is found at the transition between the vulva and the

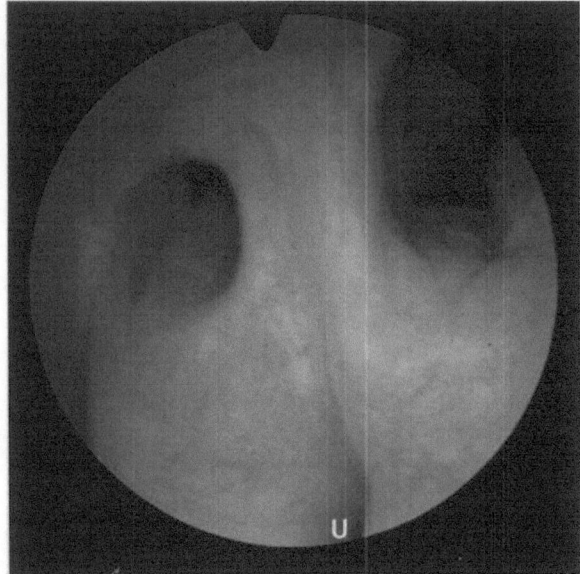

Fig. 7-35. Vaginal septum between the vestibule and the vagina in a bitch, observed during the anestrus period. (u: urethral orifice).

vestibule. Such abnormalities are easily diagnosed during vaginal palpation, which ought to be part of every pre-breeding examination. If the septum is thin it can be torn but if it is thicker it should be removed with scissors via the vaginoscope. An episiotomy is seldom necessary. Treatment may not be possible if the septum extends deep into the vagina cranially or if there are strictures.

Vaginal hyperplasia, which occurs during proestrus and estrus, can cause a breeding problem (Fig. 7–36). It may be a reason for artificial insemination. Slight hyperplasia can regress at the onset of the luteal phase but surgery is necessary for a large hyperplasia which results in protrusion of mucosal folds between the vulvar lips.[35] In such cases breeding must be postponed until the next heat.

Pseudohermaphroditism and true hermaphroditism are the result of abnormal embryological sexual development. They are accompanied by a variety of deformities of the genital tract (see Chapter 8).

7.5.4 Fertility disorders with an infectious etiology

Canine brucellosis is a contagious disease of which the clinical manifestations vary greatly. It is characterized in the bitch by generalized lymphadenopathy and by early embryonic death, abortion (mainly between the 45th and 55th day of gestation) and infertility.[36] An important characteristic is a prolonged bacteriemia which often persists 1 to 2 years or longer and which may be intermittent. Infection can occur via all mucous membranes. The most important modes of transmission are via placental tissues, vaginal discharges following an abortion, and via venereal transmission.

Canine brucellosis must be considered whenever there is a history of abortion or poor reproductive performance in either sex. The diagnosis cannot, however, be made on the basis of clinical signs alone. Serological tests for the diagnosis of canine brucellosis, such as the rapid slide agglutination

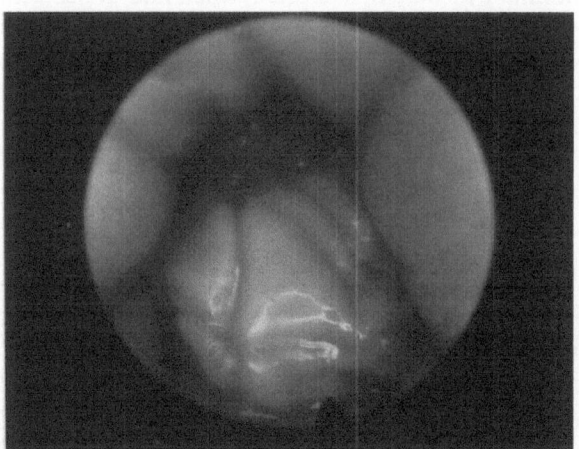
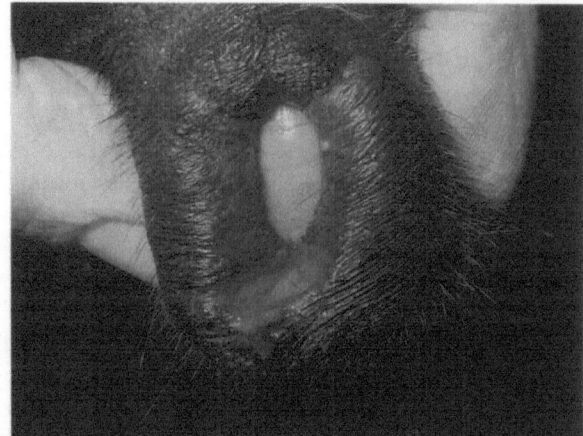

Fig. 7-36. Vaginal hyperplasia in 2 bitches during proestrus/estrus; (left) a modest hyperplasia which is observed quite often during this period of the cycle and (right) a more extensive form of hyperplasia which may cause mating problems.

153

test, the tube agglutination test, and the modified mercaptoethanoltube agglutination test, must be used to confirm the diagnosis. A useful sero-diagnostic regimen could involve the use of an agglutination test for screening in combination with an agar-gel diffusion test. Blood cultures should always be taken when canine brucellosis is suspected.[36]

There is no vaccine available. The disease is not life-threatening, but an infected animal should not be used for breeding because it will continue to be a source of infection for other dogs, and possibly humans. Treatment with antibiotics to which *B canis* is susceptible *in vitro* do not usually completely eliminate the organisms *in vivo* so that bacteriemia commonly recurs 1 to 3 months after the therapy is discontinued. Control measures in an infected kennel should therefore include the elimination of all infected animals.

Vaginitis. Conditions such as neoplasia, foreign bodies, and androgen-induced hypertrophy of the clitoris may precipitate a bacterial infection, although vaginitis may also occur without such predisposing factors. The relationship between the bacterial flora in the vagina and fertility problems is unclear. Bacteria normally inhabit the canine vagina and β-hemolytic streptococci can be present in the vagina of fertile bitches. The bacterial species isolated from bitches with vaginitis do not differ significantly from those in normal bitches, but culture usually reveals only one or two species. Specimens for bacterial culture should be taken from the cranial part of the vagina. Treatment is indicated if there are > 100 colonies per culture or if there are only one or two species. Treatment can be administered system-ically or locally, but locally applied drugs are often spermicidal and should not be used shortly before breeding.

Infection with canine herpes virus can cause a marked decrease in fertility as well as a high percentage of dead puppies in the first weeks after parturition. Infection of puppies can take place in utero, during parturition via contamination in the birth canal, by infected litter mates or by oronasal secretion from the bitch. If the fetuses are infected in utero they may be aborted or born dead. If there is a fertility problem in a kennel as a result of canine herpes virus infections it is important to stop breeding for about 6 months in order to lower the infection density.

7.6 Estrus prevention

Estrus can be prevented medically or surgically. Ovariectomy has certain advantages. It is effective after one procedure. It considerably lowers the risk of mammary cancer if performed early in life, preferably before the first luteal phase but in any case before about 2.5 years of age. It also prevents the development of pyometra and progestagen-induced growth hormone excess (see Section 2.2.3). There are, however, several disadvantages, such as the risk of anesthesia and surgery, and the irreversibility of the procedure. There is also the possibility of side-effects such as urinary in-continence. It is possible that the risk of urinary incontinence is greater if the procedure is per-formed prior to the first estrus. Incontinence occurs mainly in large breeds and particularly in the Boxer and the Doberman.

In the cat ovariectomy is the treatment of choice, for it does not induce incontinence. Furthermore, endogenous progesterone and progestagens are, as in the bitch, tumorigenic and mammary tumors in the cat are almost always malignant.[37,38]

Medical estrus prevention can be accomplished with several types of drugs, but not all available drugs are permitted in every country. The pro-gestagens are the most important drugs for estrus prevention. Androgens can also be used for this purpose but primarily for short-term prevention.

Androgens inhibit pituitary gonadotropin release, thus preventing follicular development. One orally administered synthetic androgen, mibolerone,[e] is also anabolic. It has no pro-gestational or estrogenic activity. The advantages therefore lie in the minimal influence on the endometrium. Thickening of the myometrium may occur but only when excessive doses are used. Although subsequent fertility in bitches treated with this drug appears to be good, it is not re-commended in the U.S.A. for use in breeding bitches or in bitches prior to the first estrus. It also has many side-effects, mainly related to its andro-

[e] Cheque® drops, Upjohn

154

genic properties, including clitoral hypertrophy, vaginal discharge, liver dysfunction, and weight gain. It is contraindicated in bitches with liver or kidney disease. Furthermore, the drug can induce mammary tumor development. If administered to a pregnant dog, the drug causes defects in the urogenital tract of female puppies (see Chapter 8). In addition, androgens may cause an increase in aggressiveness and a change in the urination behavior. Bitches may start to urinate like a dog and queens may develop urine spraying behavior.

GnRH agonists or GnRH antagonists administered at high doses over a long period of time also prevent estrus by down regulation of receptors on pituitary gonadotrophs. However, the early stimulatory effect of GnRH analogues, which cause estrus if administered during anestrus, and the economic and delivery problems for long-term use of GnRH antagonists make both unsuitable for clinical use.[39]

Progestagens. The mechanism of the contraceptive activity of progestagens is still unclear. In many species there is evidence that contraceptive progestagens reduce serum concentrations of gonadotropins. However, there is little information about the effects of progestagens on gonadotropic secretion in dogs. In one study high doses of medroxyprogesterone acetate (MPA) administered to beagle bitches for several months

did not reduce the increased concentrations of LH in ovariectomized bitches nor did it lower LH concentrations in intact bitches.[40] In another study high contraceptive doses of megestrol acetate (MA) did not suppress basal gonadotropin secretion during anestrus, nor was the pituitary hypersecretion of LH and FSH in ovariectomized bitches suppressed.[41] The contraceptive activity of progestagens may involve the prevention of increases in gonadotropin secretion above basal values. In addition, there may be a direct negative effect on follicle development in the ovary.[41]

The progestagens most frequently used for estrus prevention in the dog are proligestone and MPA. The single injection dosage recommended by the manufacturer for proligestone[f] ranges from 10 mg/kg for a dog of about 60 kg, to 30 mg/kg for one of 3 kg, s.c., and for MPA[g] the single injection dose is 2 mg/kg (maximum 60 mg), s.c. They should be administered during anestrus about one month before the expected follicular phase (see Fig. 7–37). The first estrus after the use of proligestone in the majority of bitches can be expected within 9–12 months; after MPA administration it may be up to 2–3 years. MPA[h] can also be administered orally, 5 mg once daily

[f] Delvosteron®, Intervet
[g] Depopromone®, Upjohn; Perlutex®, Leo
[h] Provera®, Upjohn

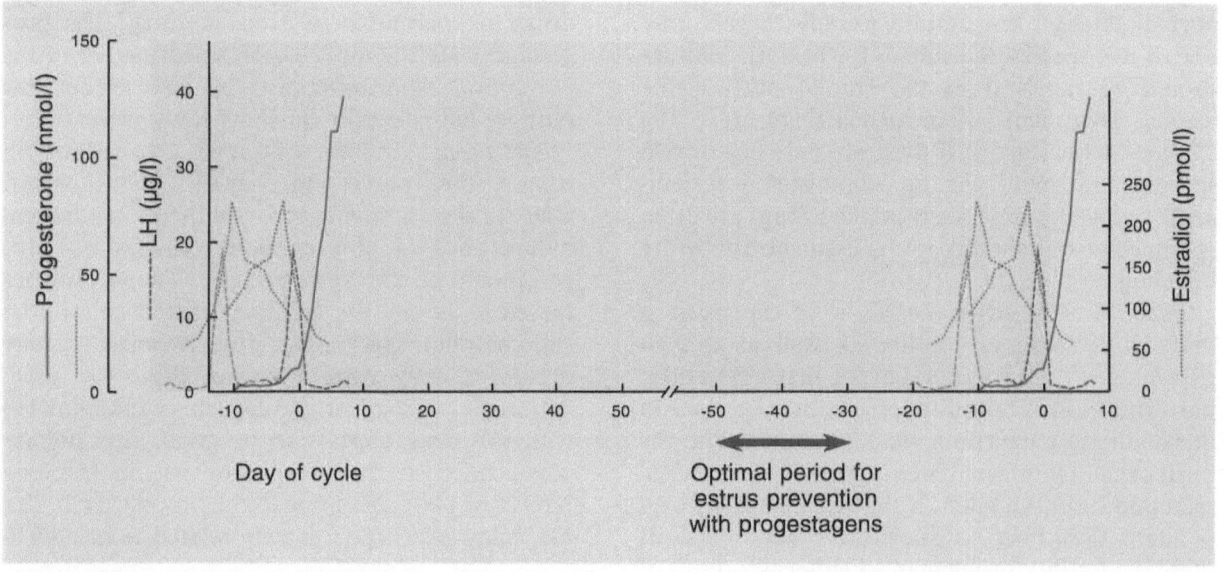

Fig. 7-37. Optimal period for progestagen treatment for estrus prevention in the bitch.

(10 mg for large dogs during the first 5 days) for as long as estrus prevention is wanted or for a maximum of 21 days. The recurrence of estrus may vary from 2–9 months. In the U.S.A. the advised dosage for megestrol acetate (MA),[i] a progestagen which probably has a stronger progestagenic effect than MPA, is 0.5 mg/kg orally once daily for 32 days starting during anestrus, or 2 mg/kg for 8 days starting at the onset of proestrus. Considering the results which are obtained with lower doses of MPA, this recommended dose appears to be quite high.

In the usual household the queen is not affected by photoperiod influences and may cycle regularly throughout the year. This can be prevented by oral administration of 5 mg MPA or 2 mg MA once a week. As an alternative, owners who can detect signs preceding proestrus may be advised to administer those drugs only on that occasion. The side-effects of oral administration of progestagens appear to be less serious than those accompaning injections. In addition, should the queen unexpectedly by found to be pregnant, the medication can be stopped and parturition can take place at the normal time. Another option is to reduce estrus frequency in the queen by inducing ovulation. This can be accomplished by mechanical stimulation of the vagina (touching the vestibulum/vagina with a cotton probe) or by treatment with a gonadotropic hormone or GnRH. The induced pseudo-pregnancy delays the recurrence of estrus.

[i] Ovarid®, Pitman Moore

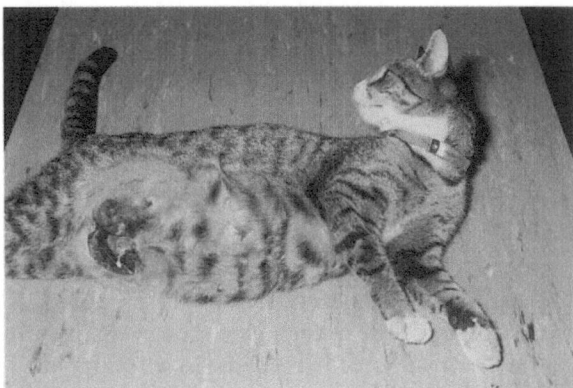

Fig. 7-38. A young queen during her first pregnancy with a large hypertrophic/fibroadenoma complex of the mammary glands.

In summary, progestagens used for estrus prevention may have the following side-effects:
– Development of CEH.
– Prolonged pregnancy. This occurs if progestagens are administered subcutaneously at the onset of the follicular phase and the bitch or queen is mated. The gestation will be prolonged and a caesarian section may be needed, unless a progesterone antagonist, mifepristone (RU 486) is given.
– Hypersecretion of GH (see also 7.3 and 2.2.3) and diabetes mellitus. In cats, the latter is usually caused by the glucocorticoid effects inherent to these progestagens.[42,43] In dogs, however, apart from direct glucocorticoid or progestagen effects, the development of dia-

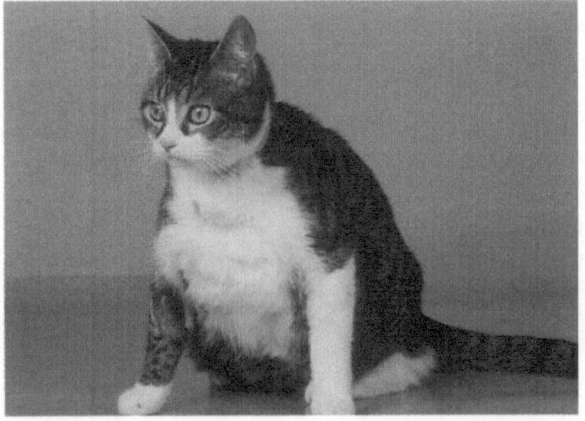

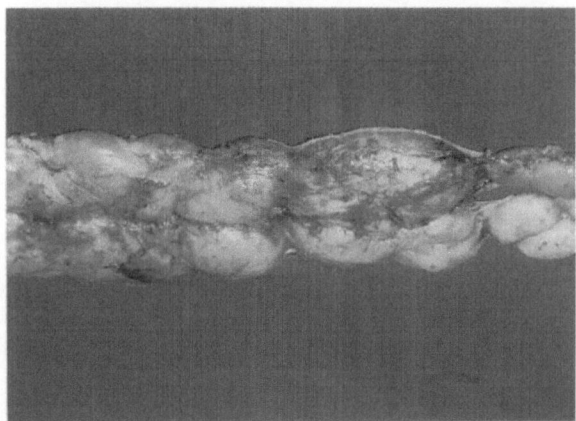

Fig. 7-39. Left: A ten-month-old queen with hypertrophic/fibroadenoma complex of the mammary glands. The queen had been treated after her first estrus with 2 mg megestrol acetate once weekly for 3 weeks. Right: The excised mammary glands of the same queen.

betes mellitus is largely due to GH excess[44] (see also Chapter 5).

- The increased risk of neoplastic transformation of mammary tissue. This ranges from hyperplasia, to adenomas and malignant tumors. The progestagen-induced neoplastic transformation of mammary tissue starts with proliferation of undifferentiated terminal ductal structures, so-called terminal end buds.[45] This proliferation increases the susceptibility of the mammary tissue to malignant transformation. However, the hyperplasia itself may also give rise to problems, especially in the queen. In young queens exogenous (but also endogenous!) progestagens may cause extensive proliferation of mammary duct epithelium and stroma, leading to a very large hypertrophic/fibroadenoma complex[46] (Figs. 7–38, 7–39).

The occurrence of these side-effects is, with the exception of "prolonged pregnancy", largely dependent upon total progestagen exposure. With the advised dosage regimens the exposure may be higher with MPA and MA than with proligestone, the latter being a rather weak progestagen.

8. Disorders of sexual differentiation

8.1 Introduction

Intersexuality in dogs and cats may be associated with a variety of clinical problems such as infertility, abnormal behavior, urinary incontinence, local irritation of abnormal external genitalia, Sertoli cell neoplasia, endometritis, and gynaecomastia. For the diagnosis, treatment, and prognosis of these disorders it is important to understand the underlying mechanisms of normal and abnormal sexual development and differentiation.

Normal differentiation of the female genital tract. In mammalian embryogenesis differentiation of the female genital tract occurs somewhat later than that of the male. Female gonadal differentiation can be recognized by the presence of female germ cells in meiosis and later by the presence of follicles.[1]

Female organogenesis is characterized by the regression of the Wolffian ducts and stabilisation of the Müllerian ducts, which later will form the oviduct, uterus, and cranial vagina (Fig. 8–1). The vagina is derived mainly from the urogenital sinus and to a very small extent also from the Wolffian ducts and the Müllerian ducts.[2] While the urethral groove remains open, part of the urogenital sinus forms the vestibule. The labioscrotal folds form the vulva. In contrast to male sexual development the formation of a female phenotype does not require the presence of gonads and the hormones they produce.[3]

Normal differentiation of the male genital tract. In the presence of a Y chromosome the undifferentiated gonad develops into a testis, which can be recognized histologically by day 36 of gestation in the dog. From this time on a glycoprotein is produced by the fetal Sertoli cells, called Anti-müllerian Hormone (AMH) or Müllerian Inhibiting Substance (MIS). This hormone is responsible for the regression of the Müllerian ducts. Regression begins at day 36 and is completed at day 46 of gestation in the dog embryo.[4]

Whereas a hormone (AMH) inhibits the development of the Müllerian ducts, the stabilisation and differentiation of the Wolffian ducts into the vasa deferentia and epidymidis is largely the result of stimulation by testosterone. Wolffian ducts cells lack the enzyme 5α-reductase, which converts testosterone to dihydrotestosterone (DHT). Therefore testosterone is responsible for the development of male duct derivatives (Fig. 8–1). In the cells of the urogential sinus, 5α-reductase converts testosterone to DHT and mediates the androgenic action necessary for the formation of the prostate[5] and masculinization of the external genitalia. Part of the urogenital sinus develops into the membraneous urethra and the urethral groove closes to form the penile urethra. The glans penis develops from the genital tubercle and the labioscrotal folds from the raphe scroti.

Abnormal sexual differentiation and development. Classification of intersexuality is often based on the histology of the gonads and the phenotype, and this is also applied in this chapter. However, the disorders may develop at the chromosome level. Errors in the constitution of the chromosomes can influence gonadal differentiation or cause gonadal dysgenesis. Nevertheless, chromosomal and gonadal sex do not always correspond, as can be seen in sex-reversed individuals.[6]

The following disorders of sexual differentiation are discussed in this chapter:
1. Gonadal dysgenesis and other sex chromosome anomalies (8.2);
2. True hermaphroditism (8.3);

157

A. Rijnberk (ed.), Clinical Endocrinology of Dogs and Cats, 157–165.
© 1996 *Kluwer Academic Publishers.*

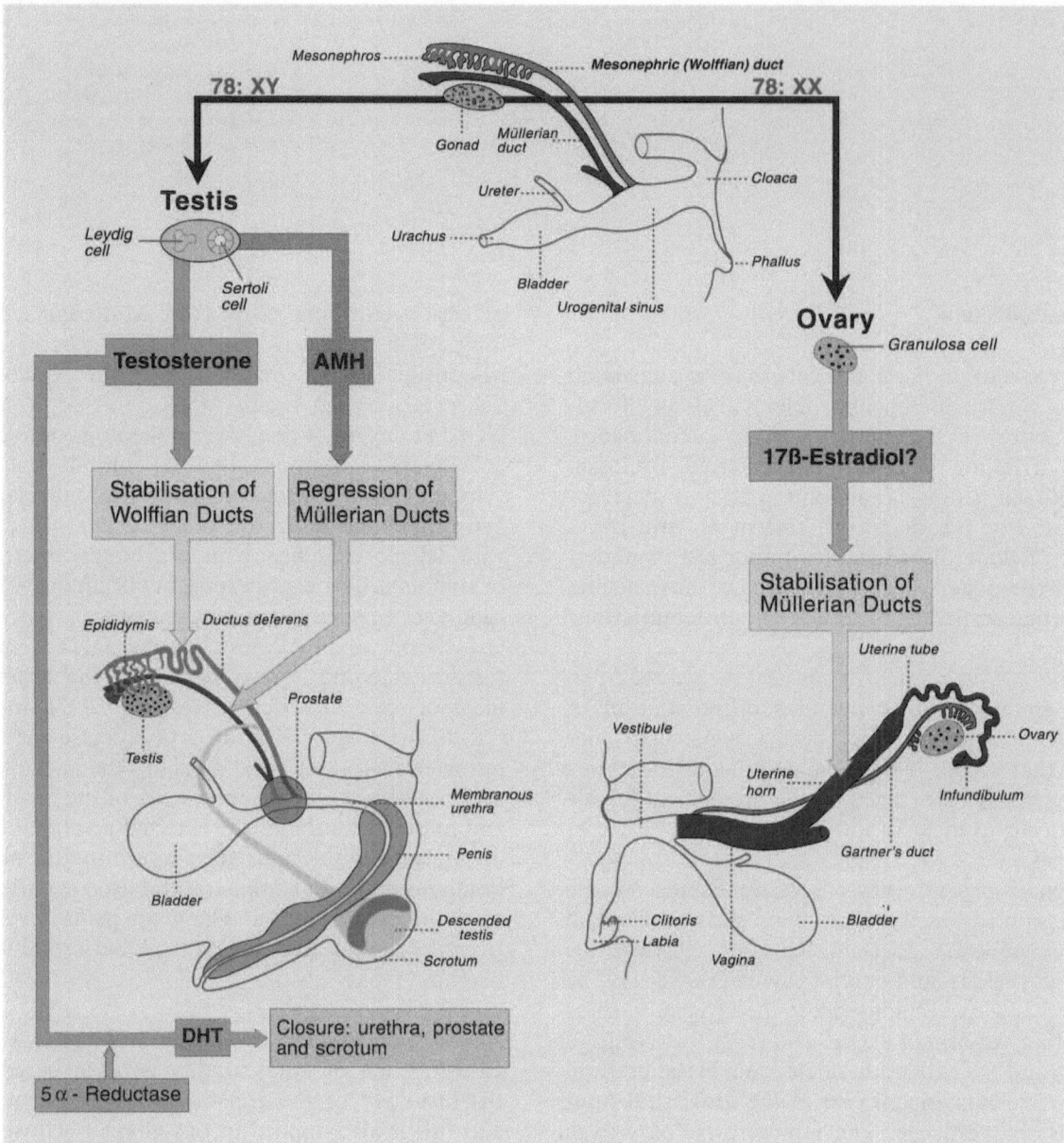

Fig. 8-1. Schematic representation of male and female differentiation and development from the undifferentiated state under stimulation and inhibition of sex steroids and regulatory peptides. The presence of a Y chromosome leads to male differentiation of the gonad with subsequent secretion of testosterone and Antimüllerian Hormone (AMH). Testosterone stabilizes the former Wolffian (or mesonephric) duct. Dihydrotestosterone (DHT) is required for the complete development of the external male genitalia and closure of the urethra. Secretion of AMH from the foetal Sertoli cells is necessary to inhibit the growth and development of the Müllerian ducts into female internal genitalia.

3. Female pseudohermaphroditism (8.4);
4. Male pseudohermaphroditism (8.5).

8.2 Gonadal dysgenesis and other chromosomal anomalies

8.2.1 Gonadal dysgenesis (XO syndrome)

Gonadal dysgenesis is the result of the absence of a second sex chromosome, most often the paternal, which is lost during spermatogenesis or after fertilisation. The X-monosomy is often associated with absence of germ cells and the gonads contain mainly fibrous tissue. In man the clinical features are characterized by small body size and facial deformities. This syndrome is named Turner's Syndrome. The absence of germ cells leads to a lack of steroidal stimulation of the female genitalia and these individuals are often infertile.

Clinical manifestations. Only two cases have been reported in the dog so far, one of which showed a paradoxical pattern of persistent prooestrus. Both dogs were presented with failure to develop oestrus and small body size, and one had facial deformities.[7] The syndrome also has been reported in a cat.[8]

Differential diagnosis. The most prominent clinical sign is primary anoestrus and therefore other possible causes such as male or female pseudohermaphroditism, oophoritis or hypothyroidism must be excluded (see also Section 7.5).

Diagnosis. Primary anoestrus in dogs and cats is defined as failure to develop oestrus before the age of 18 months (see also Section 7.5.2). Concentrations of LH and (if possible) FSH in plasma can be measured and are elevated in the absence of ovarian tissue. Histological examination of gonadal tissue obtained via laparoscopy or at laparotomy can confirm the diagnosis of gonadal dysgenesis and cytogenetic examination supports the diagnosis of X-monosomy.

Therapy. The unusual signs of persistent proestrus in an Eskimo Hound stopped after ovariohysterectomy,[7] but most dogs might not require any therapy.

Prognosis. The clinical manifestations usually do not interfere with the health of the animal.

8.2.2 XXY syndrome

Another chromosomal anomaly resulting in abnormal sexual development is the XXY Syndrome or Klinefelter's Syndrome. The presence of a Y chromosome explains the male gonadal differentiation with subsequent testosterone and AMH production and therefore the individuals are phenotypically male. The presence of an extra X chromosome causes atrophy and hyalinisation of the seminiferous tubules as well as abnormal Leydig cell structure and decreased steroid secretion by the Leydig cells.[9] Most cases in humans have been described as having testis atrophy, gynaecomastia, and penis hypoplasia. The only reported case in a dog had a normal male phenotype, small testes, and no spermatogenesis.[10] More cases have been described in cats,[11,12] associated with a tortoiseshell or calico coat pattern (Fig. 8–2). This coat can only be seen with this

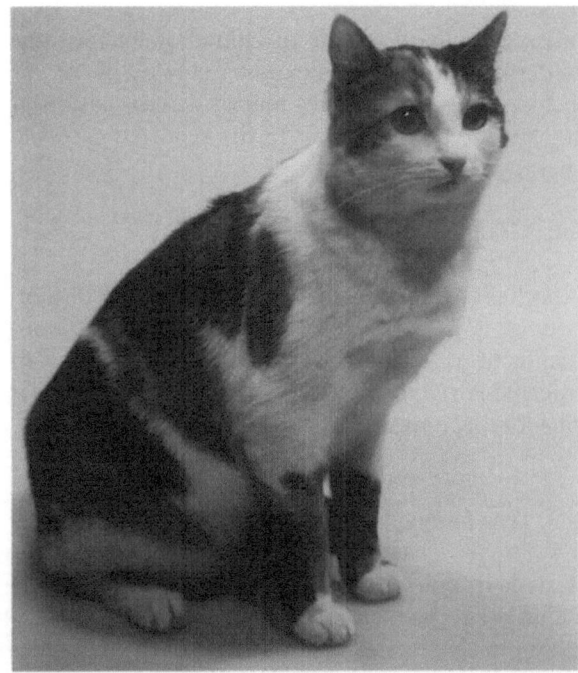

Fig. 8-2. A male cat with a tortoiseshell coat pattern, suggesting a chromosomal anomaly. (Courtesy of Dr. A.A. Bosma, Department of Functional Morphology, Faculty of Veterinary Medicine, Utrecht University; case referred by Prof. Dr. J.E. Gajentaan.)

160

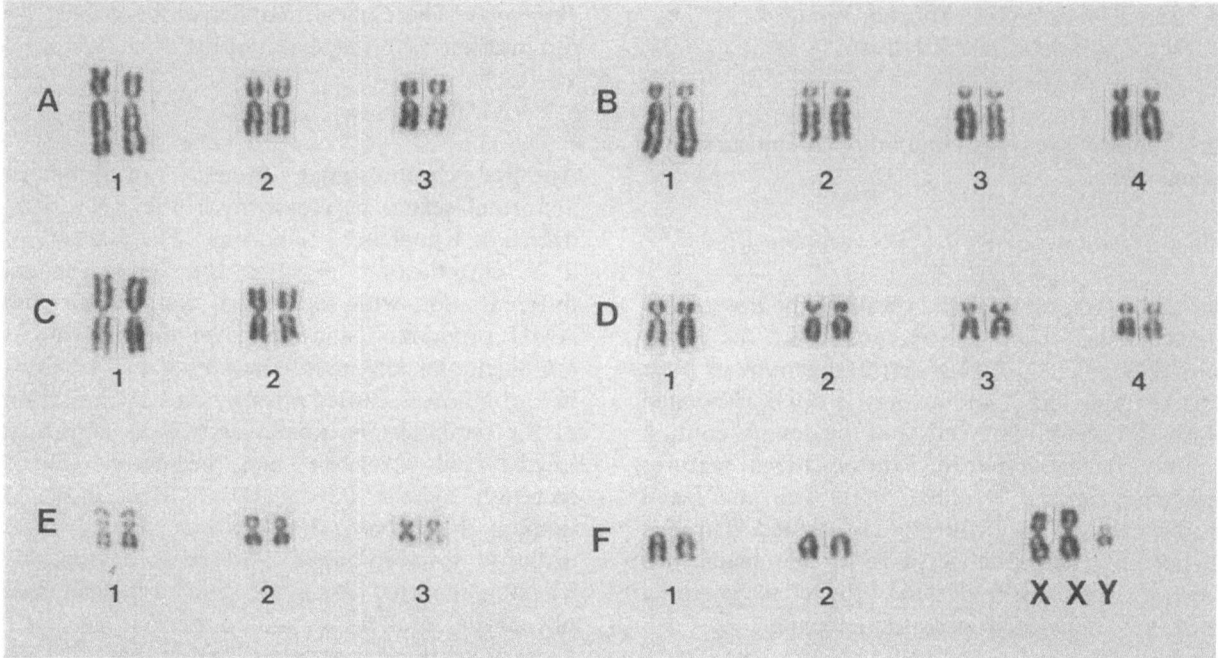

Fig. 8-3. Karyotype of the cat of Fig. 8–2, illustrating the presence of two X chromosomes and a Y chromosome (similar to Klinefelter's Syndrome of man). Chromosomes are arranged according to a standardized system developed for the domestic cat (Courtesy of Dr. A.A. Bosma, Department of Functional Morphology, Faculty of Veterinary Medicine, Utrecht University.)

disorder or with mosaic or chimeric chromosome patterns. The diagnosis can be made by histologic examination of the testes and/or determination of the karyotype (Fig. 8–3). In the reported cases no therapy was necessary.

8.2.3 Triple X syndrome

Another chromosomal anomaly, the Triple X Syndrome, is probably also a result of meiotic nondisjunction. The only reported case was an infertile Airedale bitch with a small uterus, female phenotype, and with ovaries without follicles.[13]

8.3 True hermaphroditism

True hermaphrodites have both ovarian and testicular tissue in their gonads. Abnormal differentiation in these cases could be the result of chimerism or mosaicism. Chimerism is the presence of two or more genotypes arising from different zygotes in the same individual. Mosaicism is the presence of two or more genotypes originating from a single zygote. These chromosomal ab-

normalities are usually the result of a mitotic nondisjunction or anaphase lag.

Gonadal differentiation can also lead to a phenotype opposite to the chromosomal sex. A female karyotype with an almost male phenotype is called XX sex-reversal and has been reported in dogs. The condition is inherited as an autosomal recessive trait in the American Cocker Spaniel.[14] The male gonadal differentiation in the absence of a Y chromosome is explained by the transmission and expression of the gene carrying the information for male sex determination by an XX individual.[15] Other breeds with this familial disorder are Beagle, Pug, Kerry Blue Terrier, and Weimaraner.[6]

The degree of masculinization in true hermaphrodites depends directly on the amount of testicular tissue in the gonad. Although in patients with much testicular tissue the oviducts can be absent, the uterus is always present.[16]

Clinical manifestations. Most true hermaphrodites are presented with a female phenotype with some degree of masculinization, which can vary from a small clitoric protuberance with a small os penis

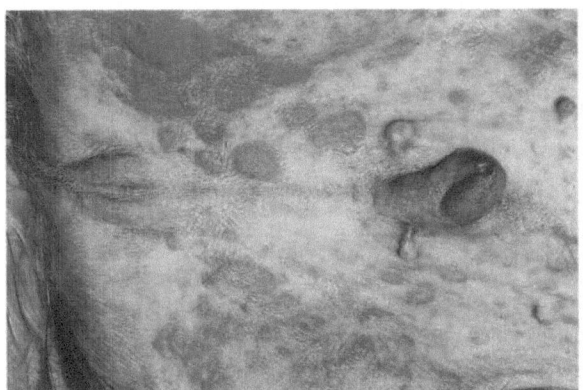

Fig. 8-4. Hypoplastic prepuce, penis, and empty scrotum in a Cocker Spaniel dog with true hermaphroditism. Note the local skin irritation caused by urinary incontinence.

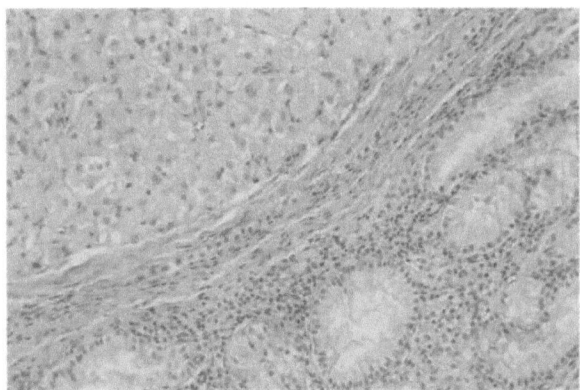

Fig. 8-6. Histologic section of an ovotestis from a dog with true hermaphroditism. The seminiferous tubules (lower right) can be recognized close to ovarian tissue with a corpus luteum (upper left).

up to a hypoplastic penis (Fig. 8–4). The clinical signs include infertility, primary anoestrus, irregular cycles, vulvar irritation, and urinary incontinence.

Differential diagnosis. A female phenotype with masculinization is also seen in male pseudohermaphrodites. Female appearance without overt masculinization requires exclusion of X monosomy, trisomy, hypothyroidism and oophoritis.

Diagnosis. Elevation of plasma testosterone after stimulation with hCG or GnRH allows a presumptive diagnosis. Retrograde contrast radiography can reveal female internal genitalia in dogs with a male appearance (Fig. 8–5). The definitive diagnosis, and especially the diagnosis of sex

reversal, requires cytogenetic examination and histologic examination of the gonads (Fig. 8–6).

Treatment. Vulvar irritation is most often caused by the presence of an os clitoris. The problem can be resolved by surgical removal of the osseous structure (Fig. 8–7). Gonadectomy and hysterectomy have been recommended, but the choice of this treatment can be a matter of debate. The risks of Sertoli cell neoplasia (see Section 6.4) and/or endometritis have to be weighed against the morbidity and mortality of a preventive abdominal surgery. Laparotomy certainly is indicated in patients which have developed Sertoli cell neoplasia and/or endometritis. Urinary incontinence due to urine pooling in the female genitalia can be resolved by radical excision of all female genital structures.

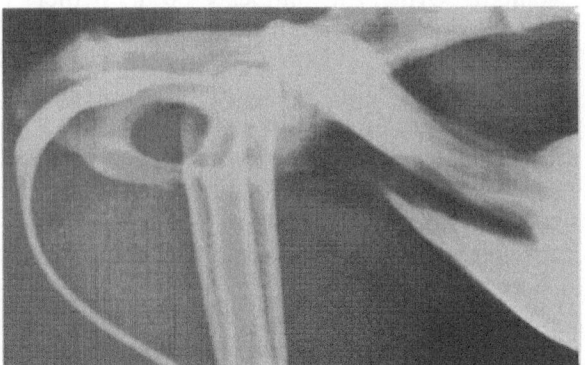

Fig. 8-5. Retrograde cystourethrography in a true hermaphrodite Cocker Spaniel with hypoplastic male external genitalia. Note the male urethra and the accumulation of contrast material in the female genitalia.

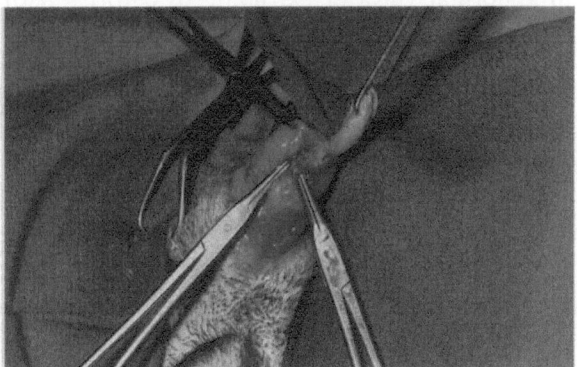

Fig. 8-7. Surgical removal of an os clitoris from a male pseudohermaphrodite dog with female external genitalia.

Prognosis. Some dogs may not require any treatment. Local irritation of the vulva usually resolves after removal of the os clitoris. Depending on the amount of ovarian tissue, affected dogs can have normal cycles. Even delivery of a normal litter has been described.[15] Breeding should be discouraged in dogs with XX sex reversal, as this can be a hereditary disorder.

8.4 Female pseudohermaphroditism

Masculinization of androgen sensitive tissues in individuals with ovaries and an XX karyotype is called female pseudohermaphroditism. This condition is dependent on exogenous or endogenous androgen exposure. In the androgenital syndrome, in which there is an inborn error in glucocorticoid synthesis, the high ACTH release causes increased concentrations of adrenal androgens. This syndrome is well known in humans but has not yet been reported in the dog or cat. Female pseudohermaphroditism was found less frequently than other forms of intersexuality in a survey of 52 canine cases.[17] Probably the few reported cases have been the result of the administration of progestagens or androgens during gestation. In some reported cases the use of androgens during pregnancy could be verified by the history[18]. The use of androgens in intact female dogs should therefore be discouraged.[19]

Clinical manifestations. Minor masculinization (Fig. 8–8) can lead to vulvar irritation caused by an abnormal vulva or extruding os clitoris. With

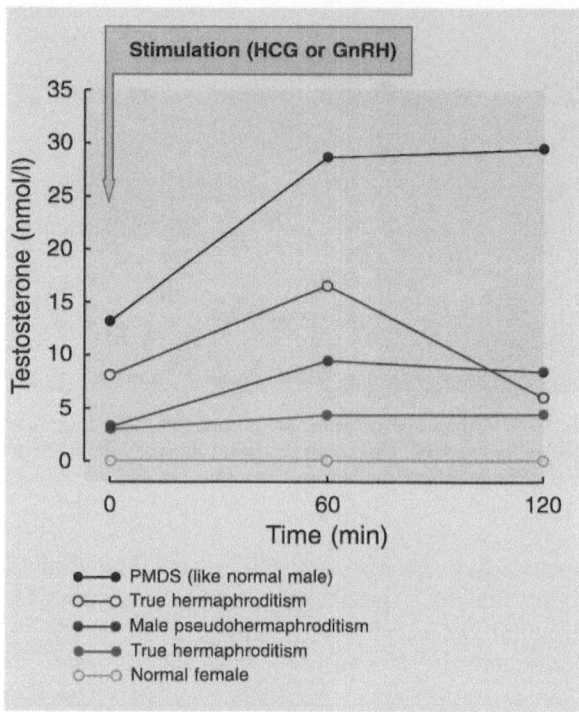

Fig. 8-9. Schematic illustration of blood testosterone concentrations before and after stimulation with hCG or GnRH (Chapter 13). The height of the basal testosterone concentration and the values after stimulation depend on the amount of functional testicular tissue; see, for example, the different values in the two cases of true hermaphroditism.

complete external masculinization signs such as hematuria, genital swelling and attraction of other male dogs can be observed, which might be the result of cyclic activity of the ovaries. Systemic illness can develop if there is endometritis/pyometra. Urinary incontinence occurs if there is urine pooling in the internal female genitalia.

Diagnosis. Low or undetectable testosterone concentrations after stimulation with hCG or GnRH indicate the absence of testicular tissue (Fig. 8–9). For the definitive diagnosis histological examination of the gonads is required and cytogenetic examination can also contribute to the diagnosis.

Treatment. Clinical signs usually disappear after ovariohysterectomy. Vulvar irritation caused by a protruding clitoris resolves after resection of the os clitoris. Plastic surgery also has been used in order to remove the masculinized external genitalia.[20]

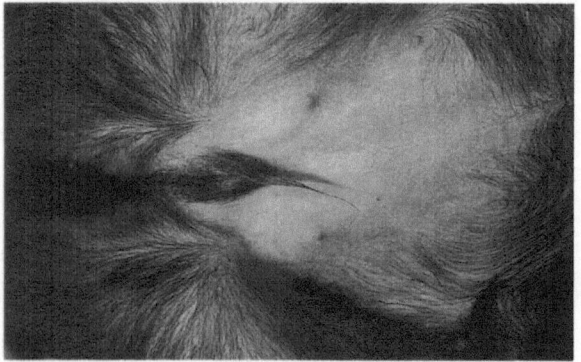

Fig. 8-8. Female pseudohermaphroditism in a dog as a result of administration of anabolic steroids to the mother during pregnancy.

8.5 Male pseudohermaphroditism

In animals with male pseudohermaphroditism there is a Y chromosome and there are testes but the genital ducts and/or external genitalia are incompletely masculinized. In principle, this can be the result of (1) defective testicular different-iation, (2) an error in the synthesis of testosterone or the release of AMH, and (3) defects in the androgen-dependent target tissues such as 5α-reductase deficiency and low or absent androgen receptor activity. In its complete form the latter is called testicular feminisation. It is characterized by bilateral testes, female-appearing external gen-italia, a blind-ending vagina, and the absence of Müllerian derivatives. It is an X-linked defect that seems to be rare; it has been described in one dog and one cat.[21,22]

A much more common form of male pseudo-hermaphroditism is the so-called Persistent Mullerian Duct Syndrome (PMDS). A defect in the mechanism of Müllerian duct regression by AMH (MIS) is responsible for the presence of oviducts, a uterus, and a cranial vagina in otherwise completely normal male dogs (Fig. 8–10). PMDS was first described in Miniature Schnauzer dogs, a breed in which an autosomal recessive mode of inheritance for this disorder has been proved by breeding experiments.[23] Even more clinical cases were detected in the Basset Hound.[24] Experimental studies in both breeds

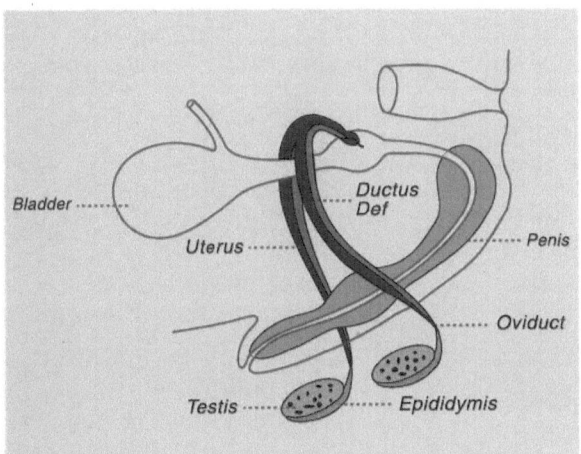

Fig. 8-10. Schematic representation of the persisting Müllerian ducts in a male dog. Note that the vasa deferentia appear to be located in the wall of the uterus.

showed that AMH is produced and is bioactive in the critical period of Müllerian duct regression.[23] Thus a defect at the receptor or post-receptor level must be responsible for the disorder.

Clinical manifestations. Animals with a predomin-ating female appearance often have vulvar irri-tation caused by a protruding clitoris. All clinical signs which can be found in dogs with Sertoli cell neoplasia and endometritis can also be present in male pseudohermaphrodites. Bassethounds with PMDS are often presented with signs suggesting lower urinary tract disease. Animals with PMDS can be fertile when the testes have descended and the epidymidis is not affected by inflammatory changes which are also found in the uterus. Endo-metritis is probably the most prominent problem and causes hematuria, abdominal pain, and systemic illness. In Miniature Schnauzer dogs the high incidence of cryptorchism has also resulted in Sertoli cell neoplasia.[25]

Differential diagnosis. True hermaphroditism and female pseudohermaphroditism can be associated with similar clinical problems. In dogs with PMDS signs of lower urinary tract diseases are often so prominent that the underlying condition can be overlooked until the appropriate studies are performed.

Diagnosis. Except in PMDS the definitive diag-nosis can be made by histological examination of the gonads, cytogenetic examination, and receptor studies. In dogs with descended testes and normal male external genitalia the finding of a uterus allows the diagnosis of PMDS. In dogs and cats with a female phenotype the measurement of testosterone after stimulation with hCG or GnRH can prove the presence of testicular tissue. Studies of the secretion of oestrogen, LH, and (if possible) FSH can contribute to the diagnosis. In Basset Hounds with PMDS the internal female genitalia cannot be detected by radiographic examinations but are easily found by ultrasonography (Fig. 8–11) or laparoscopy.[24]

Treatment. Resection of an os clitoris stops vulvar irritation. Dogs with PMDS and clinical signs were successfully treated by hysterectomy (Fig. 8–12). Most cases also required orchiectomy be-

164

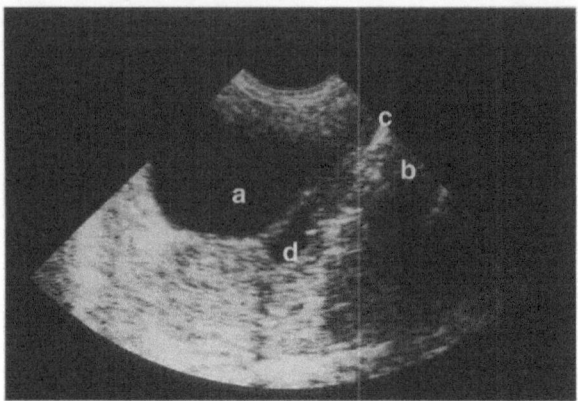

Fig. 8-11. Longitudinal ultrasonogram from the ventral abdominal wall of a male Bassethound with Persistent Müllerian Duct Syndrome. Dorsal to the bladder (a) and craniodorsal to the prostate (b) and cranial urethra (c) the persistent Müllerian duct (d) is visualized.

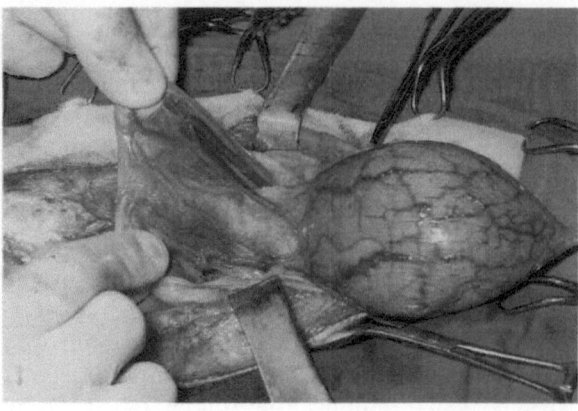

Fig. 8-12. Photograph of persistent Müllerian ducts in a male Basset Hound dog during laparotomy. The bladder is pulled caudally to reveal the uterus and uterine horns (between the fingers of the surgeon).

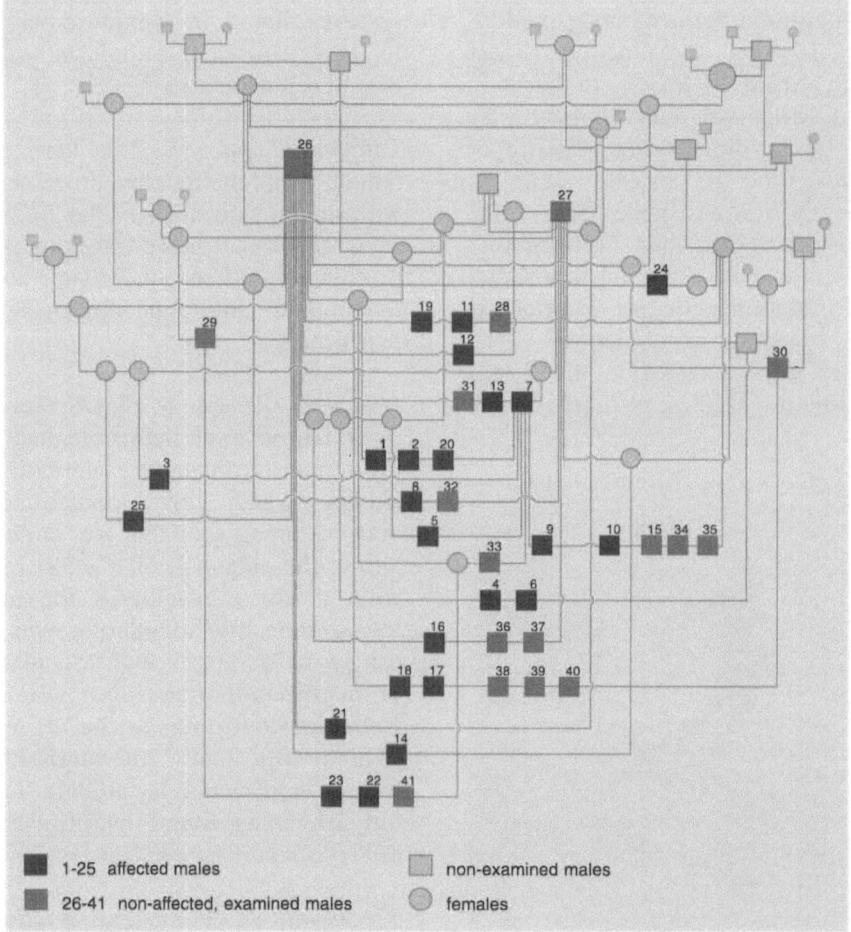

Fig. 8-13. Schematic representation of familial relations in Basset Hound dogs with Persistent Müllerian Duct Syndrome. Mating of assumed male carriers (e.g., nos. 26 and 27) with related females results in affected offspring (e.g., nos. 14 and 21). Offspring from an affected male dog (no. 7) include even more affected littermates, supporting an autosomal recessive mode of inheritance.

cause of abnormalities of the epidydimis or testis. Selective hysterectomy/vasectomy can be performed in dogs with PMDS having unaffected testes and epidydimis.

Prognosis. Surgical therapy usually solves the clinical problems. Breeding of dogs with PMDS should be discouraged. As both parents of affected animals are carriers, some advice on breeding management should be given (Fig. 8–13).

9. Parathyroids

9.1 Introduction

The parathyroid glands generally consist of four small oval disks with a diameter of 1 to 5 mm. The two largest parathyroids arise from the fourth branchial pouches and remain almost stationary during embryonic development, accounting for their final location at the cranial pole of the thyroid (Fig. 9–1). Two smaller parathyroids are usually located beneath the thyroid capsule, embedded at various depths near the caudal thyroid pole. They develop from the third branchial pouches in association with the thymus; migration with the descent of the thymus may give rise to ectopic parathyroid tissue.

The major cell of the parathyroids is the so-called chief cell, which is the parathyroid-hormone (PTH) secretory cell. These cells have clear or slightly eosinophilic cytoplasm, depending on the amounts of intracellular fat and glycogen (Fig. 9–2). The cytoplasm of active chief cells has a higher density due to the abundance of organelles and membrane-bound secretion granules, as well as to the loss of glycogen and lipid.

PTH synthesis and secretion. In the species studied PTH is an 84-amino-acid linear polypeptide, that is synthesized from pre- and pro-forms as outlined in Fig. 1–3. The intact 1–84 molecule is the major circulating form. The full biologic activity of the intact hormone resides within the amino-terminal 1–34 fragment. In the absence of a stimulus for release such as in association with hypercalcemia, intraglandular metabolism occurs, causing the release of biologically inactive carboxy-terminal fragments. Conversely, in association with hypocalcemia, degradation of PTH within the parathyroid cell is minimal, and the major product released is intact bioactive PTH.

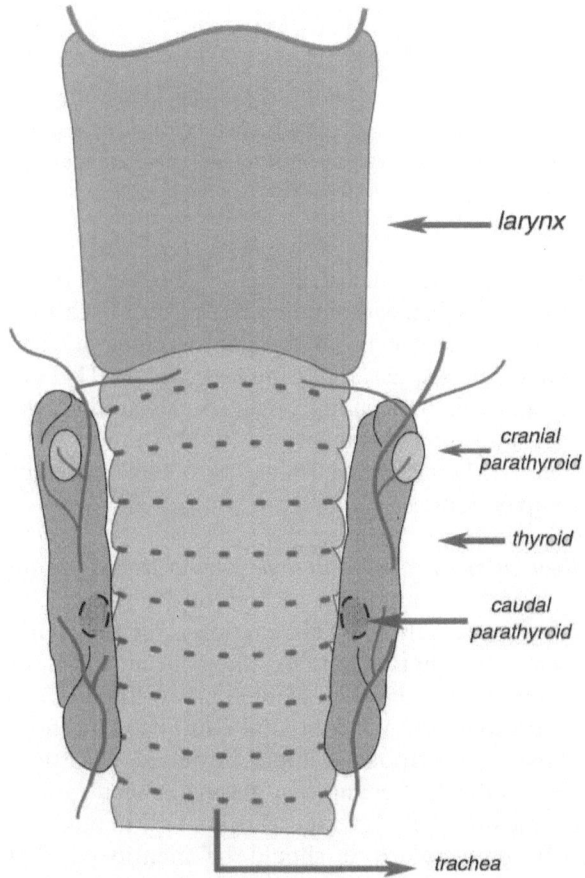

Fig. 9-1. Schematic illustration of the location of the parathyroid glands. The cranial or "external" parathyroids are loosely attached to the thyroid capsule. The caudal or "internal" parathyroids are subcapsular and usually embedded in thyroid tissue.

Circulating carboxy-terminal fragments may also be derived from peripheral (largely renal) breakdown of the intact hormone. As with the fragments of parathyroid origin, this may result in high immunoreactive PTH concentrations not

167

A. Rijnberk (ed.), Clinical Endocrinology of Dogs and Cats, 167–175.
© 1996 *Kluwer Academic Publishers.*

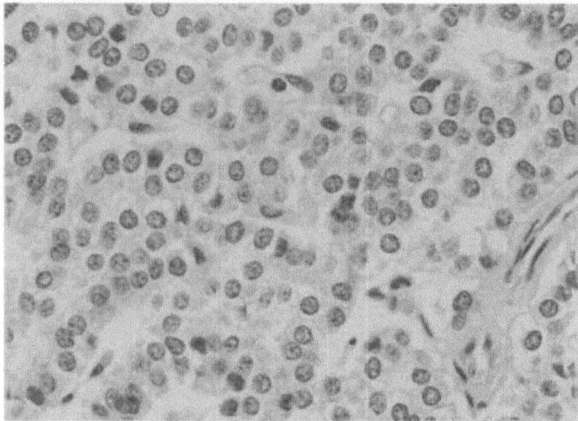

Fig. 9-2. Histologic section of the parathyroid gland of a dog with renal secondary hyperparathyroidism; note the the large pale (= active) chief cells (60×, H & E).

related to the concentrations of bioactive PTH, especially when radioimmunoassays are used that recognize the carboxy-terminal fragment. The amino acid sequences of canine and feline PTH are not known, but among other species studied the amino-terminal fragments are highly homologous, whereas the carboxy-terminal parts have different compositions.

Regulation of PTH secretion. The ionized fraction of blood calcium is the important determinant of hormone secretion. PTH secretion is regulated at a "setpoint" that maintains the concentration of plasma ionized calcium within narrow limits. Concentrations below the setpoint stimulate and those above the setpoint inhibit hormone secretion. These effects of changes in plasma concentrations of calcium on PTH secretion occur within minutes.

In this context it should be mentioned that commonly total (= bound and ionized) rather than ionized, calcium is measured. Therefore one should be aware of factors that may influence the fraction of plasma calcium that is ionized. Of these, the circulating albumin concentration is of greatest relevance, since it is the main calcium-binding protein. When in patients with hypoalbuminemia a "normal" plasma calcium concentration is found, there may actually be elevated levels of ionized calcium. Acid-base status also influences the protein binding of calcium; alkalosis decreases the ionized calcium concentration and acidosis increases it.

PTH action. Binding of PTH to a plasma membrane receptor causes a rise in cyclic 3′,5′-adenosine monophosphate (cAMP) and possibly other second messengers (see also Fig. 1–4) in cells of the main target organs: kidney and bone. In the kidney this results in (1) enhanced reabsorption of calcium from the glomerular filtrate, (2) increased excretion of phosphate, and (3) activation of 1-α-hydroxylase, the enzyme that catalyzes the formation of calcitriol [$1,25(OH)_2$ vitamin D] (see also Chapter 10).

In bone, PTH causes the release of calcium and phosphate into the extracellular fluid by changing the shape of the osteoblasts, which secondarily promotes osteoclast activity (Chapter 10, Fig. 10–4). The combination of calcium mobilisation from bone and the retention of calcium by the kidneys causes the plasma calcium concentration to rise. As mentioned above, also the formation of calcitriol is stimulated, which enhances intestinal calcium and phosphate absorption and thereby contributes to the maintenance of normocalcemia. The phosphatemic action on bone, and indirectly on intestine, tends to blunt the hypercalcemic effect of the hormone owing to the formation of calcium phosphate complexes, but this is counteracted by the phosphaturic action of PTH.

9.2 Hypoparathyroidism

Hypoparathyroidism is the state of deficient PTH secretion or action. The latter may be the result of the release of biologically ineffective hormone or unresponsiveness of target cells, but so far these abnormalities have not been observed in dogs and cats. Thus for the time being for these species the definition of the disease may be confined to deficient secretion of PTH. As with other endocrine glands theoretically a primary form and a secondary form can be distinguished. Secondary hypoparathyroidism is encountered in situations of hypercalcemia, which has an inhibitory influence on PTH release (Section 9.1). However, just because of the causative hypercalcemia, the hypofunction will not become manifest as such. In contrast, primary hypoparathyroidism has serious clinical consequences.

Pathogenesis. From a pathogenetic point of view there are two main causes of primary PTH deficiency: (1) neck surgery, and (2) idiopathic disease. The former type is especially encountered following surgical treatment of hyperthyroidism or primary hyperparathyroidism. It may be a transient or a permanent hormone deficiency, depending on the viability of the tissue left in situ at the time of surgery (see Sections 3.4.1, 9.3.1).

This section will concentrate on the second form. In this spontaneous disease the few histological studies available have revealed parathyroid atrophy, i.e., no parathyroid tissue may be found on surgical exploration.[1] In addition lymphocytic infiltrations have been found in some cases, suggesting an immune mediated cause of the atrophy.[2,3]

Clinical manifestations. In both the dog and the cat spontaneous hypoparathyroidism is rare. The disease may occur at almost any age but the occurrence appears to be highest in young adults (1–4 years of age).

The presenting signs and symptoms are directly attributable to the decreased concentration of extracelluar ionized calcium. The rate of decrease in plasma calcium is an important determinant in the development of neuromuscular manifestations. For example, signs of hypocalcemic tetany may occur in dogs after bilateral thyroidectomy when calcium values are still higher (e.g., 1.8 mmol/l) than might be found in cases of spontaneous PTH

deficiency, in which a plasma calcium concentration of 1.3 mmol/l may not be associated with clinical manifestations of tetany.

Neuromuscular signs include focal muscle twitching, rear limb cramping, generalized muscle spasms, and convulsions. The onset of these neuromuscular signs often occurs during exercise, excitement, or stress. In some cases intense facial rubbing and licking and biting of the legs may be seen, which can be interpreted as paresthesias due to increased sensory excitability, known from the disease in man.[4] In addition there may be lethargy and anorexia. On the other hand, once tetany occurs there may be an alarm reaction giving rise to restlessness and panting.

Examination reveals a somewhat anxious and panting animal that may have a stiff gait, muscle rigidity, and muscle fasciculations. The increased muscle tone may lead to hyperthermia. The cardiac manifestations of hypocalcemia may include a weak femoral pulse. In the ECG prolongation of the QT interval and T wave changes such as peaking and inversion may be seen (Fig. 9–3).

Differential diagnosis. Not completely identical but similar neuromuscular features may be observed in hypoglycemia (Section 5.3), epilepsy, and possibly tetanus. Occasionally also severe hyperkalemia may give rise to muscle twitching (Section 4.2.1). As to the cause of hypocalcemia, in principle conditions such as renal failure, puerperal tetany, ethylene glycol (antifreeze) poison-

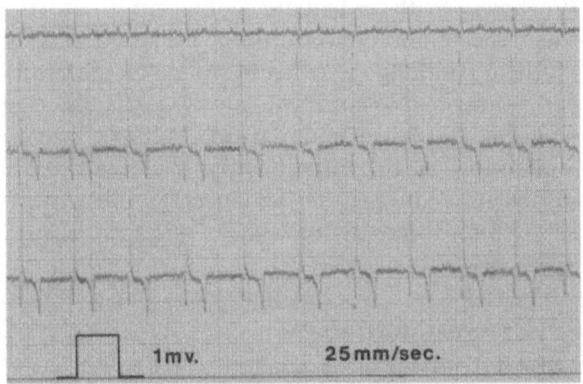
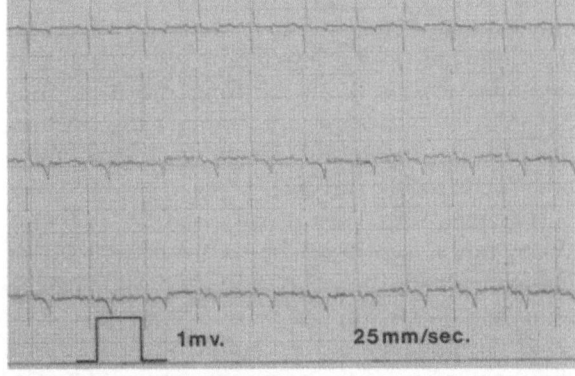

Fig. 9-3. ECG recordings (lead I, II, and III) of a 2-year-old female German Shepherd with primary hypoparathyroidism (calibration: 1 cm = 1 mV; paper speed 25 mm/s). Left: On admission (total plasma calcium concentration 1.0 mmol/l) the recordings were disturbed by muscle twitching. In addition, the T waves were deep and wide. Right: During administration of calcium these ECG changes disappeared; at the time this recording was made total plasma calcium concentration had only increased to 1.35 mmol/l (Courtesy of J.J. van Nes and A.A. Stokhof.)

ing, acute pancreatitis and hypoalbuminemia may also be considered, but usually associated signs and symptoms point to the underlying disease so that there is little chance of confusion.

Diagnosis. In the absence of renal failure, the diagnosis of hypoparathyroidism is virtually certain if hypocalcemia and hyperphosphatemia are found. The diagnosis may be further supported by measurements of basal concentrations of plasma PTH. An undetectable plasma PTH concentration confirms the diagnosis, provided the assay used is sensitive enough to measure plasma PTH in healthy animals. Commercially available assays for intact and midmolecular human PTH have been validated for use in dogs (Fig. 10–11) and cats.[6,7]

Treatment. Emergency treatment of hypocalcemic tetany, requires slow (5–10 min) intravenous injection of calcium in a dose of 0.5–1.0 mmol Ca^{++}/kg body weight (= 20–40 mg Ca^{++}/kg) as calcium gluconate (= roughly a total dose of 2–5 ml of a 20% solution). Once the signs of hypocalcemia are controlled, the calcium gluconate can be administered subcutaneously (1:2 diluted with NaCl 0.9%) every 6 h until oral medication can be started.

Oral maintenance therapy comprises supplementation with the vitamin-D compound dihydrotachysterol[a] and calcium lactate or carbonate. Dihydrotachysterol is given initially in a dose of 20–30 µg/kg body weight, together with calcium lactate (25–50 mg/kg). After about 2–3 weeks dihydrotachysterol reaches its maximal effect and the dose has to be lowered to prevent hypercalcemia (Fig. 9–4). In the long run it is often possible to omit supplementation with calcium; the calcium supply via commercially manufactured foods will be sufficient.

Hypercalcemia may reveal itself by polyuria. When this is confirmed by measurements of the plasma calcium concentration, the supplementation should be stopped to minimize the risk of renal insufficiency due to nephrocalcinosis. With discontinuation of the administration of dihydrotachysterol there is no immediate risk of hypo-

---

[a] Dihydral®, Duphar, Amsterdam and Roxane Laboratories, Columbus OH (0.2 mg dihydrotachysterol per tablet).

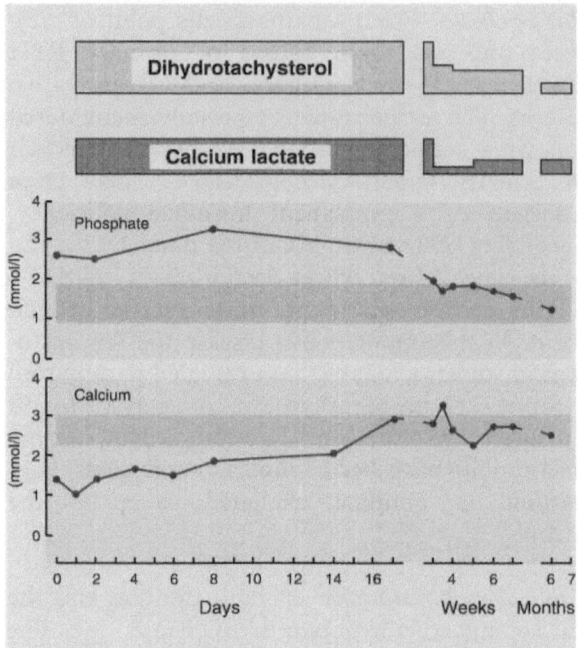

Fig. 9-4. The dog described in the legend of Fig. 9–3 was initially treated twice daily with 500 µg dihydrotachysterol and 2.5 g calcium lactate. This caused the plasma calcium concentration to gradually rise until it was within the reference range (zone). When hypercalcemia developed the doses were lowered. The dog did very well for many years on twice daily 100 µg dihydrotachesterol and twice daily 1 g calcium lactate as a supplement to the balanced commercial dog food. (Courtesy of J.J. van Nes.)

calcemia as the effect of the drug will cease only after several days.

Prognosis. With adequate monitoring of the plasma calcium concentration the prognosis is excellent. Initially the calcium should be measured daily and when less critical, weekly. Once the dog or cat is stable on maintenance therapy, two to four follow-up examinations per year are usually sufficient. With proper guidance the life expectancy is not different from that of a healthy dog.

9.3 Hyperparathyroidism

Hyperparathyroidism can be primary or secondary. Primary hyperparathyroidism is the state of autonomous hypersecretion of PTH, most commonly by an adenoma of the chief cells. Secondary hyperparathyroidism is an adaptive increase in

PTH secretion, unrelated to intrinsic disease of the parathyroids. In the latter, the increased PTH secretion is the result of chronic (tendencies to) decreases in the concentration of ionized calcium in plasma. Several conditions may lead to these events, but in dogs and cats there are only two in which secondary hyperparathyroidism produces clinically significant manifestations: chronic renal failure (Section 9.3.1) and calcium deficiency during growth (Section 10.2).

9.3.1 Primary hyperparathyroidism

Pathogenesis. A small solitary parathyroid adenoma (Fig. 9–5) is the most common cause of primary hyperparathyroidism in both the dog and

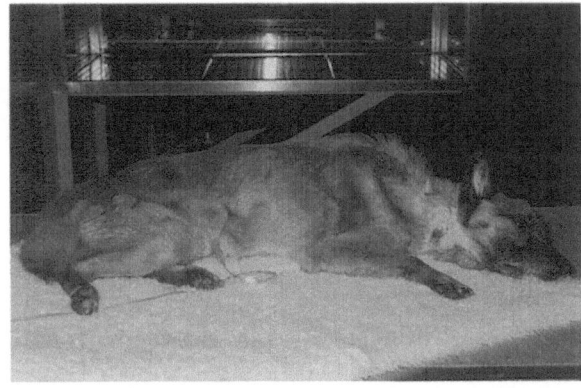

Fig. 9-6. A 9-year-old male Malines Shepherd with emaciation, dehydration, and weight loss due to primary hyperparathyroidism.

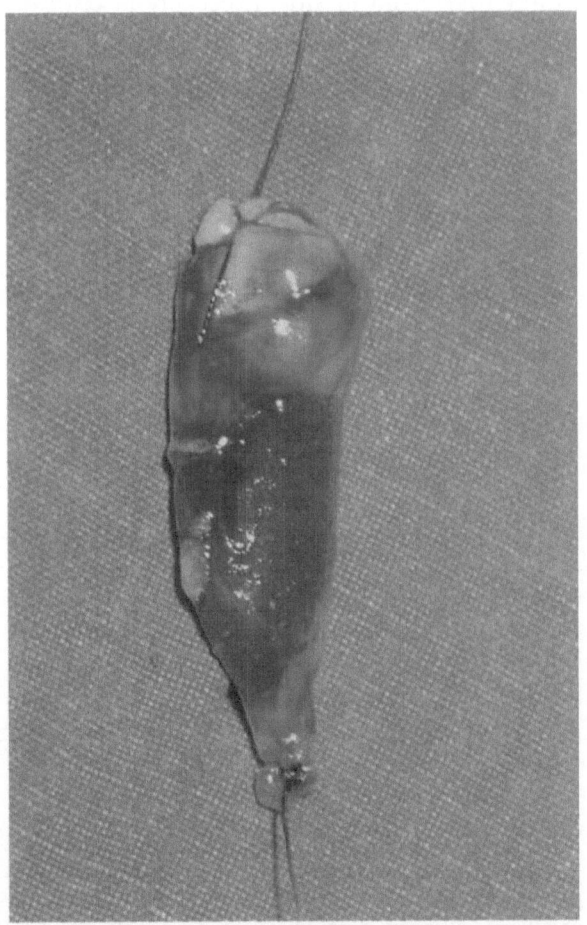

Fig. 9-5. Surgical specimen following unilateral thyroparathyroidectomy in a 9-year-old male Malines Shepherd with primary hyperparathyroidism. Note the parathyroid adenoma originating from the parathyroid tissue at the cranial pole (top) of the thyroid gland.

cat.[8,9] At surgery the other glands may appear normal or atrophied. The PTH excess may also be caused by only minimally enlarged glands with multiple nodular hyperplasias, that may be present in more than one parathyroid gland.[10] Very rarely the disease is caused by a parathyroid carcinoma.[8]

Clinical manifestations. Primary hyperparathyroidism is an uncommon disease of older dogs (≥ 7 years) and there is no pronounced sex predilection. In cats the disease is even less frequent and occurs in the same age range, possibly with a predilection for females and Siamese cats.[9]

The disease may be asymptomatic or there may be mild or severe systemic illness. Roughly three categories or stages of presentation can be distinguished. In the mildest form there may be no symptoms or signs and the disease is discovered because hypercalcemia is found by a routine laboratory examination. In the second form polyuria develops insidiously in an otherwise healthy dog; in cats polyuria is less common.[10] In the third and so far most common form the disease period may be rather short and the animals are presented with polyuria/polydipsia (dogs!) and lethargy, anorexia (and vomiting), weakness, and weight loss. Especially in cats the manifestations may be rather nonspecific and can be confined to anorexia and malaise.

When presented cases in the third category are usually characterized by weakness and lethargy (Fig. 9–6). Because of the small size of the parathyroid lesions, they are rarely palpable. If a mass is palpable, the possibility of a carcinoma should

172

be considered.[11] Radiography and routine laboratory data (other than calcium and phosphate) are usually unremarkable, unless the disease is complicated by renal failure or pancreatitis.

Differential diagnosis. The main problem in the differential diagnosis of primary hyperparathyroidism is distinguishing it from other conditions associated with hypercalcemia and specifically hypercalcemia of malignancy (Chapter 11). Other causes of hypercalcemia such as hypervitaminosis D (Section 10.3.2), (acute) renal failure and primary hypoadrenocorticism (Section 4.2.1) pose less of a diagnostic problem because of the changes associated with the primary disease.

Diagnosis. The presence of hypercalcemia is established when three measurements of total plasma calcium concentration reveal values exceeding the reference range. This, in combination with normo- or hypophosphatemia and the appropriate signs, may give rise to the suspicion of primary hyperparathyroidism. Nevertheless, the approach should be to exclude hypercalcemia of malignancy, which is more common than hypercalcemia of parathyroid origin. The exclusion procedures include careful inspection or the perianal region, thoracic radiography and cytological examination of aspirates from lymph node(s) and/or bone marrow (see also Section 10.3.2).

Definite distinction between parathyroid and nonparathyroid causes of hypercalcemia may rely on measurements of plasma PTH concentrations. As discussed in Section 9.1 this is best performed with the two-site type of assay that measures intact PTH and is unaffected by renal function. In the absence of renal failure (see also 9.3.2) an elevated PTH level confirms the diagnosis of primary hyperparathyroidism, as animals with hypercalcemia of non-parathyroid origin should have low PTH concentrations as a result of the inhibitory effect of hypercalcemia on parathyroid gland function. A serious diagnostic problem may arise when it is suspected that primary hyperparathyroidism is complicated by renal failure; for a final diagnosis a surgical exploration of the neck may be needed.

Often the results of the PTH measurements are not available at the time that treatment is required. Therefore, if the history and physical examination

are compatible with primary hyperparathyroidism, and other causes of hypercalcemia have been excluded as well as posssible, surgical exploration of the neck can be performed for a definitive diagnosis and (hopefully) treatment.

Treatment. In most cases a solitary and easily recognizable parathyroid adenoma is found at surgery. Removal results in a rapid decline in plasma calcium concentration and a rise (if lowered) in the phosphate level (Fig. 9–7). When an adenoma is not identified immediately, all four parathyroid glands should be inspected carefully for the presence of (multiple) nodular hyperplasia. In that case macroscopically suspected gland(s) are removed, thereby leaving of course at least one parathyroid gland in situ. Especially in critically hypercalcemic cases perioperative measures to

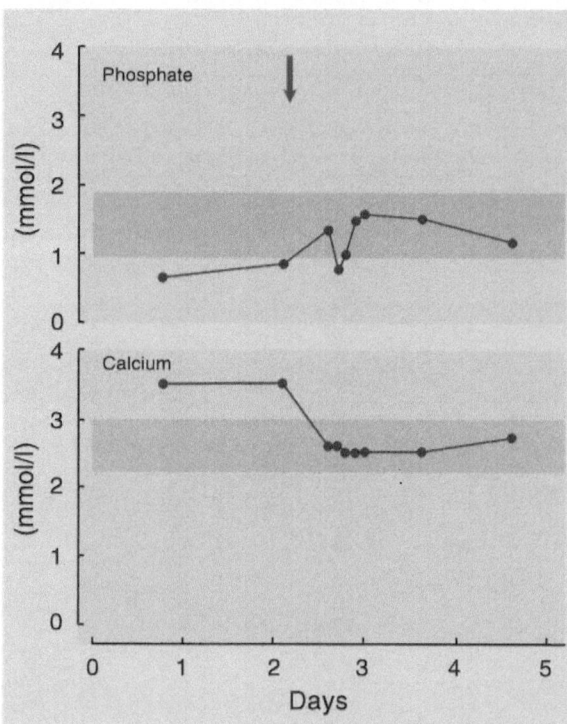

Fig. 9-7. Plasma calcium and phosphate concentrations in a 7-year-old castrated female Airdale Terrier with primary hyperparathyroidism before and after removal (arrow) of a solitary parathyroid adenoma measuring 7 × 5 × 4 mm. Plasma PTH concentrations ranged from 15 to 22 ng/l. In this dog the disease was rather mild and of short duration (polyuria lasting 3–4 weeks), and apparently had not yet caused suppression of the nonaffected parathyroid tissue and postsurgical hypocalcemia.

reduce the hypercalcemia (see also Chapter 14) should be directed at increasing urinary calcium excretion by volume expansion, i.e., intravenous therapy with isotonic saline.

Following removal of the parathyroid adenoma there is a rapid decline in the circulating PTH concentration, while the unaffected parathyroids are still suppressed from the long-term hypercalcemia. This together with the elevated calcium accretion ("bone hunger") may lead to post-operative hypocalcemia. Therefore plasma calcium concentration should be monitored post-surgically (Fig. 9–7). In order to prevent signs of hypocalcemia, administration of dihydro-tachesterol and calcium lactate (see Section 9.2) should be started when the plasma calcium concentration declines to the lower limit of the reference range. If signs of tetany have already occurred, calcium gluconate can be given intravenously and/or subcutaneously (see 9.2).

The aim is to maintain the plasma concentration in the lower part of the normal range, so that there is sufficient stimulus for restoration of the function of the remaining parathyroid tissue. It may be necessary to continue this substitution for several weeks. Once the plasma calcium concentration is stable, withdrawal of the dihydro-tachysterol can be attempted gradually by first giving it every other day and then increasing the number of days between administration. When the hypocalcemia does not recur, the calcium supplementation can also be lowered gradually. One should be careful not to induce hypercalcemia, as this is now a more serious risk than in primary hyperparathyroidism; dihydrotachysterol induces not only hypercalcemia but also (a tendency to) hyperphosphatemia, which combination much more easily leads to nephrocalcinosis (Section 10.3.2) than hypercalcemia per se.

Prognosis. When the source of the PTH excess can be removed successfully and the perioperative period can be overcome adequately, the prognosis is excellent.

9.3.2 Renal secondary hyperparathyroidism

Pathogenesis. Several factors are involved in the pathogenesis of secondary hyperparathyroidism in animals with chronic renal failure (Fig. 9–8). The

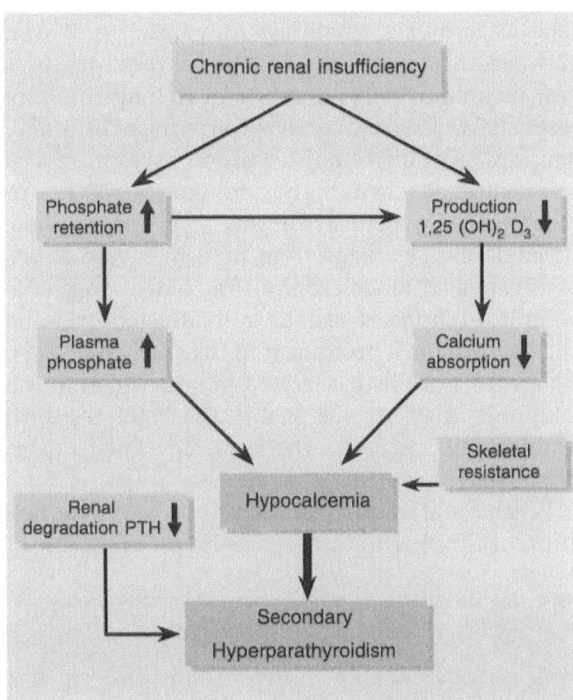

Fig. 9-8. Principal factors involved in the pathogenesis of secondary hyperparathyroidism due to chronic renal insufficiency. The main stimuli are (1) renal retention of phosphate, wich causes precipitation of calcium in soft tissues, and (2) decreased production of 1,25(OH)$_2$D.

initial stimulus appears to be chronic reduction in circulating ionized calcium because of renal retention of phosphate. High concentrations of phosphate in plasma may precipitate calcium in soft tissues and also seem to decrease the release of calcium from bone.[12] In addition, decreased production of 1,25(OH)$_2$D$_3$ in the kidney causes a reduction in the intestinal absorption of calcium. A further contributing factor to the hypocalcemia is the relative skeletal resistance to PTH. The concerted actions of these factors lead to hypocalcemia, which stimulates PTH secretion and results in hypertrophy of all parathyroid glands. Finally, the renal insufficiency contributes to the increase in PTH levels because it is associated with a decreased rate of removal of the hormone from the circulation. As discussed in Section 9.1 there is also an increase in biologically inactive PTH fragments.

Clinical manifestations. The animal may be presented with the classic signs of renal insufficiency,

174

such as anorexia, vomiting, polydipsia, polyuria, and depression, but in some cases these features may be mild or only intermittent. In long-standing cases signs of secondary hyperparathyroidism may develop. Although not common, symptoms of neuromuscular irritability and tetany similar to those of hypoparathyroidism may occur. The skeletal changes range from mild to severe forms of fibrous osteodystrophy. In older dogs the volume of bone is usually not affected and the changes are most prominent in the skull (Fig. 9–9). As a result of the accelerated bone resorption the mandibles may become pliable, for which the term "rubber jaw" is used. The jaws may fail to close properly (Fig. 9–10).

When renal insufficiency develops before maturation of the skeleton the repair by proliferation of

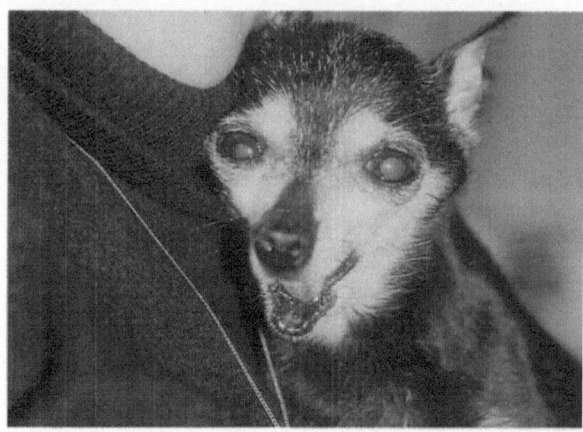

Fig. 9-10. A 14-year-old mongrel dog with chronic renal insufficiency. The associated secondary hyperparathyroidism had caused severe bone demineralization with a so-called "rubber jaw" and the inability to close the mouth.

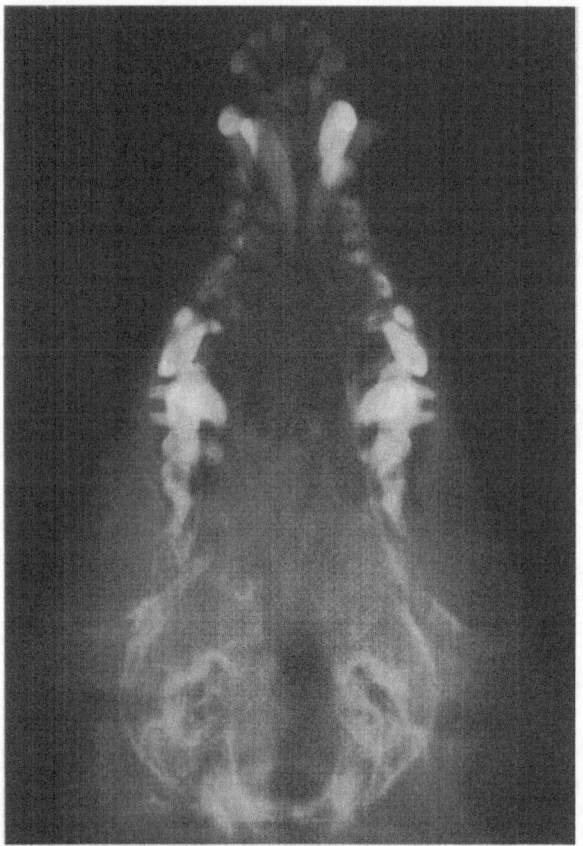

Fig. 9-9. Demineralization of all bones of the skull and mandible of a dog with advanced secondary renal hyperparathyroidism. Due to subperiosteal bone resorption the contours of the bone are hardly visible. The teeth have maintained a normal density, causing an increased contrast between teeth and bone.

connective tissue may exceed the rate of bone resorption. This results in an increase in bone volume. This hyperostotic osteodystrophy results in facial swelling (Fig. 9–11).

The laboratory findings are usually dominated by the abnormalities associated with the renal insufficiency, such as elevated plasma levels of urea, creatinine, and phosphate. Despite the often (low) normal plasma calcium values, PTH secretion increases and gradually causes the above skeletal changes.

Treatment. The most important step in the prevention and treatment of renal osteodystrophy is the restriction of phosphorus. This also has a beneficial effect on kidney function, to which an adaptation of the protein intake may also contribute.[13] The phosphate restriction may be reinforced by administering aluminum-containing antacids that prevent phosphate absorption. In cases in which there is a tendency to hypocalcemia this approach may be extended by supplementation with calcium and vitamin D sterols (Section 9.2). The associated lowering of the circulating PTH levels is said to be beneficial in the progression of the renal insufficiency, although this has not been convincingly demonstrated.[14] In addition there is evidence that administration of vitamin D analogues decreases appetite, even before hypercalcemia is induced.[15]

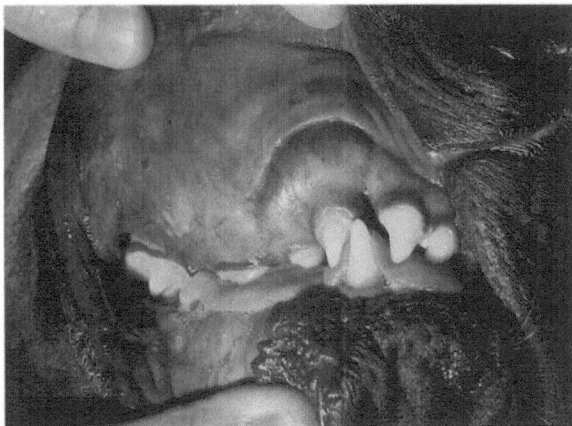

Fig. 9-11. A 7-month-old male Great Dane with renal insufficiency. In this young dog the secondary hyperparathyroidism had caused hyperostotic osteodysthrophy, which had led to facial swelling (left). Lifting of the upper lip (right) revealed that the facial swelling was due to increased volume of the maxilla.

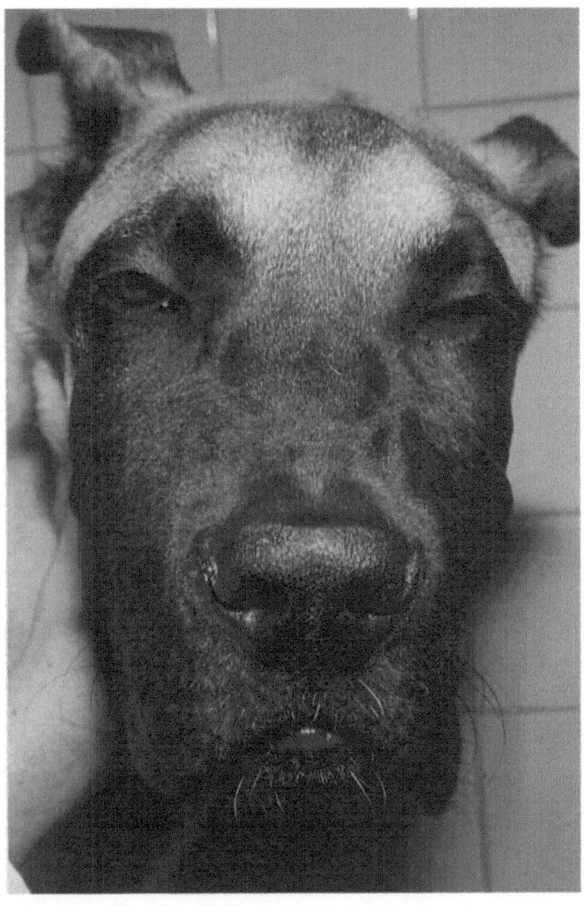

9.4 Puerperal tetany

At the peak of lactation, two to three weeks postpartum, hypocalcemia may occur in bitches and less often in queens. Little is known about the pathogenesis, but insufficient calcium supply during nursing may be a causative factor.

Clinical manifestations. Once the plasma calcium concentration has reached a critical level, the signs may proceed rapidly from restlessness, panting, and ataxia to tetany with tonic/clonic convulsions and opisthotonus. Examination usually reveals an anxious, restless animal with tachycardia and hyperthermia. The condition is fatal if left untreated. Laboratory examination will reveal hypocalcemia and usually also hypophosphatemia.

Diagnosis. The diagnosis is usually made by the recognition of the combination of a heavily lactating animal with signs of increased neuromuscular excitability.

Treatment. The treatment is begun without delay, i.e., without laboratory confirmation. As in hypocalcemia of primary hypoparathyroidism (Section 9.2), calcium gluconate is injected intravenously. The signs of tetany usually disappear within a few minutes. In order to prevent rapid recurrence a similar dose is given subcutaneously. Puppies or kittens should be removed to reduce the lactational calcium loss. When sufficiently mature, the puppies or kittens can be weaned. If not, they can be returned after 24 h and in the meantime fed a milk substitute.

Prognosis. With a nutritionally balanced diet and oral calcium supplementation (Section 9.2) during the remaining of the lactation period, there are usually no recurrences. For the next pregnancy and lactation care should given to supply the dam with a complete, well-balanced diet. Additional feeding of the litter with a milk substitute early in lactation and with food as early as possible, may also help to prevent tetany. There is no need to give extra calcium in excess of the normal requirements during pregnancy, and in line with experiences in other species it may even be contraindicated.

10. Calciotropic hormones and bone metabolism

10.1 Introduction

Functionally the skeleton can be considered as two organs: (1) a supporting and protecting framework, and (2) a reservoir of minerals. Each has its own regulatory mechanism with consequences for skeletal integrity, involving the same cellular structures. Since most cellular activity occurs during skeletal growth, most derangements of skeletal integrity are observed during early life.

Growth in width of the long bones starts when the periosteum, surrounding the cartilaginous template, forms primitive (i.e., woven) bone which organizes itself into highly organized lamellar bone.[1] Growth in length of the long bones is limited to those places in which cartilage remains during the adolescent life, namely, the juncture between the primary (diaphysis) and secondary (epiphysis) ossification centres (Fig. 10–1). The cartilage also extends to the epiphyseal ends of the long bone, allowing for the proportional growth of the epiphyses. This longitudinal growth occurs via the process of endochondral ossification[2,3] (Fig. 10–1).

In adulthood, about one quarter of bone is organic material (of which 90% is collagen) and about three quarters inorganic material. The latter is initially a poorly crystallized calcium phosphate

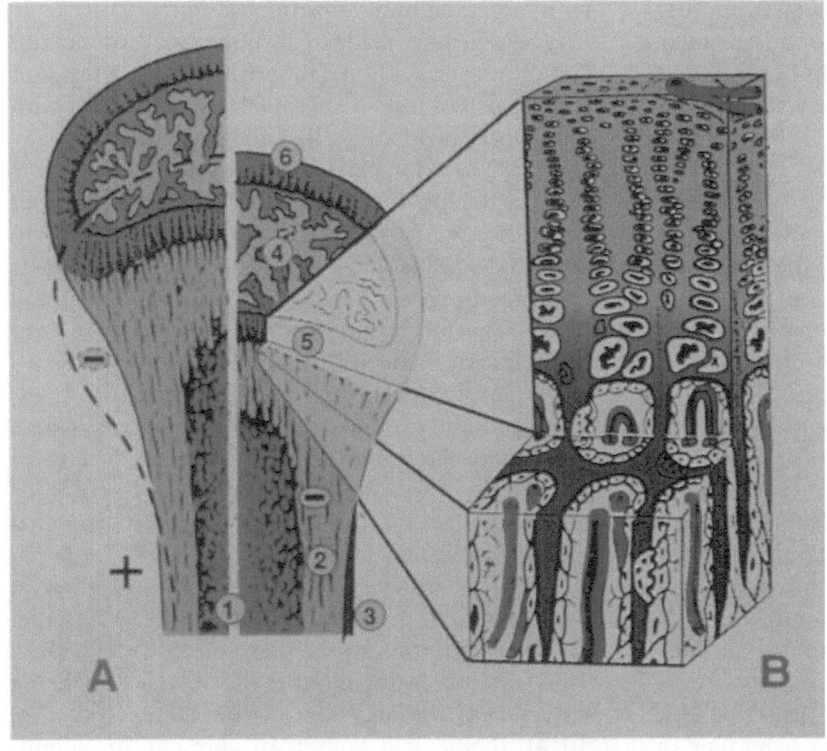

Fig. 10-1. A: Schematic representation of the proximal end of a long bone with (1) medullary cavity, (2) diaphysis, (3) periosteum, (4) secondary ossification centre (epiphysis), (5) physeal growth plate, (6) epiphyseal cartilage. During longitudinal growth (↑) periosteal bone formation (+) and bone resorption (—) in the medulla and at metaphyseal sides, maintain the bone's characteristic form as part of the remodelling process. B: The inset shows the process of endochondral ossification: chondrocytes are orientated in rows and while dividing and enlarging, they move away from their nutrient vessel. The intercellular substance mineralizes and consequently seals off the chondrocytes from nutrition, causing death of chondrocytes in their lacunae. Metaphyseal vessels grow into the empty lacunae, introducing osteoblasts which cover the mineralized cartilage with osteoid that will be bone after its mineralization. Multinucleated chondroclasts remove the remnants of mineralized cartilage to complete the process of endochondral ossification. (Modified from Nap et al., 1994.[2])

A. Rijnberk (ed.), Clinical Endocrinology of Dogs and Cats, 177–195.
© 1996 *Kluwer Academic Publishers*.

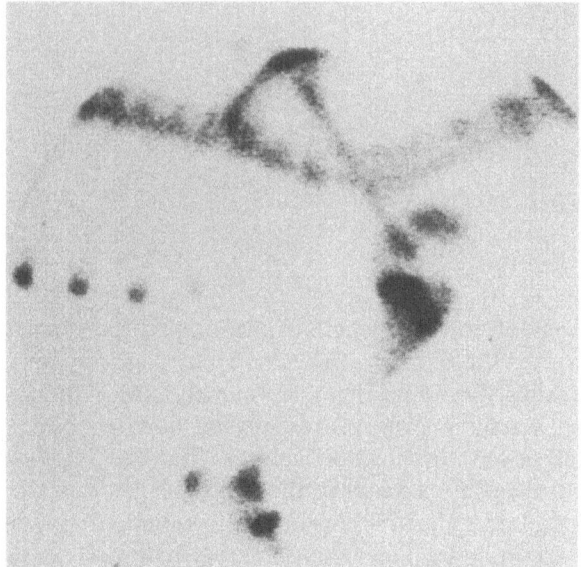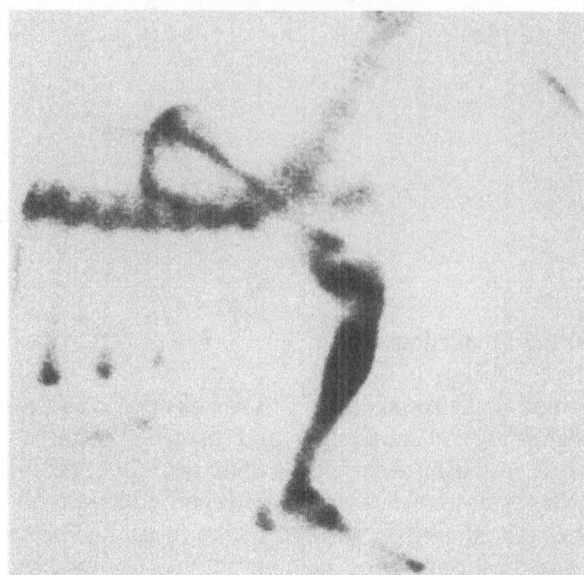

Fig. 10-2. Methylene diphosphonate is bound to newly formed bone within 2 h after its intravenous application. Labelled with $^{99m}TcO_4{}^-$, it can be used to localize physiological and pathological mineralization. Left: A bone scan of a front leg of an 8-month-old Retriever reveals high bone cell activity in the metaphyseal areas. Right: A bone scan of a 14-month-old Retriever with shifting lameness and bone pain, revealing increased bone cell activity in the medullary cavity, typical of enostosis.

and later crystalline hydroxyapatite (HA). For mineralization of bone, calcium- and phosphate-rich vesicles are extruded from osteoblasts into the extracellular matrix. In addition to this cellular regulation of mineralization, physicochemical processes of direct formation of crystalline HA and growth of HA crystals play a role in tissue mineralization. Pyrophosphate, two phosphate molecules linked through an oxygen molecule, inhibits calcium phosphate crystallization in tissues and body fluids by binding to the surface of calcium phosphate and blocking the formation and growth of HA crystals. Enzymatic degradation of pyrophosphate by alkaline phosphatase, as present in calcifying cartilage, could raise the local Ca^{2+} and $PO_4{}^{3-}$ concentration to a point where HA precipitation begins.

Diphosphonates (not normally present in biological systems and with phosphate-oxygen replaced by a phosphate-carbon binding) have the same binding and mineralization inhibiting properties as pyrophosphates and are completely stabile in an aqueous biological environment. They are used as a coating of certain implants (e.g., heart valve replacements) to prevent their mineralization and they are used as a marker of tissue mineralization.[4] By labelling diphos-phonates with ^{99m}technetium, increased radio-nuclide accumulation can be found at skeletal sites with increased mineralization[4] (Fig. 10–2).

Osteoblasts embedded in bone, i.e., osteocytes, communicate with neighbouring osteocytes and surface osteoblasts by cytoplasmic extensions running through canaliculi, allowing for ion exchange. These ion exchanges play a significant role in transducing mechanical loading in organized bone cell work, via the piezo-electric effect, to structural adjustments (Fig. 10–3). Osteoblasts covering bone surface, the so-called bone lining cells, separate multinucleated osteoclasts from bone matrix. The osteoclasts are able to resorb mineralized bone at their brush border (Fig. 10–4) and are mainly found in metaphyseal areas, where they shape the funnel, and on the inner surface of the diaphysis at the endosteal side, where they adapt the medulla to hemopoetic and mechanical demands (Fig. 10–1).

In physiological states including growth, osteoblast and osteoclast activity is coupled (Fig. 10– 4). In addition to the piezo-electric effect (Fig. 10–3), an increasing number of substances is being recognized (biologically active factors in Fig. 10–4). These substances are present in demin-eralized bone and may have the ability to attract

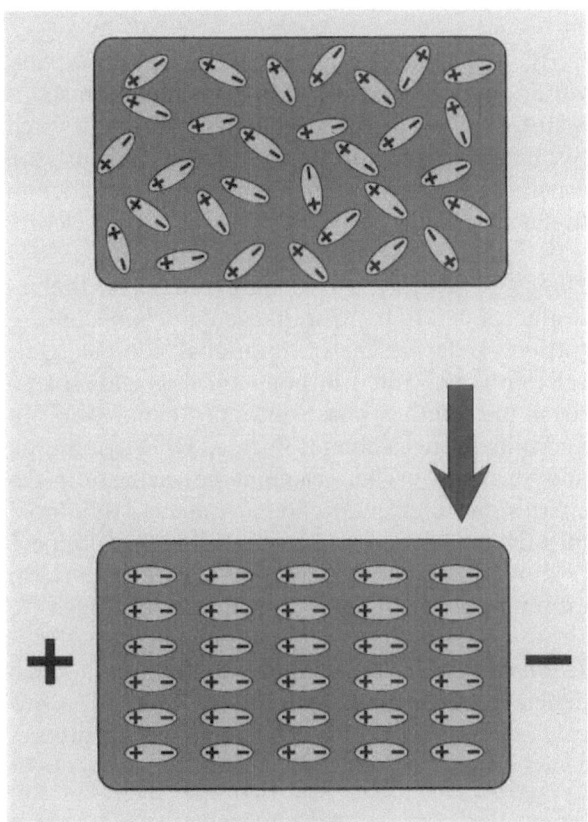

Fig. 10-3. A: Bone will adapt itself to mechanical forces. Due to the piezoelectric effect in crystals like hydroxyapatit, electrical orientation occurs under pressure with a negative loading at one side as net effect. This will stimulate osteoblasts to form bone, resulting in a decrease of pressure (closed feedback loop), whereas osteoclasts are more active at the opposite side. B: Its clinical relevance is demonstrated with a radiograph of the tibia of a 10-month-old Dachshund with severe varus deformity and thickening of the concave cortex, being more under pressure than the convex cortex. Following corrective osteotomy, fixation with a bone plate was performed, which neutralized the forces acting on the bone. The radiograph after plate removal 6 months later revealed disuse osteoporosis, i.e., osteoporosis due to lack of external forces.

A

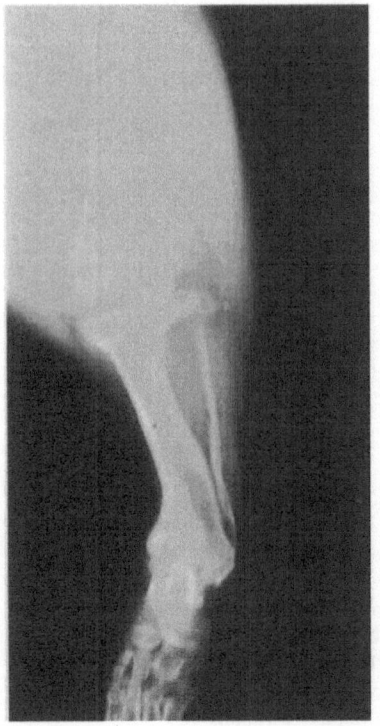 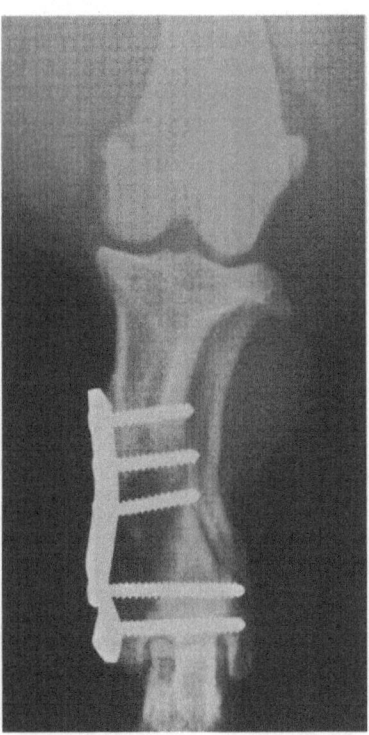 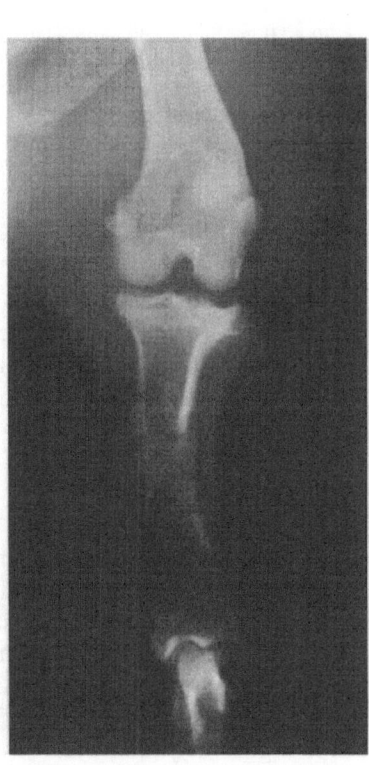

B

180

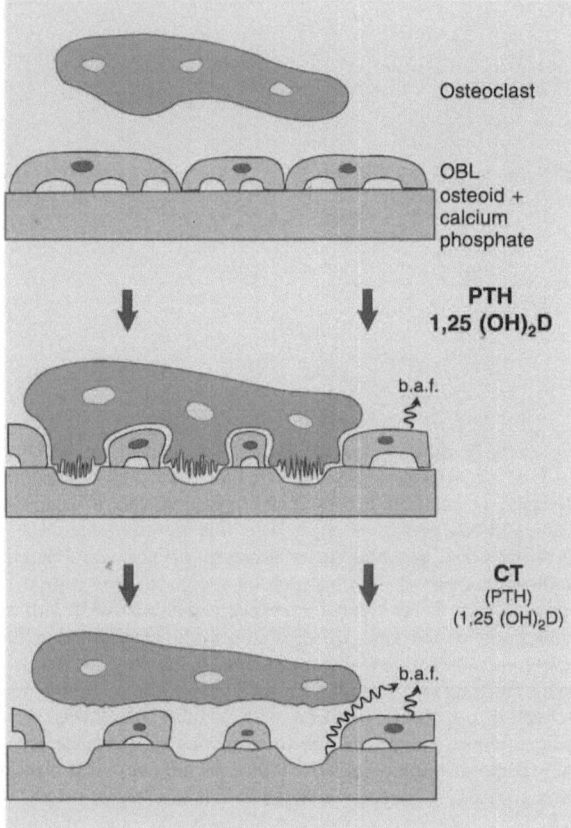

Fig. 10-4. Bone lining cells, osteoblasts (OBL), separate bone from nonresorbing osteoclasts (OCL). PTH and 1,25 (OH)₂vit D change the shape of the OBL, allowing OCL to resorb bone. CT prevents bone resorption by promoting the retraction of the brush border of the OCL; this occurs even in the presence of PTH and/or 1,25(OH)₂D. Biologically active factors, (b.a.f.) released by OBL and from the bone during resorption, have chemotactic and mitogenic actions on bone cells.

and activate bone cells.[1] The capacity of these factors is used in orthopedic surgery, when transplants of cancellous bone are placed in defects in order to accelerate bone healing.

10.2 Calcium metabolism

About half of the circulating calcium is loosely bound to plasma proteins (mostly albumin). Ten percent is bound to other ions and the remainder comprises the biologically significant ionically active fraction. In healthy states total plasma calcium concentration varies within narrow limits and is higher in young than in adult dogs, but is

fairly constant even under extreme dietary variations (Fig. 10–5). Calcium homeostasis is maintained by direct mechanisms and is assisted by calciotropic hormones.[5] Three organs are especially involved in maintenance of the calcium homeostasis: the gut, the kidney, and the skeleton.

Direct. When calcium is absorbed from the intestine, it tends to raise plasma calcium concentration. Independent of hormonal control some calcium is deposited in bone and less is dissolved from the soluble phase into the circulation. In addition, more calcium is filtrated by the glomeruli and excreted. When calcium concentration decreases, more calcium enters from the labile pool into the circulation and less is lost via the kidneys (Fig. 10–6). In both situations endogenous fecal excretion does not seem to be much influenced.

Hormonal control. In animals living in a calcium deficient environment and eating food with a low calcium content (Table 10–1), such as carnivores

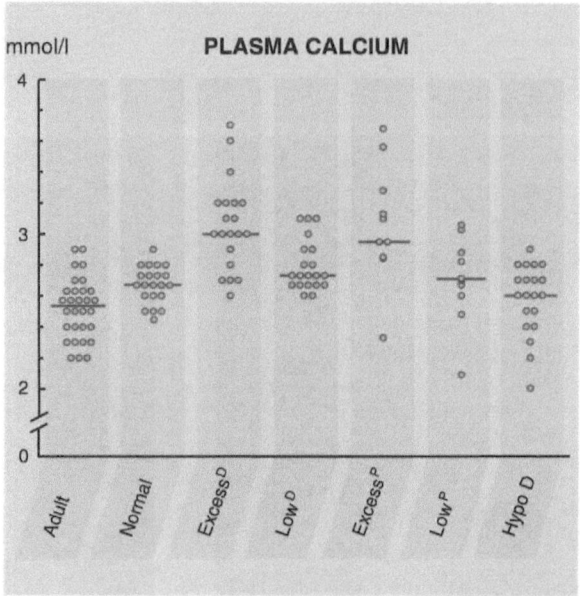

Fig. 10-5. Plasma calcium concentrations (with median values) are given for adult dogs and young dogs (all younger than 6 months) receiving food containing 1.1% calcium (normal), young Great Danes[13] fed 1 month a diet with 3.3% Ca (excess^D) or 0.55% Ca (low^D), young Poodles[23] fed 1 month a diet with 3.3% Ca (excess^P) or 0.33% Ca (low^P), and mongrel dogs on standard food only without vitamin D (HypoD). Despite 6–10× difference in daily calcium intake, the median plasma calcium concentrations vary within narrow limits.

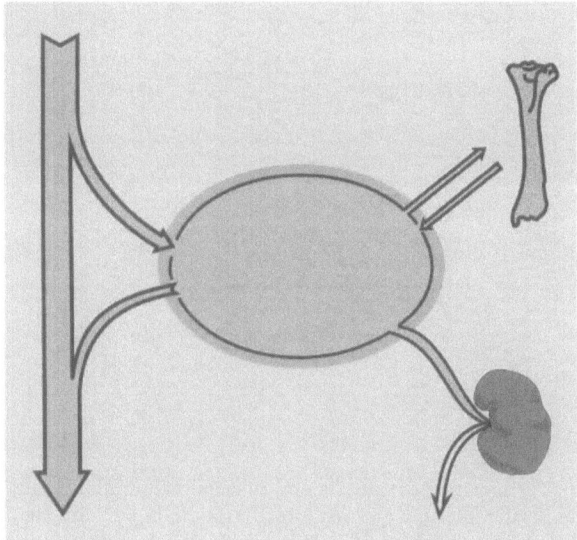

Fig. 10-6. Three organs are especially involved in calcium homeostasis: intestines, kidneys and skeleton. When calcium is absorbed from the intestine, the calcium concentration in the extracellular fluid will tend to increase. Due to *direct regulation* more calcium will be stored in the labile phase of the skeleton and more calcium will be filtered in the glomeruli, which contributes to the normalization of the calcium concentration in the extracellular fluid.

Table 10-1. Analysis of foodstuffs for carnivores.

	dry matter*	calcium*	phosphorus*	Vit D*
Horse meat	25.5	0.03	0.18	4IU
Heart	24.8	0.01	0.20	4IU
Rumen	23.3	0.11	0.14	n.k.
Liver	27.1	0.01	0.36	80 IU
Poultry by-product	30.1	0.02	0.20	n.k.
Egg	25	0.04	0.15	100 IU
Cat fish	20	0.02	0.18	20 IU
Minimal requirements for growth (NRC 1985)	100	0.59	0.44	40 IU

* = grams per 100g product   n.k. = not known

+ = IU per 100g product (1 IU vit D = 0.025µg)

Absolutely and relative to phosphorus, the calcium content of animal foodstuff is too low to fulfill the requirements, when bones are not included.

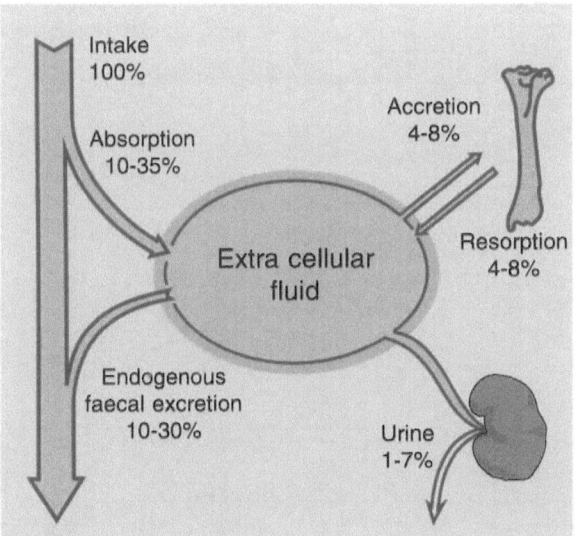

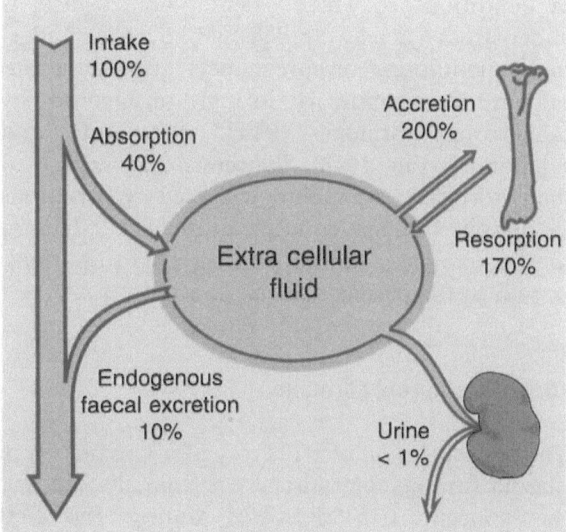

Fig. 10-7. The relative calcium fluxes in adult and young growing dogs. a: In adult dogs a calcium intake of 100 mg per kg body weight per day covers all losses. b: In young dogs calcium metabolism is characterized by high calcium turnover in the skeleton and more efficient absorption; the requirements in absolute amounts depend on the size and growth rate of the dog, and may vary from from 50–350 mg/kg body weight.

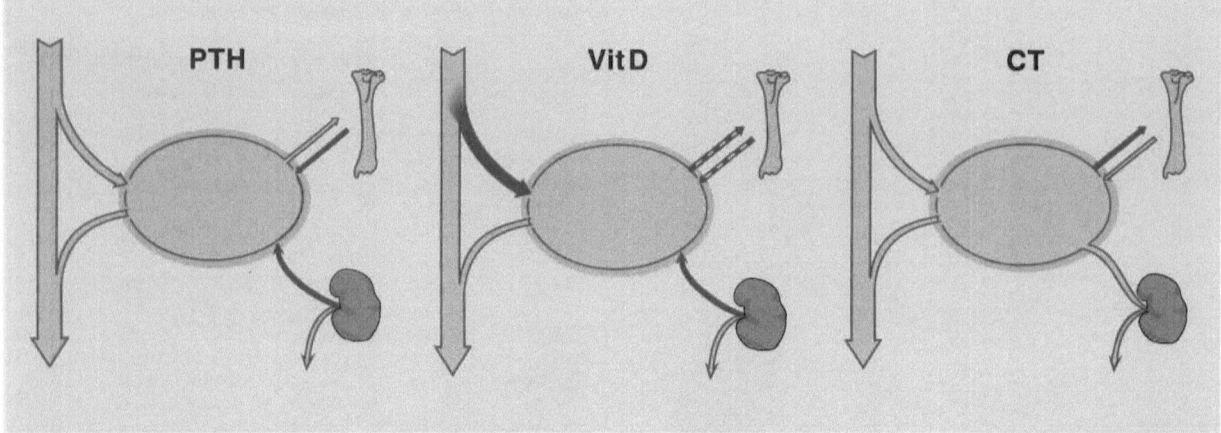

Fig. 10-8. Influences of calciotropic hormones on calcium metabolism. *PTH* increases osteoclasia and calcium reabsorption in the renal tubules. *Vitamin D* metabolites increase active calcium absorption in the intestine and renal reabsorption; in addition they activate osteoclasia and osteoid and cartilage mineralization. *CT* decreases osteoclastic activity and thus increases bone mineralization.

may when bones are not part of the meal, an efficient hormonally controlled system helps to retain calcium from the food. In adult animals, a low calcium intake may be sufficient to replace the losses in urine and feces (Fig. 10–7a). Growth presents a formidable challenge for maintaining plasma calcium concentration in the normal range, since large amounts of calcium are transferred to the growing skeleton (Fig. 10–7b). This is especially so in young dogs of large breeds.[2] In conditions in which calcium homeostasis is under stress (such as rapid growth, over- or under-supplementation, or pregnancy and lactation) calcium metabolism is strongly influenced by calciotropic hormones (PTH, vitamin D, and calcitonin) (Fig. 10–8). Synthesis and release of these hormones are mainly triggered by variations in plasma calcium concentration. The effect of these calciotropic hormones is directed to normalization of the plasma calcium concentration.[5]

10.3 Parathyroid hormone

The concentration of PTH (see also Chapter 9) in plasma in dogs depends on the animal's age, for the concentration decreases during the first months of life (Fig. 10–9) and thereby parallels bone cell activity during skeletal growth. The effects of PTH on bone can be either catabolic or anabolic, depending on the mode of secretion.

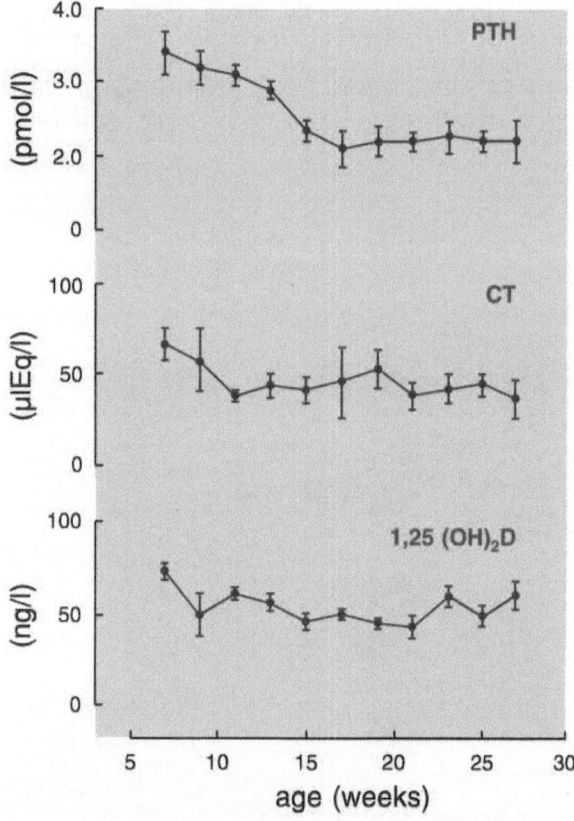

Fig. 10-9. Plasma concentrations (mean ± SEM) of immunoreactive PTH, CT, and 1,25(OH)$_2$D in growing Great Danes from 6–26 weeks of age. Both PTH and CT, but not 1,25(OH)$_2$D, are significantly negatively correlated with age.

High concentrations of PTH cause catabolic actions: osteoblasts shrink and change their shape, allowing osteoclasts to come into contact with bone-matrix surface and to resorb bone.[6] Osteoclasts are recruited and activated by local biologically active factors (b.a.f. Fig. 10–4) originating from osteoblasts and resolved from bone matrix. Intermittent low doses of PTH cause anabolic actions in bone: increases in the number of osteoblasts, alkaline phosphatase concentration and collagen synthesis.

10.3.1 Nutritional secondary hyperparathyroidism

In growing dogs, especially of the larger breeds, and in cats a substantial amount of calcium is laid down as calcium phosphates in newly-formed osteoid and cartilage. If insufficient calcium is available in the food, the calcium concentration in plasma will tend to decrease, initiating hyperparathyroidism. Since in carnivores nutritional secondary hyperparathyroidism (NSH) is especially seen in animals fed an unbalanced food mainly based on meat or meat by-products (Table 10–1), this entity is also known as the *all meat syndrome*.

In NSH, PTH production and secretion increase, leading to increases in calcium reabsorption in the kidney, osteoclasia, and $1,25(OH)_2D$ synthesis. The former two effects result in a rapid normalization of plasma calcium concentration (Fig. 10–8), whereas the latter effect requires a few days but eventually will lead to an augmentation of the absorption efficiency of calcium and phosphorus (Fig. 10–10). The circulating concentration of phosphate will increase due to augmented intestinal phosphate absorption and increased bone resorption with liberation of phosphates. Concomitantly and due to the hyperparathyroidism, the tubular maximum for phosphate will decrease, causing hyperphosphaturia and preventing further elevation of the plasma phosphate level. Depending on the growth velocity of the animal (and thereby its calcium requirement) and the severity of the calcium deficiency, the increased bone resorption will cause clinical problems within 1–3 months.[7]

Clinical manifestations. Cancellous bone in the epiphyseal and metaphyseal areas may become so thin that spiculae will collapse, causing compression fractures. Osteoclasts at the endosteal side will remove cortical bone to such an extent that the cortex will bend under the influence of body weight and muscle tone, causing folding (i.e., greenstick) fractures and deformed skeletal protuberances.

On presentation, the patient will be alert and have a good hair coat, and a disproportionally enlarged abdomen due to the fact that the growth of the skeleton lags behind that of the soft tissues (Fig. 10–11). The animal will be reluctant to walk due to bone pain and pathological fractures. There may be fractures and abnormal alignment of bones and bones may be painful upon palpation. In severe cases there may be paresis posterior due to compression fractures of vertebrae (Fig. 10–11). As explained earlier, plasma calcium concentration is very effectively regulated and its measurements do not contribute to the diagnosis (Fig. 10–5). Plasma and urinary concentrations of phosphate may be elevated.

In adult animals the calcium requirement is

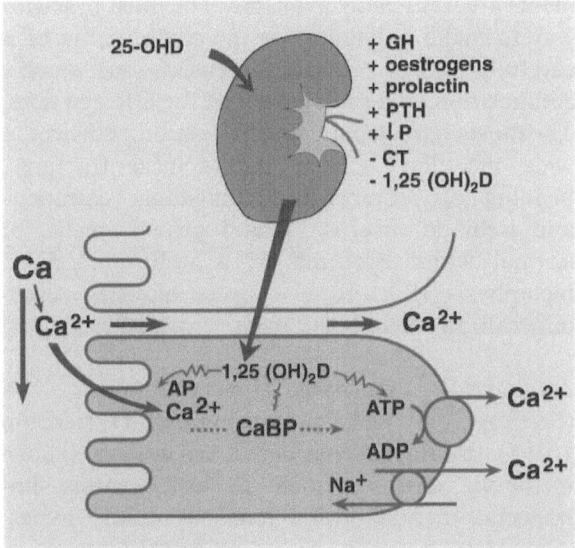

Fig. 10-10. Intestinal calcium absorption is the sum of passive and active absorption. Passive paracellular calcium absorption occurs under the influence of the concentration gradient between the intestinal lumen and the interstitium. Transcellular active absorption is influenced by $1,25(OH)_2D$. This hormone is formed in the kidney and its synthesis is regulated by a variety of hormones as well as plasma phosphorus. In the intestinal cell synthesis of alkaline phosphatase (*AP*), calcium binding protein (*CaBP*), and ATP-ase are stimulated and thereby cellular absorption, transport, and expulsion of calcium.

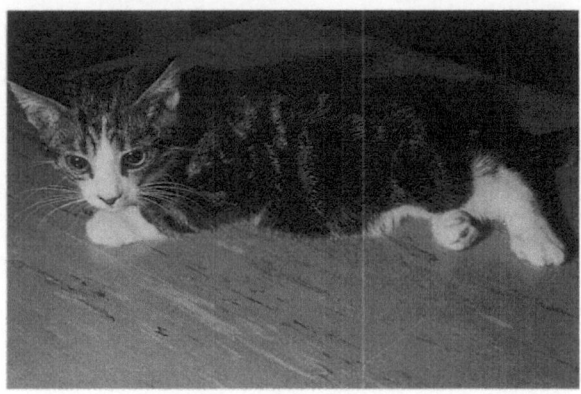
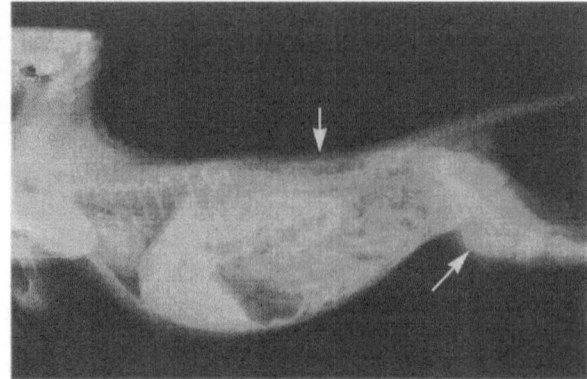

Fig. 10-11. Left: Kitten, 3 months of age and fed chicken meat almost exclusively, was in good general condition but unable to stand. Right: The radiograph revealed the disproportionally enlarged abdomen, thin cortices and wide medullae of the long bones, pathological fractures of both femurs and compression fractures of vertebrae (arrows).

lower than in young growing animals. Nevertheless, very prolonged dietary calcium deficiency may cause problems that become manifest by loosening of teeth due to alveolar resorption.

Diagnosis. PTH and $1,25(OH)_2D$ concentrations will be elevated (Fig. 10–12), but these measurements are not readily available. The most practical way to make a diagnosis is the combination of a carefully taken history, focused on dietary composition, and radiographs of the affected sites. The most characteristic features are thin cortices, a wide medullary cavity, pathological fractures, bending of protuberances (including calcaneus and ischiatic tuberosity), and growth plates of normal width bordered by a well mineralized metaphysis (Fig. 10–11). Bone biopsies reveal mineralized osteoid with massive osteoclasia.

Differential diagnosis. Hypervitaminosis A (Section 10.6) and hypovitaminosis D (Section 10.4.1) should be considered, as well as inborn metabolic diseases such as osteogenesis imperfecta. In adult dogs, renal secondary hyper-

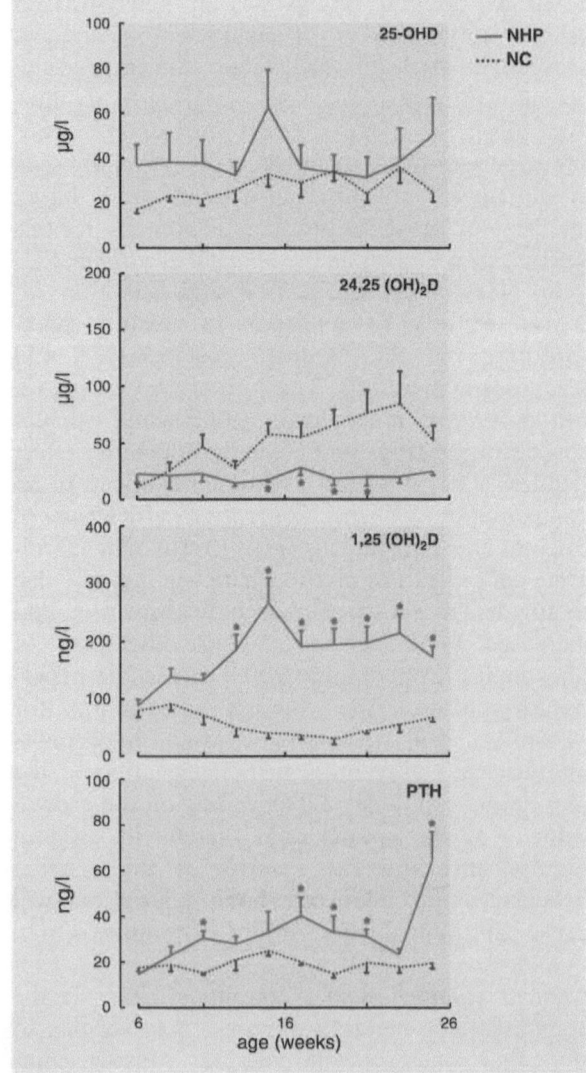

Fig. 10-12. Plasma concentrations of the vit D metabolites and of PTH in Poodles with nutritional hyperparathyroidism (NHP) compared with normally fed dogs (NC) (0.05% and 1.1% Ca, respectively). The vit D content of the food was the same for both groups, reflected in no differences in 25-OHD concentrations in the plasma of both groups. In NHP, PTH increases $1,25(OH)_2D$ synthesis at the expense of hydroxylation into $24,25(OH)_2D$. This illustrates the reciprocal relationship between the synthesis of these metabolites. (Modified from Nap, 1993.[23]) (* $p < 0.05$.)

parathyroidism (Section 9.3.2) and parodontal diseases should be taken into account.

Treatment. In the severe stage of NSH the pathological fractures of the long bones cannot be treated by splinting, since the bone will break just proximal to the splint, nor by osteosynthesis, because of the weakened nature of the bones. Therapy is limited to good nursing to prevent additional damage to the skeleton – especially the vertebrae – and food with a normal calcium content (i.e., 1.1% on a dry matter basis).[7] This will improve skeletal mineralization in three weeks. Extra calcium as calcium carbonate (50 mg Ca/kg body weight per day) can be prescribed during this period. Since the endogenous 1,25(OH)$_2$D concentration in the plasma (Fig. 10–12), and thus its effects on intestines and bone cells, is highly increased (Fig. 10–8), additional administration of vitamin D is contraindicated.

Prognosis. The prognosis depends on the severity and the extent of pathological fractures. Compression fractures of vertebrae can (but do not always) have a bad prognosis. Healed greenstick fractures and bent long bones will not always cause locomotion disturbances. Narrowing of the pelvis may cause repeated constipation although in less severe cases in which treatment is begun soon enough, constipation may not remain a problem.

10.4 Vitamin D

The D vitamins (calciferols) are steroid molecules in which one of the four rings has been opened (Fig. 1–2). In dogs and cats (unlike omnivores and herbivores) vitamin D is an essential vitamin because these animals are not able so synthesize vitamin D in their skin under the influence of UV-B radiation[8] (Fig. 10–13). Following absorption from the gut, vitamin D (cholecalciferol = vit D$_3$ of animal origin, or ergocalciferol = vit D$_2$ of plant origin) is hydroxylated in the liver to 25 hydroxyvitamin D (25-OHD). The concentration of this metabolite varies with dietary intake. A second hydroxylation takes place in renal mitochondria, catalyzed by 1α-hydroxylase or 24-hydroxylase. The 24-hydroxylation is reciprocally

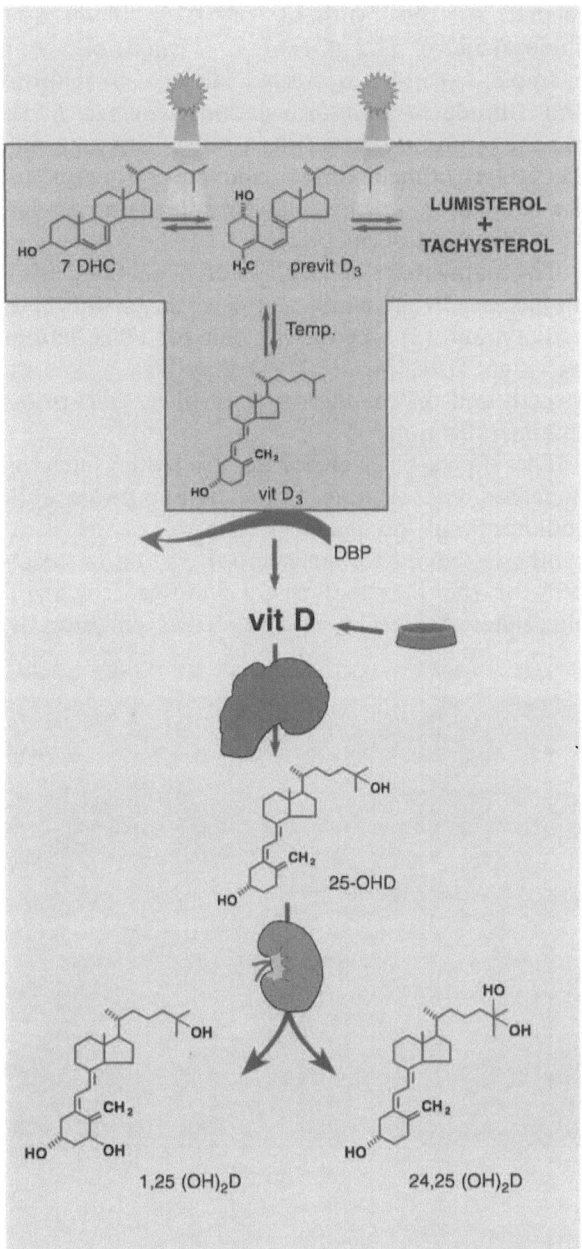

Fig. 10-13. In the skin (beige area) of most mammals,[8] but not the dog and cat,[7] 7 dehydrocholesterol (7 DHC) is photosynthesized under the influence of sunlight (UV-B) into previtamin D$_3$ followed by a temperature-dependent isomerisation into vit D$_3$. Other isomers including lumisterol and tachysterol can be formed under prolonged radiation. When synthesized or absorbed with the food, vit D is bound to vit D binding proteins (DBP) and transported to the liver for its first hydroxylation into 25-OHD, followed by a second hydroxylation in the kidney into 24,25(OH)$_2$D and the biologically most active metabolite, 1,25(OH)$_2$D. (Modified from How et al., 1994.[8])

related to the synthesis of 1,25 dihydroxy-cholecalciferol (1,25(OH)$_2$D = calcitriol); for example, calcitonin decreases calcitriol formation and stimulates 24-hydroxylation, whereas PTH has the opposite effects (Fig. 10–12). Although the 24,25(OH)$_2$D metabolite is abundantly present in the circulation, its physiological role is not as well defined as that of calcitriol.

The main effects of calcitriol on bone include (1) an increase in the number of osteoclasts and their activity, and (2) a permissive role for PTH action on osteoblasts. 24,25(OH)$_2$D may play a role in growth and differentiation of cartilage cells prior to mineralization.[5]

The effects of calcitriol on the kidney include increased reabsorption of calcium, phosphate, and sodium, and the feedback control of its own synthesis (closed feedback loop). In the mucosal cells of the proximal small intestine, calcitriol stimulates the uptake, transport, and extrusion of calcium (Fig. 10–10). In the distal part of the small intestine, phosphate absorption is promoted similarly, although independent of calcium absorption.

10.4.1 Hypovitaminosis D

Dogs and cats are dependent on the dietary vitamin D content to fulfill their requirement.[8] Prey, home-made diets containing animal fat, or commercial pet foods contain sufficient vit D (Table 10–1). Only when extremely deficient diets are fed (i.e., only lean meat or only vegetables) vitamin D deficiency may develop, and then especially in pups or kittens which have not had the chance to store enough vit D in their body fat.[7] Hypovitaminosis D in young animals (*rickets*) occurs rarely, but may be mentioned by the owner because it is a classic bone disease. Hypovitaminosis D in adults (*osteomalacia*) does not cause clinically

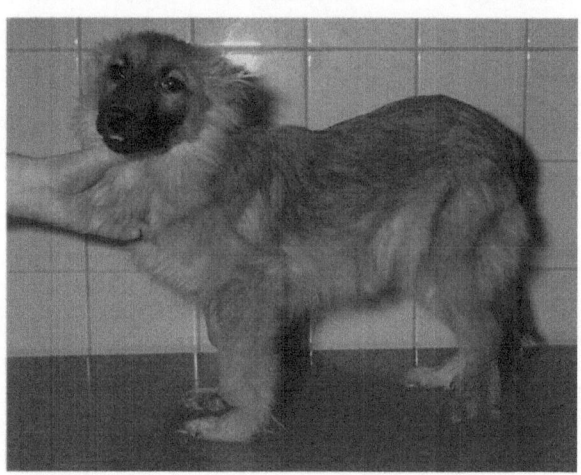

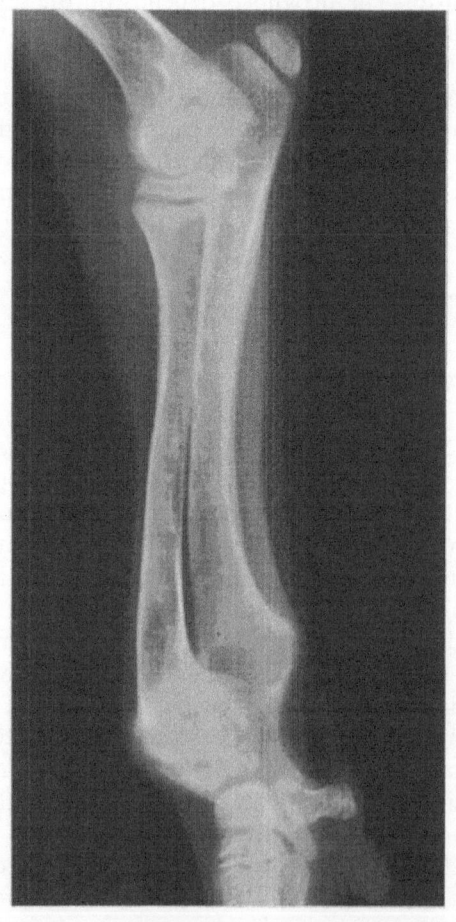

Fig. 10-14. Left: Young mixed breed dog with clearly noticeable bulging metaphyseal areas of the distal radius and ulna, as well as pronounced palpable areas near the growth plates of all ribs. Right: The radiograph of the radius and ulna revealed thin cortices, large diameters of the medullary cavity, and increased width of the growth plates with a mushroom appearance, typical for hypovitaminosis D.

relevant disturbances in bone metabolism. This chapter will therefore focus on rickets.

When there is a low vit D intake, insufficient $1,25(OH)_2D$ is formed. This leads to insufficient calcium and phosphate resorption from the intestine, low osteoclastic activity and renal reabsorption of calcium and phosphate. As a result, the calcium concentration in plasma tends to decrease. This in turn stimulates the parathyroid glands to hypersecretion, thereby increasing calcium reabsorption and osteoclastic activity (Fig. 10–8) and decreasing the renal tubular maximum for phosphate. Due to hypovitaminosis D, newly formed osteoid is not mineralized. The mineralized bone is therefore sealed off by non-mineralized osteoid, making it inaccessible to the osteoclasts for resorption and remodelling. The newly-formed cartilage will not mineralize and this prevents the cascade of events in endochondral ossification (Fig. 10–1) to be completed.

Clinical manifestations. The animal is alert, its coat may be in poor condition, and its body conformation may be disproportional due to the fact that growth of bones lags behind that of the soft tissues. The animal is reluctant to walk and palpation of the bones causes pain. The legs are bent and the metaphyseal areas of long bones and ribs are enlarged (Fig. 10–14). The plasma concentration of calcium is low to normal (Fig. 10–5), whereas the phosphate concentration is low in plasma (< 1 mmol/l) and high in urine (> 20 mmol/l), the latter due to the concomitant hyperparathyroidism.

On radiographic examination the cortex of the long bones is thin and may be folded or there may be pathological fractures. The growth plates are extremely wide for the chronological age of the animal (Fig. 10–14).

Diagnosis. The plasma concentrations of 25-OHD and $24,25(OH)_2D$ are very low and the concentration of calcitriol is < 20 pg/ml. The radiological abnormalities are quite typical of hypovitaminosis D. A biopsy of the greater tubercle, in order to harvest cancellous bone and growth plate cartilage without disturbing growth in length, will reveal osteoid seams covering poorly mineralized trabeculae and an extremely widened growth plate.

Differential diagnosis. This entity can be confused with or be complicated by nutritional secondary hyperparathyroidism, depending on the mineral content of the food. However, the plasma concentration of vit D metabolites and the radiological appearance of growth plates will be different. With regard to the latter, hypertrophic osteodystrophy (Fig. 10–15) and congenital diseases such as chondrodysplasia[9] have to be considered.

Treatment. The dog or cat must be fed with a normal food, containing 400 IE vit D per kg,[7] as

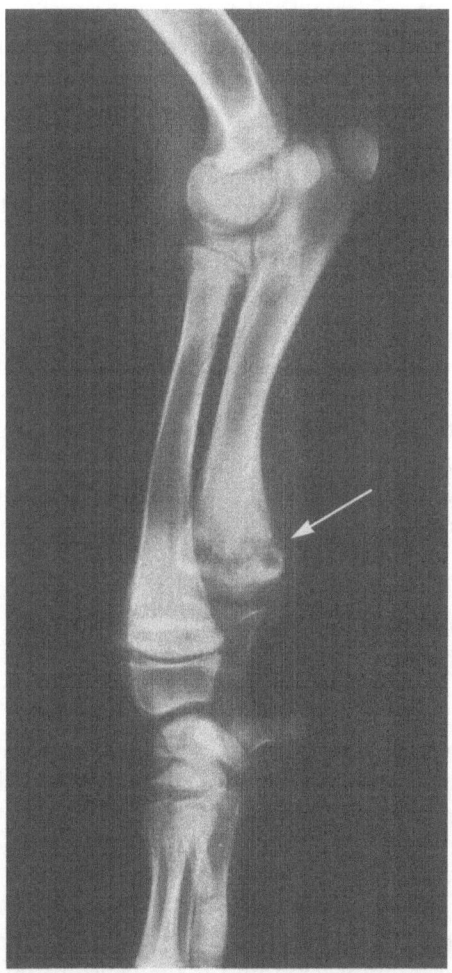

Fig. 10-15. Radiograph of a 4-month-old Boxer with hypertrophic osteodystrophy. A pathognomonic radiolucent area (arrow) parallels the growth plates and is separated from it by a thin mineralized area. In addition, the well mineralized cortex differs considerably from what is seen in case of hypovitaminosis D (see for comparison Fig. 10–14).

soon as possible. Within 4 weeks, mineralization of cortices, growth plates and callus will occur to such an extent that corrective orthopaedic surgery can then be performed if necessary.

Prognosis. The prognosis for mineralization of bone and cartilage is good, but the functional recovery depends on the severity of the skeletal abnormalities.

10.4.2 Hypervitaminosis D

Hypervitaminosis D may result from excessive supplementation of vit D in the diet, overdosage of vit D in the treatment of hypoparathyroidism, or intoxication with cholecalciferol containing rodenticides.[10] It leads to increased formation of 25-OHD, augmented calcium and phosphate absorption from the intestine, and increased calcium and phosphate reabsorption in the kidneys. The resulting hypercalcemia causes hypoparathyroidism, which prevents osteoclasia but, due to the increase of the tubular maximum for phosphate, this cannot compensate for the increased absorption and retention of phosphate. The elevated plasma concentrations of calcium and phosphate also lead to increased urinary excretion of both elements. Eventually calcification of soft tissues will occur, including vessel walls and heart valves as well as kidney tubules with renal failure as a consequence.

Clinical manifestations. The clinical picture may be dominated by one or more of the signs of hypercalcemia such as polydipsia/polyuria, dehydration, weakness, and anorexia.[10] If complicated by renal insufficiency, there may be vomiting and other signs of azotemia. Routine laboratory investigations will reveal that calcium and phosphate concentrations in plasma and urine are elevated. The circulating concentration of PTH is low and that of 25-OHD metabolites is high, whereas the plasma concentration of $1,25(OH)_2D$ is low (except when that metabolite has been administered and is the cause of intoxication).

Diagnosis. The diagnosis can be made on the basis of the history and the finding of elevated concentrations of calcium and phosphate in plasma and urine. Especially humoral hypercalcemia of malignancy (Section 11.4) and primary renal disease should be ruled out.

Differential diagnosis. For the differential diagnosis of hypercalcemia, the reader is referred to Sections 9.3 and 11.2.

Treatment. The aim of the treatment is to minimize nephrocalcinosis by increasing renal calcium excretion and by decreasing intestinal calcium absorption. In mild cases glucocorticoids can be prescribed to reduce intestinal absorption and to increase renal excretion of calcium. In addition, a diet without calcium should be given to minimize intestinal calcium absorption.

In cases with severe hypercalcemia (> 4.0 mmol/l), general weakness, and anorexia, fluid therapy should be given, since dehydration contributes to increased ionized calcium concentration. Mild volume expansion together with furosemide will promote calciuria. It has been recommended to treat hypercalcemia with injections of calcitonin in order to reduce calcium release from the bone by osteoclasts.[10] However, osteoclasia is not the main cause of hypercalcemia in hypervitaminosis D. In addition, the use of heterologous calcitonin may cause antibody formation and contribute to the feeling of sickness. For the use of bone resorption inhibiting substances the reader is referred to Chapter 14.

Once started, treatment with prednisone, furosemide, and the special diet, this regimen should be continued for at least one month, since the release of the vitamin D stores in body fat may take several weeks.[10]

Prognosis. Neuromuscular disturbances and encephalopathy due to rapid development of severe hypercalcemia may occur and death may ensue. If there is renal damage, the prognosis is guarded. In milder cases, treatment can be successful.[10]

10.5 Calcitonin

In the dog calcitonin (CT) is synthesized mainly in the parafollicular or C-cells in the thyroid glands (Fig. 3-1). Recently the amino-acid sequence of canine calcitonin (cCT) was elucidated (Fig.

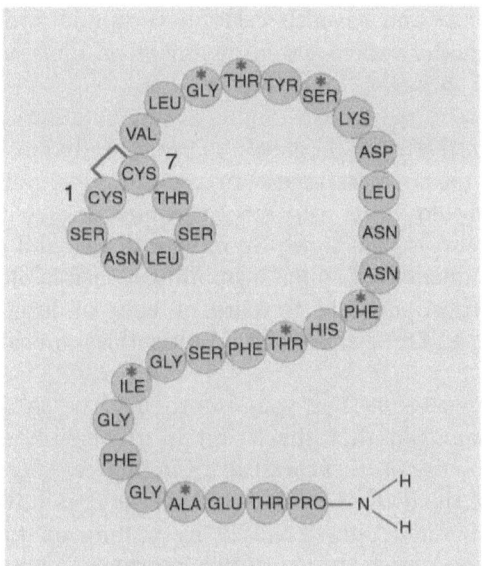 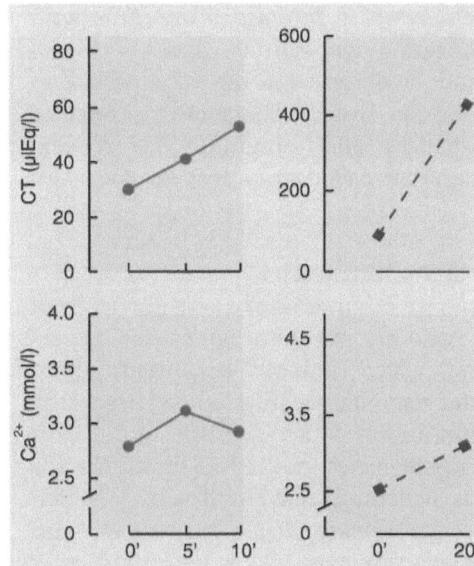

Fig. 10-16. Left: canine calcitonin (CT) consists of 32 amino acids with a disulfide bridge between cysteine in positions 1 and 7, and only differing in 7 amino acids (*) from bovine CT.[12] Right: Effects of a calcium load on plasma CT concentrations. The left panels illustrate the effect of the oral administration of 5 mg calcium per kg body weight on plasma calcium and CT concentrations of a healthy dog. The right panels depict the effect of the infusion of 1 mg calcium per kg body weight.

10–16), which allowed the development of a homologous radioimmunoassay for CT in the dog.[11,12] The circulating concentrations of CT decrease during the first three months of life (Fig. 10–9). Both the synthesis and the secretion of CT are stimulated by calcium infusion as well as by calcium ingestion[13] (Fig. 10–16).

During calcium ingestion, CT concentration is raised directly (by calcium) and indirectly (e.g., by gastrin[11]), causing osteoclasts to retract their brush border (Fig. 10–4). As a consequence, calcium concentration in plasma is prevented from rising (and therefore the PTH concentration does not fall) and thus calcium is routed to the bone and not lost via the kidneys (Fig. 10–8). CT has no direct effects on the intestine or the kidney in the dog but influences the hypothalamic satiety centre and influences 1,25(OH)$_2$D synthesis[11] (Fig. 10–10).

10.5.1 Nutritional secondary hypercalcitoninism

Supplementation of balanced commercial foods and the use of home-made unbalanced diets are common errors. Especially young dogs of large breeds are often given extra mineral and vitamin mixtures. Studies in giant and miniature dogs have revealed that in large-breed dogs overfeeding of a balanced diet or supplementing an otherwise balanced diet with calcium causes hypercalcitoninism, with severe consequences for skeletal development.[2,7]

Calcium ingestion stimulates CT release and consequently plasma calcium concentration does not rise, which prevents the effect of a decreasing PTH release on calcium excretion by the kidney (see also Section 9.1). Calcium is routed primarily to the bone, ready to be used at a later stage or added to the mineral content of the bone (Fig. 10–8).

Chronic high intake of calcium causes C-cell hyperplasia in young dogs.[13] Persistent hypercalcitoninism causes decreased osteoclastic activity and hypermineralization of the skeleton.[11] The imbalance of the calciotropic hormones and the (direct or indirect) effect of calcium on chondrocytes may lead to disturbed endochondral ossification. In this situation the chondrocytes do not mature, the intercellular substance does not mineralize, and the chondrocytes continue to live and prevent blood vessels from invading (Fig. 10–1). The disturbed cartilage maturation is characterized by thickened cartilage and is known as osteochondrosis.[2]

190

The consequences of *decreased osteoclasia* with hypermineralization as well as signs of *osteochondrosis* may be observed in the same patient in varying gradations. However, in some cases one of these disturbances may dominate the clinical features. Therefore each entity will be discussed separately.

10.5.1.1 Decreased osteoclasia

Chronic excessive calcium intake (with or without a constant ratio to phosphorus) causes hypercalcitoninism, which induces decreased osteoclastic skeletal remodelling (Fig. 10–8). Especially foramina, that do not widen in proportion to soft tissue growth, may cause noticeable hindrance for both nervous structures and blood vessels, which may lead to the *Canine Wobbler syndrome* and *enostosis*, respectively.

Canine Wobbler syndrome. Retarded skeletal remodelling of the spinal canal at the cranial vertebral orifice may cause irreversible damage to the spinal cord. This occurs especially in the cervical region and may give rise to an atactic gait, thereby being one of the causes of the so-called Wobbler syndrome.

Diagnosis. The clinical findings include uncoordinated gait in young dogs (approximately 6 months old) of a giant breed (e.g., Great Dane), with pain in response to extension of the neck, hyperactivity of the reflexes of the pelvic limbs, and positive crossed extensor reflexes of the pelvic limbs. Radiographs of the cervical vertebrae may reveal narrowing of the cranial orifices of the fifth,

sixth and seventh cervical vertebrae and myelography will reveal impignment on the spinal cord at these locations (Fig. 10–17).

Differential diagnosis. Discospondylitis, meningitis, and traumatic or congenital abnormalities should be considered in young dogs with these neurological signs. Spondylolisthesis and the consequences of spinal instability as seen in older dogs (approximately 6 years of age) of large breeds (e.g., Doberman) can give identical clinical signs.

Treatment. The spinal cord may be so seriously damaged that the lesion is irreversible and any treatment unsuccessful. In milder cases correction of the diet, glucocorticoid therapy, and avoidance of microtrauma caused by pulling on the collar may lead to clinical improvement. Surgical decompression is indicated in young dogs with progressive signs.[14]

Prognosis. In mild cases improvement will follow after 4 weeks of conservative treatment, but the prognosis in more severe cases should be guarded.

Enostosis. In dogs with enostosis (which is also known as canine panosteitis and eosinophilic panosteitis), a delay in remodelling of the nutritional foramen is present. Consequently, edema occurs in the medullary cavity and eventually underneath the sensitive periosteum. Later there is extra bone formation, both in the medullary cavity on organized fibrous tissue and subperiosteally due to the elevation of the periosteum by the edema.[7]

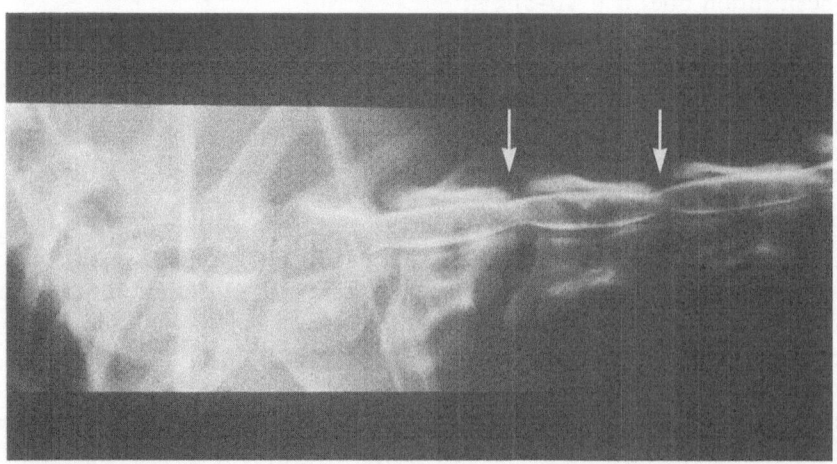

Fig. 10-17. Myelography of the cervical region of a 6-months-old Great Dane with an uncoordinated gait, pain reaction upon hyperextension of the neck, and positive crossed extensor reflexes of rear limbs. The radiograph revealed impingement of the spinal cord at the cranial orifice of the 5th, 6th and 7th cervical vertebra (arrows), typical of the Canine Wobbler Syndrome.

Diagnosis. Dogs of larger breeds not older than 2 years of age develop shifting lameness of varying severity. Physical examination may reveal an elevated body temperature, severe lameness in one or more legs, and a painful reaction to deep palpation of the long bones. Routine laboratory investigations are not conclusive. In the subacute phase (at least 3 weeks after the start of the initial signs) radiographic examination of long bones may reveal medullary new bone formation (Fig. 10–18). In the more severe cases there may be noticeable subperioseal new bone. Other causes of lameness of one or more legs in these young dogs (including osteochondritis dissecans, fragmented coronoid process, ununited anconeal process) can occur solely or together with enostosis and may confuse the results of the physical examination. Bone scanning (Fig. 10–2) and other imaging techniques may help to make the diagnosis.

Differential diagnosis. Disturbances of skeletal mineralization including NSH, painful conditions such as hypertrophic osteodystrophy, and even infectious diseases may be included in the list of differential diagnoses of shifting lameness with elevated temperature.

Treatment. Treatment should be directed at augmentation of osteoclastic activity, for example by providing foods low in calcium, such as meat (Table 10–1). Although this might theoretically be logical, there are no studies proving that this will have a beneficial effect. In periods of pain, the dog can be treated with nonsteroidal anti-inflammatory drugs (e.g., aspirin, 25 mg per kg body weight 3 times per day) or with a low dose of corticosteroids (0.5–1.0 mg per kg body weight, decreasing to an alternate-day regimen), provided that joint cartilage damage has been excluded.

Prognosis. The prognosis of enostosis is good in the long term, since periods of severe and shifting lameness disappear after the age of 2 years, although they may occur repeatedly prior to that age.

10.5.1.2 Osteochondrosis

Osteochondrosis is a disturbance of endochondral ossification. Osteochondrosis can be localized at any site where growing cartilage is present during the growth period (Fig. 10–1) but especially at sites and moments of high growth velocity.[15] In particular, it can occur in the growth plate of the distal ulna (which accounts for 90% of the growth in length of the ulna). It can be present temp-

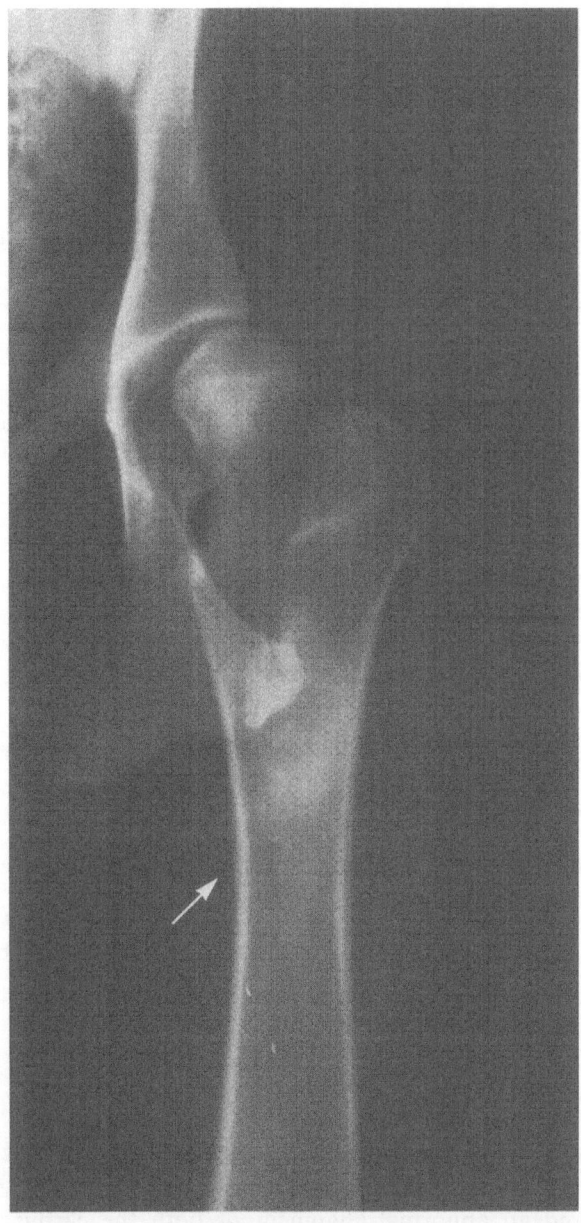

Fig. 10-18. German Shepherd dog, 9 months of age, suffering from enostosis with shifting lameness, pain upon palpation of the long bones, and radiopaque areas due to new bone formation in the medullary cavity. These confluencing dense areas are first present near the nutritional foramina (arrow) of the long bones.

192

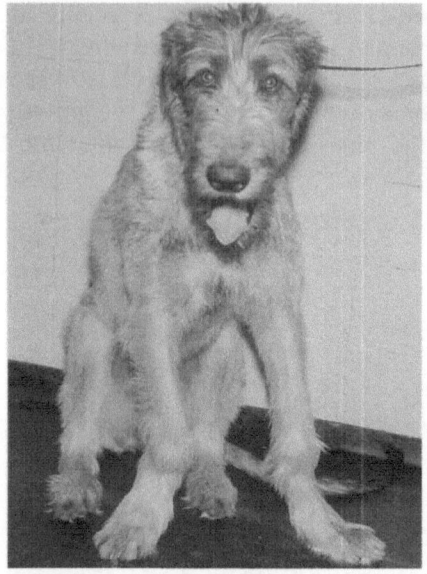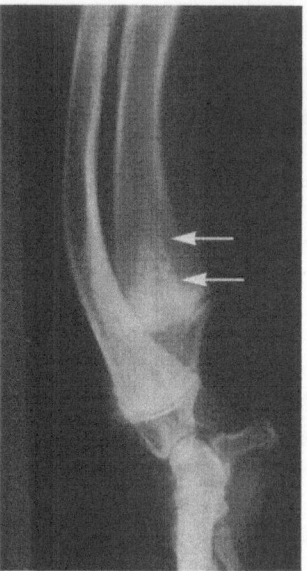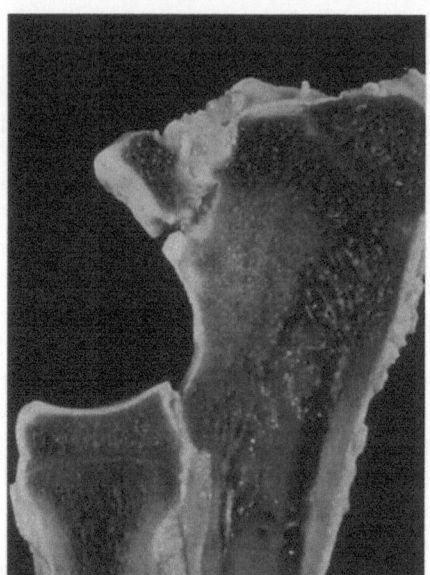

Fig. 10-19. Left: Deerhound, 8 months of age, with bilateral valgus deformation due to radius curvus syndrome,[7] with a retained cartilage cone (arrows) in the distal ulnar metaphysis (middle). Right: The radius may push the humerus proximally against the anconeal process, which breaks off in its growth plate, causing an ununited anconeal process.

orarily in dogs of large breeds without becoming clinically significant.[16] When present to such an extent that it causes a decrease in the growth in length of the ulna, it influences also the growth in length of the radius, causing the *radius curvus syndrome* (Fig. 10–19). When present in joint cartilage, microtrauma can cause fissure lines and eventually separation of diseased cartilage, now called *osteochondritis dissecans*.

Radius curvus syndrome. This abnormal development of the front legs can develop in dogs 4–6 months of age and especially in dogs of large breeds, raised on excessive amounts of food or raised on lesser amounts but with excess of calcium.[7]

There will be bilateral valgus deformity with cranial bowing of the radius. Radiographs will demonstrate a cartilage cone at the distal growth plate of the ulna, together with a curvature of the radius and a thickened concave cortex (Fig. 10–19) and an abnormal alignment of both the carpus and the elbow joint. Due to elbow incongruity, the anconeal process can be loosened in its growth plate[15] (Fig. 10–19).

Diagnosis. The bilateral valgus deformity with

retained cartilage cones on the radiographs will suffice to make the diagnosis.

Differential diagnosis. Dogs with chondrodysplasia as prescribed in breed standards (such as Basset Hounds) or as in inherited disease (as in Alaskan Malamutes)[9] are physically similar in the front legs, but also short in the rear legs. Traumatic injury to the growth plates of the distal radius or ulna may cause early closure of the affected (part of the) growth plate and consequently valgus deformation; mostly this affects only one front leg and no cartilage cone is present.

Treatment. Restriction in food and calcium intake alone can lead to normalization of the endochondral ossification.[7,16] When the valgus deformity is severe, conservative treatment will not normalize the stance nor will it prevent secondary effects, such as incongruity of the elbow joint, detachment of the anconeal process, valgus deformity, and carpal abnormalities. Additional corrective surgery will be needed in these cases.

Osteochondritis dissecans (OCD) designates osteochondrosis in joint cartilage whereby thickened cartilage is detached and the inflammation of subchondral bone and joint capsule causes pain.[15] It can occur in a variety of joints (i.e., shoulder, elbow, stifle, and tibiotarsal joint) and is very often bilateral. Recent studies have shown that the genotype of the dog also plays an important role in the occurrence of this disease, but that of all the environmental factors calcium intake is the most important.[17]

The dogs, being approximately half a year of age, of medium or large breed, and often fast growing, are lame or have a stiff gait in one or more legs.[17] Joints are overfilled and painful upon hyperextension or hyperflexion, and crepitation may be present. With radiographs or other imaging techniques an indentation of the contour of the subchondral bone can be seen, or even a mineralized cartilage flap (Fig. 10–20A).

Diagnosis. Clinical and radiological investigation will help to make the diagnosis. Arthrography, computed tomography, and arthroscopy may precede arthrotomy.

Treatment. In mild cases no treatment may be needed or nonsteroidal anti-inflammatory drugs can be given when needed. Large cartilage flaps can be removed and lesions curetted to induce early healing[15] (Fig. 10–20B). Thickened cartilage (i.e., osteochondrosis) in other joints can be prevented from detachment by decreasing overload (by reducing body weight and by rest) in order to diminish microtrauma of the unmineralized cartilage.

Prognosis. The prognosis depends on the severity of the lesion, the secondary arthrotic changes, and the joint affected. The lesion in the proximal shoulder can heal completely, whereas lesions in the talus may continue to interfere with joint stability and cause severe arthrosis.[15]

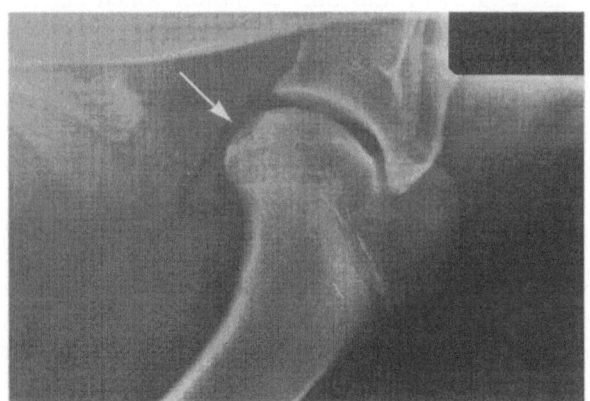
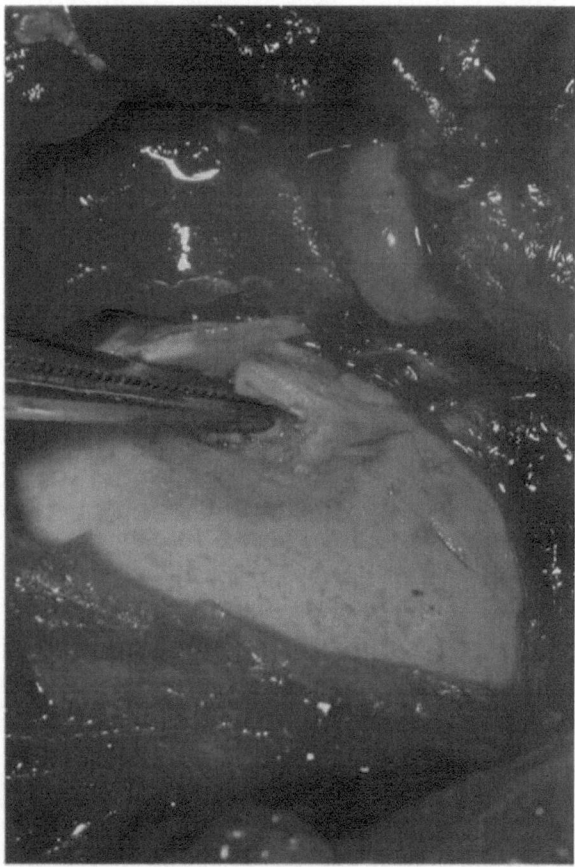

A | **B**

Fig. 10-20. A: Radiograph of shoulder joint of a 7-month-old Bouvier de Flandres with lameness of both front legs and pain reaction on hyperflexion of the shoulder joint. There is an indentation of the contour of the subchondral bone at the caudal aspect of the humeral head (arrow), indicating osteochondrosis. B: Based on the concomitant clinical manifestations, arthrotomy was performed and revealed osteochondritis dissecans with a cartilage flap. Removal of the flap was followed by curettage of the cartilage defect.

10.6 Miscellaneous

In addition to the calciotropic hormones, other hormones and nutritional factors may play a significant role in bone metabolism. Clinically relevant hormonal aspects have been covered already in previous chapters, especially Sections 2.2, 3.2 and 4.3. Their influences on bone or cartilage cells and clinical significance are summarized as follows.

Growth hormone (GH). GH promotes the differentiation and (via IGF-I) the proliferation of the chondrocytes of the growth plates[2,3] (Fig. 10–1). Deficiency of GH during the growth period causes proportional dwarfism (Fig. 2–9).

Thyroid hormone. Thyroid hormone influences maturation of the distal cells in the chondrocyte sequence, and probably also the promotion of activity of chondrocyte progenitors. Thyroid hormone deficiency in the young dog (Fig. 3–8) and cat leads to retardation of growth and maturation of the skeleton[18] (Figs. 3–10, 10–21A).

Glucocorticoids. Glucocorticoids are known to impair the effect of IGF-I on cartilage growth. This may lead to stunted growth in height when given for a prolonged period to young animals[3]. Since glucocorticoids increase PTH release and decrease calcium absorption from the intestine, the effect of glucocorticoids on bone is generalized osteoclasia, resulting in osteoporosis (Fig. 10–21B). However, chronic excess of either endogenous or exogenous glucocorticoids only rarely leads to pathological fractures in dogs and cats.

Gonadal (sex) steroids. Testosterone causes an increase in bone growth, whereas estrogens inhibit longitudinal growth[3] due to decreased IGF-I activity. Castration of immature male dogs and cats results in greater height at the shoulder[19] (Table 10–2), whereas exogenous gonadal steroids may stunt growth after an initial growth spurt.

Osteoporosis is a major problem in anestrogenic women. Also in dogs cessation of ovarian function causes bone loss,[20] but not to the extent that it leads to clinical problems.

Vitamin A (vit A). Vit A (or retinol) is formed

Table 10-2. Effects of prepubertal gonadectomy on skeletal growth in dogs.[12]

age at gonadectomy (n=number dogs)	physeal closure of distal radius-ulna	radial length
controls (n=10)	41.6 ± 1.2 weeks	16.8 ± 0.9 cm
7 weeks (n=14)	59.4 ± 3.1 weeks	18.6 ± 0.7 cm
7 months (n=8)	54.6 ± 1.2 weeks	17.6 ± 1.0 cm

Early gonadectomy leads to eunuchism: later physeal closure and taller stature.

in the gut of dogs by the reversible reduction of retinaldehyde originating from carotene. Cats require retinol (as present in a variety of foodstuffs[7]), since cats lack carotenase in their intestinal mucosa. Vit A is oxidized in its target cells to retinoic acid. Retenoic acid interacts via nuclear receptors with the genome, to regulate cellular growth and differentiation which can be considered as hormone activity.[21,22] Vit A is important for normal osteoblastic, chondroblastic, and osteoclastic activity. High doses of vit A inhibit chondrogenesis in growth plates and inhibit collagen synthesis by osteoblasts in both dogs and cats. Since cats are not able to form retinyl esters in order to excrete the excess of this fat-soluble vitamin, chronic vit A intoxication is more likely to be diagnosed in cats than in dogs.

Hypervitaminosis A in cats is characterized by new bone formation without osteolysis, starting at the points of insertion of ligaments, muscles and joint capsules which causes narrowing of the intervertebral foramina in the vertebrae bodies and ankylosis of vertebrae and larger joints. This causes pain, lameness, and stiffness (Fig. 10–21C). Plasma vit A concentration or liver biopsy can support the diagnosis. Although ankylosis is irreversible, the cat will improve with aspirin (25 mg per kg per day) and feeding a low vit A-containing food for several weeks.[7]

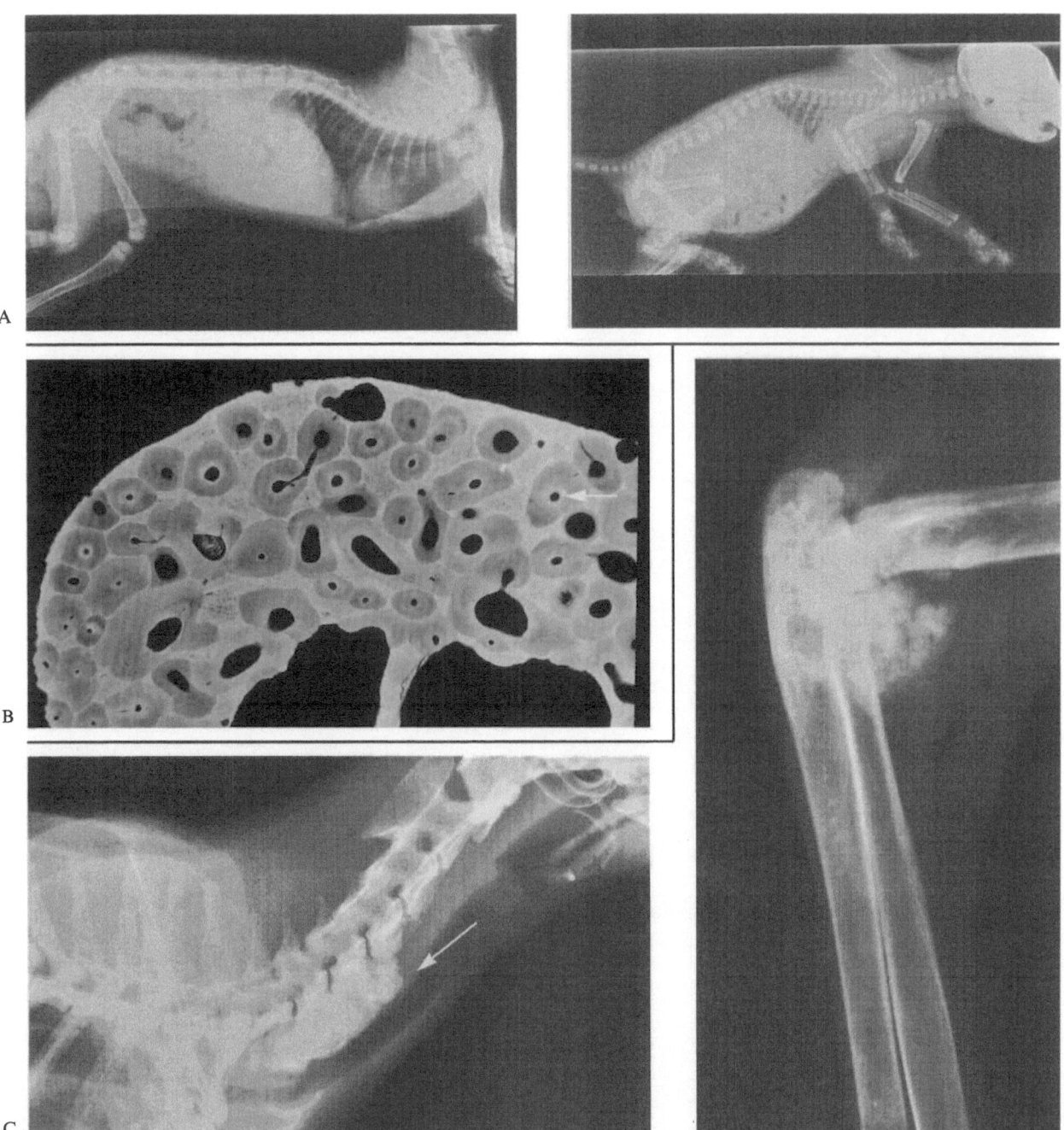

Fig. 10-21. A variety of influences on bone metabolism: A: Radiographs of two tomcats (see also Fig. 3–10), littermates, at the age of 8 weeks, one healthy (left) the other congenital hypothyroid, revealing retarded skeletal growth and development. B: Microradiogram of transverse section of the rib of a dog with hyperadrenocorticism. Osteoporosis characterized by widened Haversian canals as compared normal (arrow). (Courtesy Department of Pathology, Free University, Berlin.) C: Hypervitaminosis A in a 3-year-old cat, which according to the history ate almost exclusively cat food and raw liver and was referred because of lameness of both front legs and an inability to groom itself. The radiographs revealed new bone formation without bone loss on the vertebrae and around the elbow joint, causing ankylosis.

11. Tissue hormones and hormonal manifestations of cancer

11.1 Introduction

As discussed in Chapter 1 the capacity to synthesize and to secrete hormones is not confined to endocrine glands. In the last two decades it has become clear that body functions are also strongly influenced by diffuse hormonal secretion emanating from many cellular sources. Initially it was thought that these cells, although occurring in different anatomical sites, shared a common embryologic origin and common functional properties. Because of some common biochemical characteristics the acronym APUD (*amine precursor uptake and decarboxylation*) was coined for these cells, and because of the presumed common embryogenesis from the neural crest, the term neuroendocrine was introduced.

More recently it has become apparent that, although some of these cells are indeed derived from the neural crest, others do not originate from neural crest or ectoderm. For example, cells producing gastrointestinal and pancreatic hormones are derived from endoderm. Therefore it has been proposed to deemphasize the embryologic origin and to rename this widespread endocrine/paracrine/autocrine system as "diffuse neuroendocrine system" (DNES), of which neuroendocrine cells with APUD characteristics are a constituent.[1] A preeminent example of this system has been presented in Chapter 2, i.e., GH-producing cells in the mammary gland (Fig. 2–18).

Part of the relevance of these tissue hormones or the DNES is in the recognition of the wide distribution of peptide-secreting cells that may exert autocrine and paracrine actions (Fig. 1–1) for vital processes such as epithelial growth. In the gut there is a functional convergence of tissue hormones and the nervous system. DNES cells and local peptide-containing neuronal cells and ganglia coordinate local neuroendocrine regulatory functions.

In addition to these important roles in physiology, the cells of the DNES may give rise to excessive secretion. This may occur under the influence of exogenous or endogenous stimulation such as in the case of the progestin-induced GH excess (Section 2.2.3). It may also happen as a result of neoplastic transformation of these cells. Such hormone excess syndromes, arising from tumors in tissues that do not normally secrete that hormone in significant amounts, have been termed "paraneoplastic endocrine syndromes" or "ectopic hormonal syndromes". From the above it will be evident that these ectopic syndromes are not truly ectopic. It is rather a tumor-induced amplification of a property that is normally present in the cells from which the neoplasm originated.[2] A common feature in these syndromes is the elaboration of peptide hormones. In general, steroid synthesis by neoplasias requires an origin in adrenal or gonadal tissue. Complete synthesis of steroid (and also thyroid) hormones by tumors originated from nonendocrine tissue has not been described in dogs or cats and seems to be extremely rare in man.

In this chapter three peptides will be discussed briefly, because they have been studied in dogs or cats to some extent and/or are known to give rise to a humoral syndrome of cancer.

11.2 Atrial natriuretic peptide

Within the walls of the cardiac atria, there are myoendocrine cells having granules containing the prohormone of atrial natriuretic peptide (ANP). When stimulated these cardiocytes release the biologically active forms of the 28 amino acid

A. Rijnberk (ed.), Clinical Endocrinology of Dogs and Cats, 197–202.

198

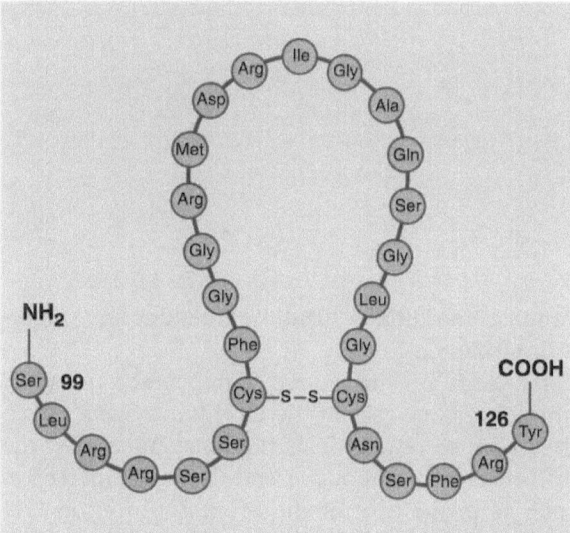

Fig. 11-1. Schematic illustration of the amino acid sequence of canine ANP. The disulfide bond is critical for biological activity.

containing ANP (Fig. 11–1), together with various N- and C-terminally extended and shortened forms of ANP. Outside the atrium synthesis of natriuretic peptides has also been found, for instance, in the brain. These natriuretic peptides (BNP, CNP) are derived from distinct genes that closely resemble the gene encoding ANP.[3]

ANP is released by stretching of the atrial wall (Fig. 11–2) and plays an important role in the regulation of volume homeostasis (Fig. 11–3). Therefore it may expected to be involved in the pathogenesis of conditions of volume overload. A sixfold increase in plasma ANP concentrations has been found in dogs with congestive heart failure.[4] In a study in dogs with variable severity of mitral valve insufficiency, plasma ANP levels did not increase until there was decompensation with severe enlargement of the left atrium.[5] In dogs with congestive heart failure, both ANP(99–126), and the unprocessed precursor of ANP are detectable in the circulation.[4]

11.3 Erythropoietin

Erythropoietin is a glycoprotein with a molecular mass of 39 kD. It is primarily produced in the kidney, most probably in interstitial or capillary endothelial cells. Extrarenal sources account for less than 10% of the production, of which the liver may be the main site.

The regulation of the release of erythropoietin follows the classic feedback control. It is secreted in response to renal tissue hypoxia, whereas hyperoxia decreases its production. This includes not only systemic hypoxia, but also local changes in renal blood flow such as in the presence of renal cysts or tumors that compress the surrounding renal parenchyma.

Eyrthropoietin acts on several steps of red cell production by the bone marrow. It also promotes hemoglobin synthesis and release of reticulocytes into the circulation. The erythroid marrow can increase production 6–10 times basal rates in response to prolonged stimulation by erythropoietin.[6]

With progressive loss of renal parenchyma, such as in chronic renal insufficiency, a relative erythropoietin deficiency may develop. Indeed, in dogs with chronic renal failure, circulating concentrations of erythropoietin were in the low normal range, despite mild to moderate anemia.[7]

Increased production of erythropoietin may originate from renal tumors. This causes inappropriate erythrocytosis and may lead to the syndrome of polycythemia. In this syndrome signs

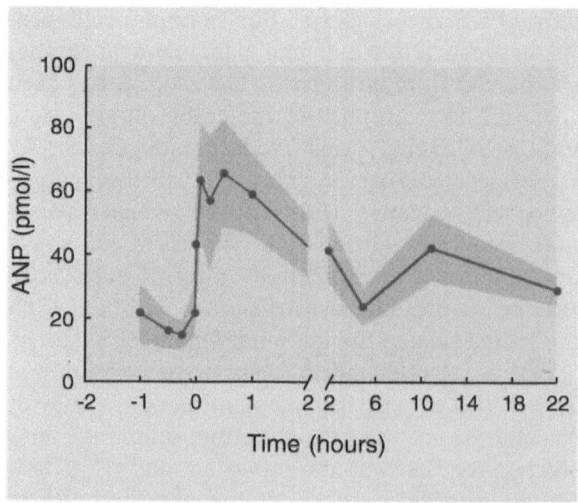

Fig. 11-2. Plasma ANP concentrations (mean ± SEM) in 11 dogs with pericardial effusion, as influenced by pericardiocentesis (at time zero). This illustrates that it is not the pericardial/atrial pressure but rather the atrial stretch that causes ANP release. (Adapted from Stokhof et al., 1994[23].)

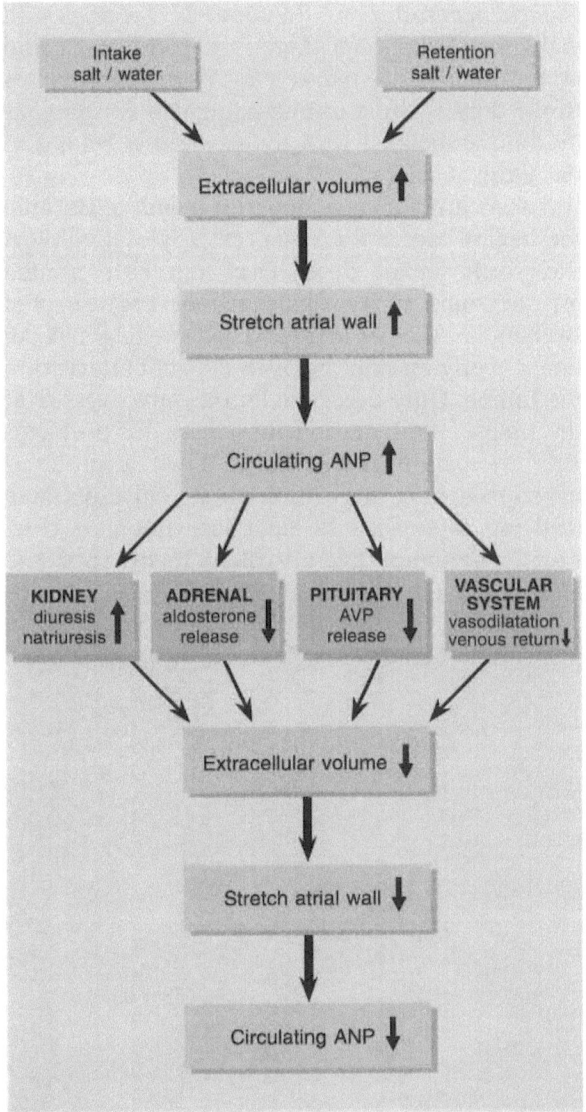

Fig. 11-3. Role of ANP in volume homeostasis; ↑ = increase, ↓ = decrease.

and symptoms can be related to hyperviscosity and include lethargy, disorientation, tremors, ataxia, (episodic) weakness, and seizures. The sludging of blood cells may result in thrombosis and hemorrhagic diathesis. Treatment of polycythemia consists of temporary alleviations by repeated phlebotomies and replacement of the removed volume by colloidal and electrolyte solutions.[8]

Polycythemia has also been observed in dogs with tumors of nonrenal origin, such as testicular tumors and hemangiosarcoma.[9] In addition to these secondary forms of polycythemia there is the so-called polycythemia vera. In this syndrome the circulating concentrations of erythropoietin are low. The excessive erythropoiesis is the result of a population of abnormally replicating erythroid progenitor cells that fail to respond to inhibitory signals. The mechanism or cause of this myeloproliferative disorder with characteristics of malignant transformation is unknown.[10]

Measurements of circulating levels of erythropoietin in dogs and cats have thus far been performed by radioimmunoassays employing antibodies to the human hormone. Crossreactivity with canine and feline erythropoietin has not been reported in detail, so that at this stage it is hard to judge whether some of the observed overlaps between categories of patients[9] are a reflection of only slight pathobiological differences or in part due to lack of specificity of the assay. The human hormone is also used for therapeutic purposes. Dogs and cats with chronic renal failure have been treated with injections of recombinant human erythropoietin (r-HuEPO). This resulted not only in significant increases in the hematocrit value, but also in improvement of well-being, i.e, improved appetite, weight gain, and increased strength. Unfortunately, the immunogenicity of r-HuEPO for dogs and cats has dampened the initial expectations and enthusiasm for its therapeutic use.[11] The antibody production results in hypoplastic anemia.

11.4 Parathyroid hormone-related protein

The parathyroid hormone-related protein (PTHrP) was initially identified as the protein responsible for humoral hypercalcemia of malignancy. Later it became apparent that parathyroid hormone (PTH) and PTHrP genes have arisen form a common ancestral gene and represent two members of a small gene family. PTHrP is larger than PTH (139–177 vs 84 amino acids), but shares 70% sequence homology with PTH in the N-terminal region. The posttranslational processing of PTHrP is extremely complex and appears to be analogous to that of proopiomelanocortin (Fig. 4–5), in that it is processed into a series of peptides with potentially different functions.[12] Peptides containing the first 34 amino acids of both PTH or PTHrP bind with equal affinity to PTH/PTHrP receptors.

The PTH and PTHrP genes are regulated quite differently. Physiological control of the PTH gene is limited to calcium and $1,25(OH)_2$vit D. In contrast, a wide variety of agents (e.g., vitamin D, prolactin, and estrogens) have been reported to influence transcription of the PTHrP gene.[13]

PTHrP is expressed in a wide spectrum of normal tissues, including muscle, lactating mammary gland, brain, and neuroendocrine cells. The physiological roles are only beginning to be explored, but there is evidence that PTHrP and PTHrP-derived peptides function in an autocrine and/or paracrine fashion in processes such as fetal growth and neonatal development, cellular growth and differentiation, reproduction and lactation, transepithelial calcium transport, and smooth muscle relaxation.[12]

11.4.1 Hypercalcemia of malignancy

Although awareness of physiological roles of PTHrP is of recent origin, it was already speculated in the 1940s that in man certain tumors might produce a substance similiar to PTH. The condition was called pseudohyperparathyroidism and first described in canine and feline malignant lymphoma in the 1970s.[14,15] In addition, the condition was found to be associated with adenocarcinomas originating from apocrine glands of the anal sac region.[16]

Pathogenesis. In principle, malignancy-associated hypercalcemia may arise through three mechanisms: (1) local osteolysis, (2) secretion of PTHrP, and (3) production of $1,25(OH)_2$vit D. The first possibility may be expected especially in hematological malignancies that produce substances that act locally in the bone marrow to mobilize calcium and phosphate.[17] Increased PTHrP concentrations in plasma have consistently been found in dogs with adenocarcinomas derived from apocrine glands of the anal sac[18]. In dogs with malignant lymphoma PTHrP concentration by itself may not be high enough to cause hypercalcemia and thus other factors such as the production of $1,25(OH)_2$vit D may interact synergistically or additively.[18]

Clinical manifestations. In about 20% of dogs with malignant lymphoma there is hypercalcemia and in this there is a marked overrepresentation of Boxer dogs.[19] Most canine malignant lymphomas that are associated with hypercalcemia belong to the T-cell subclass.[19]

Adenocarcinomas of apocrine glands of the anal sac region occur in older ($\geq$ 9 years), almost exclusively female dogs. They may be presented for the signs of hypercalcemia or because of a swelling in the perineum. This swelling has an intact overlying skin that is usually not attached to the tumor. Only occasionally they are so large at the time of presentation that there are problems with defecation (Fig. 11–4). When a probe is introduced into the orifice of the corresponding anal sac, it appears to enter into the mass (Fig. 11–5). The tumors are invariably malignant[20] and already at the first examination there may be

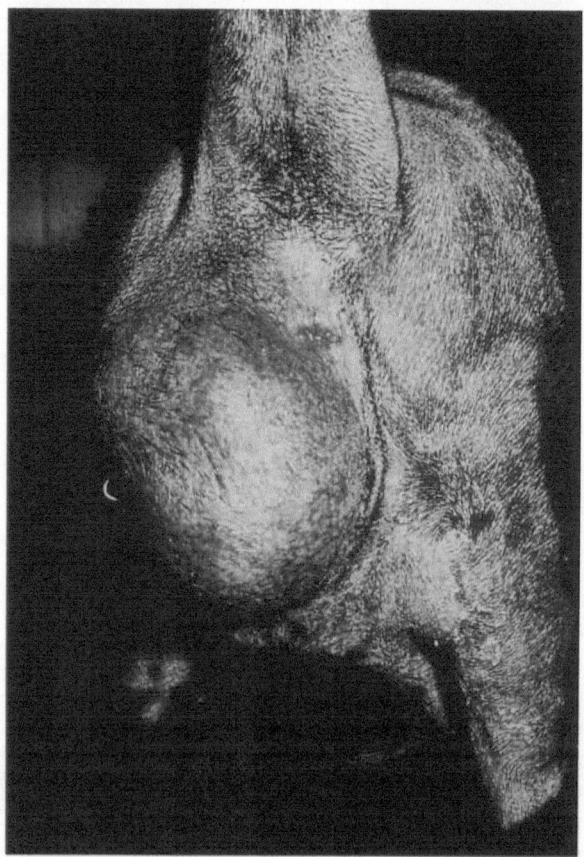

Fig. 11-4. Perineum of a female 12-year-old Cocker Spaniel with a large adenocarcinoma of apocrine glands of the anal sac region, which caused hypercalcemia.

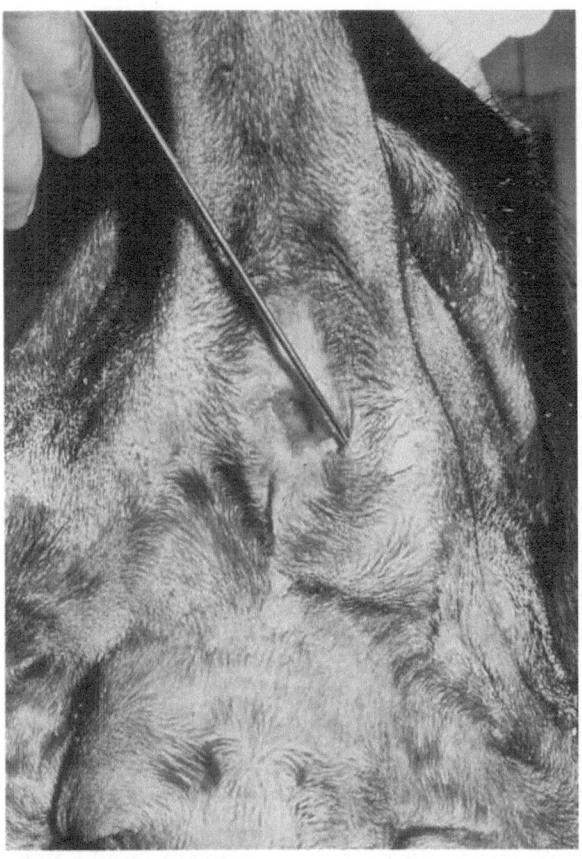

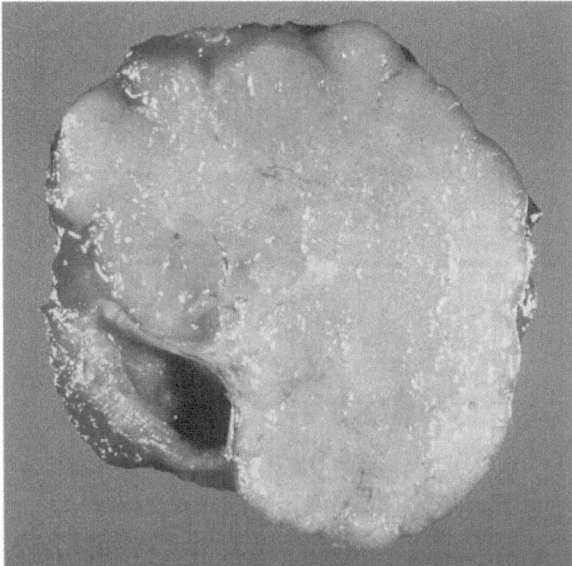

Fig. 11-5. Perineum of a 9-year-old female German Pointer with an adenocarcinoma of the aprocrine glands of the right anal sac region. A probe has been introduced into the natural orifice of the anal sac (left). The cross section of the surgerical specimen illustrates the intimate relationship between anal sac and tumor.

evidence of metastases to regional lymph nodes (internal iliac/lumbar) or distant metastases (e.g., liver, lungs, kidneys).

As in primary hyperparathyroidism the hypercalcemia of both malignancies gives rise to polyuria, polydipsia, anorexia, weight loss, and lethargy. In keeping with the concept that the hypercalcemia associated with adenocarcinoma of the anal sac is due to an excess of PTHrP, laboratory examination often reveals the combination of hypercalcemia and hypophosphatemia. As mentioned above, in malignant lymphoma most probably also other factors contribute to the hypercalcemia. As a consequence hypophosphatemia is found less often, which may be the reason that malignant lymphoma in a high frequency is associated with nephrocalcinosis and renal insufficiency.

Differential diagnosis. The differential diagnosis of hypercalcemia has been discussed briefly in Section 9.3.1.

Diagnosis. In many instances the cause of the hypercalcemia will be apparent because there is malignant lymphoma or an anal sac tumor. However, it may happen that hypercalcemia is found and that only with procedures such as thoracic radiography, abdominal ultrasonography and/or cytological examination of aspirates from lymph nodes or bone marrow the diagnosis malignant lymphoma can be secured.

In cases in which nonparathyroid malignancy is suspected but cannot be proven, measurements of PTHrP in plasma may be helpful. Assays for such measurements are becoming available.

Treatment. Surgical removal of an adenocarcinoma of the anal sac may abolish hypercalcemia if there are no metastases or there are metastases that have lost the capacity to produce PTHrP (Fig. 11–6). This decrease in circulating calcium concentration is associated with a decrease in PTHrP concentration.[18] Chemotherapy for malignant lymphoma may also decrease both calcium and

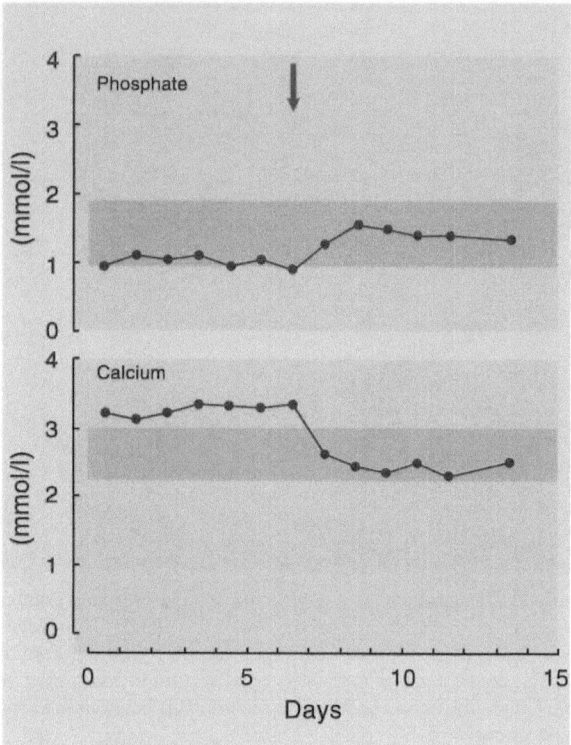

Fig. 11-6. Plasma calcium and phosphorus levels in a 12-year-old female longhaired German Pointer. Removal of the anal sac tumor led to normal calcium and phosphate values.

PTHrP concentrations in plasma.[18]

Especially if there is dehydration, plasma calcium concentration may reach critically high values. Therefore volume expansion with fluid therapy is an important supportive measure before treatment can be started that will result in elimination of the cause(s) of the increased bone resorption (see also Chapter 14).

Prognosis. In dogs with malignant lymphoma that is associated with hypercalcemia, the prognosis for response and survival with chemotherapy is worse than in dogs with malignant lymphoma and normocalcemia. This may be related to the fact that hypercalcemia is especially encountered among lymphomas of the T-cell immuno-phenotype, which have a much less favourable prognosis than the B-cell lymphomas.[21]

In the absence of metastases the prognosis after surgical removal of a perianal adenocarcinoma is excellent. However, there are often metastases to regional lymph nodes. If it is possible to resect metastases to iliac/lumbar lymph nodes, there may be a definite cure if there are no distant metastases.

11.5 Humoral manifestations of cancer

Malignant tumors originating from the testes, ovaries, adrenal cortices, or thyroid often retain the capacity to synthesize and secrete steroid or thyroid hormones (see previous chapters). Synthesis of steroid or thyroid hormones by non-endocrine tissue has not been described.

Apart from malignancies of endocrine glands that secrete peptide hormones (e.g., insulinomas) there are cancers arising from tissue other than the "classic" endocrine glands that have the capacity to produce peptide hormones. Examples have been given in the previous section. The secretion of peptides by cancers is not confined to well-known peptide hormones but may also include antibodies. Thymomas most probably give rise to myasthenia gravis by the production of antibodies against the acetylcholine receptor.[22]

Then there is the hypothesis that tumor necrosis factor (TNF) or cachectin causes the anorexia and weight loss often observed in cancer. However, most published reports of studies in man have indicated that TNF is not detectable in such patients.[2] Cancer can also be associated with fever, without any evidence of infection. This type of fever may be caused by tumor stimulation of host white blood cell pyrogen production or by production of a pyrogen by the tumor. The latter seems to be the case with malignant lymphoma.[2]

12. Obesity

In healthy animals food intake is matched to energy expenditure by coordinated activity of "feeding" and "satiety" center in the hypothalamus. When energy intake exceeds the needs for physiologic funtions at rest (resting metabolic rate) and physical activity, the energy excess is stored as triacylglycerols in adipose tissue.

The term obesity is used when the excess of body fat leads to a body weight > 20–25% of ideal weight. The reported figures for the prevalence of obesity vary widely, but there is general agreement that the condition is common in both dogs and cats. Among purebred dogs, certain breeds are more prone to obesity than others. Breeds likely to become obese are: Labrador Retriever, Cairn Terrier, Shetland Sheepdog, Basset Hound, Cavalier King Charles Spaniel, and Beagle.[1]

Pathogenesis. The positive energy balance leading to obesity results from excessive intake, decreased expenditure, or from a combination of the two. Only very rarely can this imbalance be explained by a specific underlying defect. For example, hypothyroidism decreases energy expenditure, although it should be pointed out that obesity is usually mild, for appetite usually decreases accordingly. Glucocorticoid excess most probably leads to disturbed hypothalamic control of food intake and polyphagia may develop. Also hyperinsulinemia increases appetite. Gonadal steroids and specifically estrogens seem to inhibit appetite; ovariectomy results in an increase in food intake.[2]

In the great majority of cases obesity has to be regarded as a condition in which several less specific causative factors may play a role, and some may even co-exist in one individual animal. Of these factors genotype, differences in energy expenditure and owner behavior are the most important. Genetic involvement has not yet been analyzed in dogs or cats, but the above mentioned higher incidence in certain dog breeds suggests that genetic factors play a role. Energy expenditure at rest may vary among individual animals by as much as ± 15% and it is therefore not surprising that different animals maintain weight on widely differing intakes. With energy expenditure by activity the inter-individual differences are even greater. The wide variation in exercise is partly genetically determined, but the exercise pattern is also dependent upon owner behavior. For example, in a dog that joins the owner for long walks or jogging the energy expenditure may be considerable, whereas under-exercised dogs easily may gain weight. Other influences from the owner that may contribute to obesity are additional feeding of treats and encouraging appetite.

Clinical manifestations. In regular obesity the extra adipose tissue is more or less diffusely distributed over the trunk. The ribs can no longer be palpated easily and the indentation caudal to the last ribs disappears. In some cases there is a more local accumulation of the fat mass. In the lumbar area bilaterally localized fat deposits may occur, causing some owners to think of the possibility of tumor development. It may also happen that the fat is largely distributed over the dorsal part of the trunk and has an abrupt end at the base of the tail.

Obesity is associated with increased risk of other problems. Of these joint and locomotor problems may be the most severe. In addition, there is the increased risk of metabolic problems such as hepatic dysfunction due to fatty liver and the syndrome of hepatic lipidosis in cats, as well as diabetes mellitus. The large amounts of subcutaneous fat may also lead to heat intolerance.

A. Rijnberk (ed.), Clinical Endocrinology of Dogs and Cats, 203–204.
© 1996 *Kluwer Academic Publishers.*

Differential diagnosis. Obesity has to be distinguished from endocrine diseases that may be associated with an excess of body fat, such as hypothyroidism and hyperadrenocorticism. For descriptions of these conditions and diagnostic tests the reader is referred to Chapters 3, 4 and 13.

Diagnosis. Usually obesity is easily recognized by observation and palpation. Nevertheless, it is often desirable to exclude hypothyroidism and hyperadrenocorticism (Chapter 13) before treatment is started. Of the methods for assessment of obesity, measurements of subcutaneous fat by skinfold caliper lack sufficient accuracy because the skinfold is lifted off the underlying subcutaneous fat layer. Reliable estimations of the amount of subcutaneous fat in dogs can be made with ultrasonography,[3] although this method is not yet widely used for this purpose.

Treatment. In dogs rapid weight loss can be achieved with total starvation. No severe physical or biochemical changes are observed in dogs, even when starvation is continued for 8 weeks. In about 5–6 weeks a weight loss of about 25% is achieved.[4] Although it may be considered as an option when "emergency" weight reduction is required,[1] it is not commonly used because of the need for hospitalization and insufficient owner involvement. Especially because of the latter it is often difficult to prevent recurrence.

In the long term, better results are usually obtained when owner and veterinarian together make a program for weight reduction. This should include a rough estimate of the final target weight, strict instruction of food intake, and a gradual increase in exercise. In addition, the owner should keep a record of the changes in body weight.

Currently there are several commercial pet foods with a high fiber content. Inclusion of these raw materials in a low energy diet does not seem to have a beneficial effect on satiety. In addition, a high intake of insoluble fiber is associated with gastrointestinal signs such as bloating, flatulence, and loose stools.[1]

For dogs a satisfactory approach has been the use of canned green beans. The owner is asked to feed only commercial dry food, to fix the amount exactly and then to replace half the amount by canned green beans. This approach results in a slow but steady decrease of body weight. In severe cases initially only green beans can be given for a few weeks.[5] When the target weight has been reached the dog can be fed only dry food again. However, some owners have found it easier to continue feeding a mixture of canned green beans and commercial food, adjusting the proportion as required.[5]

In cats restriction of food intake is the only means of weight reduction. Because of the risk of liver disease (lipidosis) it should be introduced and monitored very carefully. Feeding of about 60% of the maintenance requirement has been successful without any adverse effect on hepatic function or general health.[8] Especially dietary protein has been demonstrated to reduce hepatic lipid accumulation in restricted fed obese cats.[9]

So far results of pharmacological approaches have not been very encouraging. In the absence of hypothyroidism the administration of thyroid hormone is not effective. Anorectic drugs such as fenfluramine or adrenergic compounds have not found wide acceptance. Recently the administration of the adrenocortical steroid dehydroepiandrosterone (DHEA) was reported to result in significant weight loss without concomitant measures to restrict food intake.[6,7] Further long-term studies will reveal whether this promising result can be substantiated.

Prognosis. With good mutual understanding between veterinarian and owner, and good adherence by the owner to the program and regular weighing, good long-term results can be obtained.

13. Protocols for function tests

13.1 Pituitary; anterior lobe

13.1.1 CRH test

Indication. Suspicion of decreased secretory capacity of corticotropic cells, which may be due to (1) pituitary lesion by tumor or surgery, or (2) suppression by exogenous or endogenous (adrenocortical tumor) glucocorticoid excess.

Performance. At —15, 0, 5, 10, 20 and 30 min, 2–3 ml blood is collected in EDTA-coated tubes for measurements of ACTH and cortisol. At time zero 1 µg oCRH/kg body weight (Peninsula Laboratories) is injected intravenously.

Interpretation. Depending on the assay, basal ACTH values in control dogs range from 10 to 70 ng/l[1] or 20 to 125 ng/l.[2] Following CRH administration the ACTH concentrations usually peak at 5 minutes with increments ($\pm$ SEM) of 166 ± 47[3] – 279 ± 41[2] ng/l and absolute values ranging from 93 to 372 ng/l.[4] The cortisol values peak at 20 min with increments ($\pm$ SEM) of 344 ± 26 nmol/l)[2] and absolute values ranging from 220 to 543 nmol/l. In dogs with autonomously hypersecreting adrenocortical tumor, CRH causes virtually no release of endogenous ACTH or cortisol.[2]

13.1.2 GHRH test

Indication. Suspicion of decreased secretory capacity of somatotropic cells, which may be due to (1) pituitary lesion (cyst, tumor, surgery), or (2) progestin-induced GH secretion by the mammary gland.

Performance. Blood sampling before and after the intravenous administration of 1 µg hGHRH (Peninsula Laboratories) is done as in the CRH test.

Interpretation. In healthy (anestrous) dogs basal GH levels ($\pm$ SEM) between pulses are 1.3 ± 0.3 µg/l. GHRH administration causes a rise in the circulating GH levels ($\pm$ SEM) ranging from 23 ± 7 to 35 ± 14 µg/l[5] with absolute values at 10 min ranging from 5 to 28 µg/l.[4]

In dogs with congenital pituitary dwarfism there is usually no rise in GH levels. In dogs with GH excess of mammary origin, the more or less elevated GH levels cannot be further stimulated.[5] In dogs with hyperadrenocorticism, including some conditions that probably in part erroneously have been named acquired GH deficiency (Section 2.2.2), the increased endogenous somatostatin tone prohibits GH release in response to hGHRH administration.

Comments

Because of the rapid proteolytic degradation of some pituitary hormones, blood samples should be collected in EDTA-coated ice-chilled tubes and be centrifuged in a cooled centrifuge. Plasma should be stored at or below —20 °C. Thus preferably the samples should be collected in laboratories where the measurements are performed. If not, the frozen samples should be shipped on dry ice using an overnight mail service.[a]

Very recently a combined function test has been introduced. In this test the anterior pituitary is stimulated with four hypothalamic releasing hormones (oCRH, hGHRH, TRH and GnRH)

[a] For homologous GH assay: Biochemical Laboratory, Department of Clinical Sciences of Companion Animals, Yalelaan 8, P.O. Box 80.154, 3508 TD Utrecht, The Netherlands. Fax: 31–30–518126

205

A. Rijnberk (ed.), Clinical Endocrinology of Dogs and Cats, 205–212,
© 1996 *Kluwer Academic Publishers.*

206

with measurments of ACTH(+cortisol), GH, PRL, and LH.[4] There appears to be little interference as compared with the single administration of these secretagogues, except for the LH response, which is lower in the combined test than following single GnRH administration.[4]

As far as alternatives for the hypophysiotropic hormones is concerned, it should be mentioned that lysine-vasopressin (LVP) can stimulate the pituitary-adrenocortical axis. However, in contrast to CRH it is not suited for distinguishing pituitary-dependent hyperadrenocorticism from hyperadrenocorticism due to adrenocortical tumor, because cortisol release from adrenocortical tumors can be directly stimulated by LVP.[2]

Instead of GHRH, the α_2-agonist clonidine[b] can be administered at a dose of 10 µg/kg body weight. Increments ($\pm$ SEM) tend to be somewhat higher than following 1 µg GHRH/kg and range from 30 $\pm$ 7 to 45 $\pm$ 14 µg/l.[5] Also another α_2-agonist may be used, i.e., xylazine.[c] Following a dose of 0.3 mg/kg, GH concentrations (mean $\pm$ SEM) in plasma rises to 71 $\pm$ 16 µg/l[6] at 15 min, although a lower dose (0.1 mg/kg) is also a sufficient stimulus.

13.2 Pituitary; posterior lobe

13.2.1 Modified water deprivation test

Indication. Suspicion of disturbance of vasopressin release.

Priniciple. In this indirect test for vasopressin secretory capacity, plasma osmolality (Posm) is increased by water deprivation to stimulate vasopressin release. The effect is measured indirectly by measurements of urine osmolality (Uosm) during the test.

Performance. Following 12 h of fasting, water is withheld and plasma and urine are collected every hour or every two hours, depending on the severity of the polyuria. In both fluids osmolality (Posm and Uosm) is measured. When the weight loss approaches 5% of initial body weight, the test

[b] Catapresan®, Boehringer Ingelheim
[c] Rompun®, Bayer

should be stopped. When, in the presence of an adequate osmotic stimulus (Posm $\geq$ 310 mOsm/kg), urine concentration is maximal (less than 5% increase in Uosm between consecutive collections), 2 U lysine vasopressin are administered subcutaneously. Uosm is measured again 1 h later.

Interpretation. In both nephrogenic diabetes insipidus and central diabetes insipidus Uosm will remain low during water deprivation. In complete diabetes insipidus Uosm will rise by 50% or more following the injection of vasopressin, whereas in the partial forms of central diabetes insipidus the rise will be $\geq$ 15%, and in nephrogenic diabetes insipidus there will be very little or no rise in Uosm (Figs. 2–29, 2–30)[7]. Because of the indirect character of the test, the results may not always be conclusive.[8]

13.2.2 Vasopressin measurements during hypertonic saline infusion

Indication. Suspicion of deficient vasopressin release or inappropriate vasopressin secretion.

Performance. The euhydrated animal is infused for 2 h via the jugular vein with 20% NaCl solution at a rate of 0.03 ml/kg body weight per minute. Samples for plasma AVP and Posm are obtained at 20-min intervals. Especially in the severely polyuric animal there is the risk of inducing critical hypertonicity; the samples should be checked for Posm immediately and at values of about 360 mOsm/kg the infusion should be stopped.

Interpretation. The slope of the regression line for Posm and Pavp is used as a measure of the sensitivity of the osmoregulatory system. In the nomogram developed by Biewenga et al.,[8] the 90% range for sensitivity was 0.24–2.47 pmol/ml per mOsm/kg. The 90% range for the threshold of the system was 276–309 mOsm/kg. See also Figs. 2–28, 2–30, 2–31).

Comment
The test requires very close observation and monitoring of Posm. This, and the fact that vasopressin is very sensitive to proteolytic breakdown, makes it advisable that the test is performed

in institutions that have developed experience with this test.

13.3 Thyroids

13.3.1 TSH-stimulation test

Indication. Suspicion of hypothyroidism.

Performance. Plasma (EDTA or heparin) for plasma T_4 measurements is collected immediately before and 4 h after the intravenous injection of 5 IU of TSH.

Interpretation. In healthy dogs, plasma-T_4 concentrations are 20–46 nmol/l and increase to 39–80 nmol/l at 4 h after TSH administration. Classically in primary hypothyroidism the plasma-T_4 concentration is < 5 nmol/l and there is little (< 5 nmol/l) or no increase after TSH administration.

Some nonthyroidal diseases (e.g., hyperadreno-corticism and chronic renal failure) and administration of certain drugs (e.g., glucocorticoids, nonsteroidal anti-inflammatory drugs, and anti-convulsive drugs) may lead to low T_4 levels, but the increase following TSH is parallel to that in normal dogs.

In dogs with secondary hypothyroidism, plasma-T_4 concentrations are reduced and after TSH administration they increase until within the lower part of the reference range for basal values. The only very occasionally occurring mild (and nonprogressive) forms of primary hypothyroidism may pose a problem and for definite diagnosis a thyroid biopsy may be needed (Fig. 13–1).

Comment

As long as there is no assay for measurements of endogenous levels of canine TSH,* the TSH-stimulation test will be needed. However, since the introduction of assays for measuring TSH in

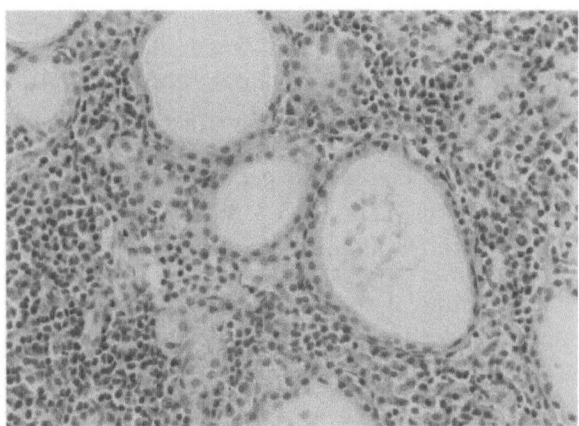

Fig. 13-1. Responses of plasma-T_4 concentrations to be expected in healthy dogs (blue), dogs with drug-induced lowering of basal T_4 and secondary hypothyroidism (red), and dogs with primary hypothyroidism (green), together with the results of basal T_4 measurements in a 9-year-old spayed female Heidewachtel dog that was presented for a dull coat and some weight gain since about a year. On three occasions (May, September and October) a TSH-stimulation test was carried out. The responses seemed to suggest the possibility of secondary hypothyroidism. However, a thyroid biopsy in October revealed focal and diffuse lymphoplasmacytic thyroiditis (right). The course of the disease, the basal T_4 values, the responses to TSH and the results of the biopsy indicated that there was mild primary hypothyroidism with little or no progression.

*) See also addendum at page 212.

Thyroxine (nmol/l)

Months

human plasma, the bovine TSH for the stimulation test has become less available. Although in some parts of the world it is still on the market,[d] in several European countries it is no longer available. Therefore the Veterinary Pharmacy of the Utrecht University has been providing a bovine TSH preparation for TSH-stimulation tests.[e] It is delivered as freeze-dried powder (5 IU/vial) together with vials containing 2 ml 5% dextrose as the solvent.

As an alternative the TRH test may be used. At 4 h after intravenous administration of 200 μg TRH[f] in healthy dogs there is a significant increase in plasma-T_4 concentration.[9,9a] Because of its indirect character the test may have less discriminatory power than the TSH-stimulation test.

13.4 Adrenal cortex

13.4.1 ACTH-stimulation test

Indication. Suspicion of decreased adrenocortical reserve capacity: (1) primary adrenocortical insufficiency (Addison's disease), and (2) (iatrogenic) secondary adrenocortical insufficiency.

Performance. Plasma (heparin or EDTA) for cortisol measurements is collected immediately before and 90 min after intravenous administration of 0.25 mg synthetic ACTH.[g] In cases in which treatment for adrenocortical insufficiency was already started, on the morning of the test the cortisone administration is postponed until after completion of the test. When dexamethasone is used instead of cortisone, it may not be necessary to omit the glucocorticoid substitution as in most cortisol assays there is no cross reactivity with dexamethasone.

Interpretation. In healthy dogs, the cortisol concentrations rise to 270–690 nmol/l. In Addison's

disease the control value is usually low and there is no increase following ACTH administration. In animals with secondary adrenocortical insufficiency the basal cortisol values may be low as well, and, depending on the severity (duration) of the ACTH deficiency, the cortisol rise is subnormal or absent.

Comment
When in doubt about the differentiation between primary or secondary adrenocortical insufficiency, ACTH concentrations in plasma should be measured. These will be extremely high in primary hypoadrenocorticism and (unmeasurably) low in secondary hypoadrenocorticism.

13.4.2 Low-dose dexamethasone suppression test (LDDST)

Principle. The sensitivity of the hypothalamus-pituitary-adrenocortical axis for the suppressive effect of glucocorticoids is tested by administering a low dose of a potent glucocorticoid that suppresses the system in normal animals but not in animals with hyperadrenocorticism.

Indication. Suspicion of hyperadrenocorticism.

Performance. In the morning 0.01 mg dexamethasone per kg body weight is administered intravenously. Blood for cortisol measurements is collected immediately before and at 4 h and 8 h after dexamethasone administration.

Interpretation. A plasma cortisol concentration exceeding 40 nmol/l at 8 h after dexamethasone adminstration may be regarded as diagnostic for hyperadrenocorticism with a diagnostic accuracy of 0.83 (95% confidence limits 0.76–0.88).[10] The measurements at 0 and 4 h are not needed for the diagnosis of hyperadrenocorticism but may be informative in the differential diagnosis. It is not uncommon that the high value at 8 h is preceded by a lower value at 4 h.[11] Thus, at 8 h the system escapes from the suppression by dexamethasone. If the value at 4 h is at least 50% lower than the basal value, the disease may be regarded as pituitary dependent.

---

[d] Thyropar®, Rorer Pharmaceuticals Corporation, Fort Washington, PA, USA

[e] Veterinary Pharmacy, Faculty of Veterinary Medicine, Yalelaan 6, 3584 CM Utrecht, The Netherlands. Fax: 31–30–532065

[f] TRH®, Hoffman-La Roche, Basel, Switzerland

[g] Cortrosyn®, Organon (0.25 mg tetracosactide per ampoule)

13.4.3 High-dose dexamethasone suppression test (HDDST)

Principle. Although in the great majority of cases of pituitary-dependent hyperadrenocorticism the sensitivity of the pituitary-adrencortical system is found to be decreased with the low-dose dexamethasone suppression test, the system usually is still suppressible with a high dose of dexamethasone. Since the circulating cortisol levels cannot be suppressed with high doses of dexamethasone in hyperadrenocorticism due to adrenocortical tumor, this test often allows differentiation between the two forms.

Indication. Once the diagnosis has been established by the low-dose dexamethasone suppression test, the high-dose dexamethasone suppression test is performed to distinguish between pituitary-dependent hyperadrenocorticism and hyperadrenocorticism due to adrenocortical tumor.

Performance. Blood for cortisol determination is collected immediately before and 3 h after administration of 0.1 mg dexamethasone per kg body weight.

Interpretation. If the plasma cortisol concentration declines by more than 50%, the diagnosis pituitary-dependent hyperadrenocorticism is justified. A decrease of less than 50% can be due to an adrenocortical tumor or to a dexamethasone-resistant form of pituitary-dependent hyperadrenocorticism.

13.4.4 Urinary corticoid/creatinine ratios with high-dose suppression test (C/C+Dex)

Principle. By measuring cortisol in morning urine an "integration" of the production over a period of about 8 h is achieved, thereby adjusting for the wide and rapid fluctuations in plasma cortisol levels. The values are related to the creatinine concentrations to correct for differences in urine concentration.

Indication. Suspicion of hyperadrenocorticism and differentiation between pituitary-dependent hyperadrenocorticism and hyperadrenocorticism due to adrenocortical tumor.

Performance. The owner is instructed to collect morning urine samples at the same time (e.g., 7 a.m.) on three consecutive days. On the preceding evenings the animal should have its last walk at identical times (e.g., 11 p.m.). After collection of the second urine sample, oral administration of dexamethasone is begun. The owner administers 0.1 mg dexamethasone per kg body weight at 8-h intervals.

Interpretation. C/C ratios exceeding 10×10^{-6} can be regarded as compatible with hyperadrenocorticism with a diagnostic accuracy of 0.91 (95% confidence limits 0.85–0.95).[10] When the ratio of the third urine sample is > 50% lower than the mean of the first two ratios, the diagnosis of pituitary-dependent hyperadrenocorticism is justified. A lesser decrease may be due to either adrenocortical tumor or dexamethasone-resistant pituitary-dependent hyperadrenocorticism.

Comments
For reasons of finances, convenience, and diagnostic accuracy in the dog the combination of LDDST and HDDST is increasingly replaced by the C/C+Dex test,[12,13] or the latter is at least regarded as a sensitive screening test.[14,15] In the meantime the C/C+Dex test has also been introduced for cats, where it seems to be applicable as well. In cats the reference values vary more widely ($2–36 \times 10^{-6}$) than in the dog, but in 7 cats with independently confirmed hyperadrenocorticism the C/C ratios were significantly higher (median 139×10^{-6}, range $50–270 \times 10^{-6}$).[16] In cats, even more than in dogs, stress during or prior to the urine collection (e.g., hospitalization) should be avoided as much as possible, since this easily activates the pituitary-adrenocortical axis and thus elevates cortisol excretion.

Urinary corticoid/creatinine ratios are also very useful for monitoring the result of treatment, i.e., following hypophysectomy or adrenalectomy, or after/during adrenocorticolysis with o,p'-DDD.[17,18] When such animals are substituted with glucocorticoids and/or mineralocorticoids, the administration of these drugs should be omitted the night before the urine sample is collected. Immediately after collection of the sample the owner should continue the substitution therapy as before (Fig. 4–36). Complete ablation of the adrenal

210

cortices or the pituitary gland results in C/C ratios $< 2 \times 10^{-6}$.

An example of a client instruction for the collection of urine and the administration of the dexamethasone tablets is given as Appendix 1 to this chapter.

13.5 Ovary, testis

13.5.1 GnRH-stimulation test

Indication. Search for ovarian or testicular tissue, i.e., in primary anestrus and suspicion of anorchism, cryptorchidism, and hermaphroditism. In addition, the test may be used when there is suspicion of incomplete ovariectomy, although usually finding of plasma progesterone concentration (> 3 nmol/l) is sufficient to detect such a remnant.

Female dog
Performance. Two ml EDTA-plasma is collected prior to, and 60 and 120 min after intravenous injection of 10 µg GnRH[h]/kg body weight for measurements of estradiol. If LH can also be measured, extra samples are collected at 10, 20 and 40 min. For sample handling and storage see 13.1.

Interpretation. In six healthy female dogs mean basal LH concentrations (+ SEM) were 1.8 ± 0.2 µg/l in early anestrus and 2.1 ± 0.4 µg/l in advanced anestrus, and estradiol concentrations were 20.2 ± 4.4 pmol/l in early anestrus and 21.6 ± 8.4 pmol/l in advanced anestrus. Following stimulation, peak LH concentrations of about 42 µg/l (early) and 50 µg/l (advanced) occurred after 5 to 20 min (Fig. 13–2). Stimulation induced a moderate increase in estradiol concentrations that did not return to pretreatment values during 160 min after stimulation (Fig. 13–2).

The LH and estradiol responses in advanced anestrus were greater than those in early anestrus.[19]

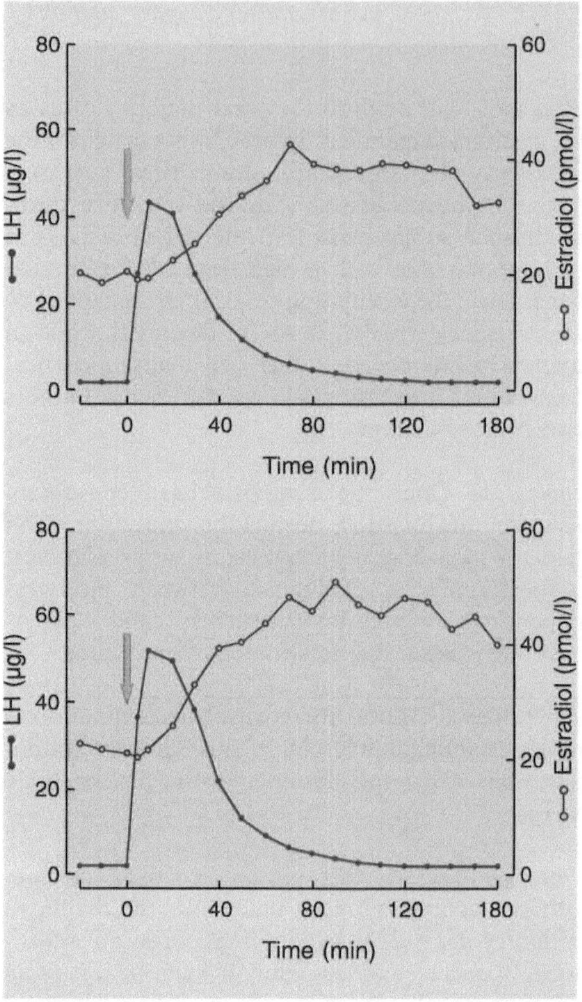

Fig. 13-2. Mean responses of LH (blue) and estradiol (green) in six healthy female dogs during early (upper panel) and advanced (lower panel) anestrus. (Adapted from Van Haaften et al., 1994.[19])

Male dog
Performance. Two ml EDTA-plasma is collected before and 40 minutes after intravenous injection of 10 µg GnRH[h]/kg body weight for measurements of testosterone. For LH measurements see female dog.

Interpretation. In six healthy male dogs mean basal LH and testosterone concentrations (± SEM) were 4.6 ± 0.5 µg/l and 9.7 ± 1.7 nmol/l,[20] respectively. Following stimulation the mean LH concentration (± SEM) at 20 min was 57 ± 13 µg/l and the mean testosterone concentration (± SEM)

[h] Fertagyl®, Intervet

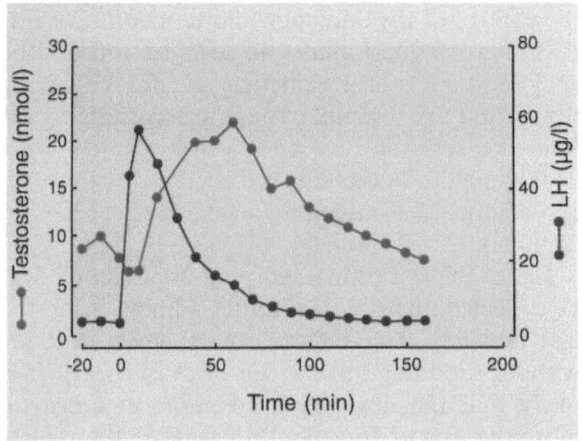

Fig. 13-3. Mean responses of LH (blue) and testosterone (red) in six healthy male dogs to the administration of 10 µg GnRH/kg body weight. (Adapted from Knol et al., 1993.[20])

at 40 min was 16 ± 4 nmol/l (Fig. 13–3). In female dogs and castrated male dogs the testosterone concentrations are low and do not change after GnRH administration.

Comments

For the detection of testicular tissue, stimulation with 500 IU human chorionic gonadotropin (hCG)[i] can also be used.[21,22] Sampling at 40 min is appropriate but may also be done at 60 and/or 120 min (Fig. 8–9) as the testosterone concentrations decline slowly over a period of 24 h.[22,23]

If remnant ovarian tissue is suspected after ovariectomy of a *queen*, 10 µgGnRH[h]/kg body weight is injected during estrus behavior. Plasma can be collected after 7–10 days for the measurement of progesterone; a value > 3 nmol/l indicates the presence of ovarian tissue.

13.6 Carbohydrate metabolism

13.6.1 Glucose tolerance test

Indication. Suspicion of decreased glucose tolerance in animals with normoglycemia after an overnight fast.

Performance. After an overnight fast 1 g glucose/ kg body weight is injected intravenously as a 50% dextrose solution over a period of 30 s. Blood for glucose measurements is collected immediately before and at 5, 15, 30, 45, 60, and 90 min after the glucose administration.

Interpretation. In healthy dogs the plasma glucose concentration usually reaches the initial values at 45 min.[24] In cats glucose disappearance is slower and the glucose value may not return to within the reference range until 90 min of more.[25]

Plotting the glucose values on semi-logarithmic coordinates allows an estimate of the half-time (t), i.e., the time required for the plasma glucose concentration to fall by one-half. Subsequently also the fractional turnover rate (k) can be calculated from the well-known relationship: $k = \ln 2/t \times 100 = 0.693/t \times 100 = \%$ disappearance per minute. Reported t and k values (mean ± SD) for dogs range from 20 ± 6 to 25 ± 8 min and 2.8 ± 0.9 to 3.8 ± 0.9%/min, respectively.[26,27] For cats the values (mean ± SEM) are 40.9 ± 1.6 min and 1.7 ± 0.1%/min,[25] illustrating more quantitatively the relative slow disappearance rate of glucose in cats.

Comments

Apart from individual variation, the results of glucose tolerance tests also vary because of factors such as the period of fasting, stress, and the carbohydrate content of the previous diet.[28,29] Chemical restraint by anesthetics or sedatives also strongly influences the result of the test.[30,31]

For optimal results strict standard conditions are required, that are not often met under clinical conditions. Therefore the value of the test may lie primarily in (clinical) research, where the glucose measurements can also be combined with those of insulin. The test is rarely used in our clinic for diagnostic purposes.

[h] Fertagyl®, Intervet
[i] Chorulon®, Intervet

212

Client information for CC+Dex test

Your dog has signs that could be due to an excessive production of the hormone cortisol by the adrenal cortex. In order to evaluate the cortisol production, we need to make measurements using morning urine samples.

We would like you to collect a sample from the dog's first morning urination on three successive days. The dog should be taken out to urinate fairly late in the evening preceding each of the three morning collections and the collection should be made at about the same time on each of the three mornings.

Place the sample in the tube, numbered 1, 2 or 3, respectively. Fill the tube only half-full (to the mark) and then place it in the freezer or freezer compartment of the refrigerator until all three samples can be mailed or brought to the address below. The tubes can be filled to less than the mark, but please do not fill them above this level, since the stopper can be forced out when the urine is frozen. The samples should not be allowed to remain unrefrigerated for more than a day, and so should not be mailed just before the weekend.

The samples are used to determine whether cortisol production is abnormal but also to assess the control of the adrenal gland function. For this reason we request that you also administer the enclosed tablets of dexamethasone after collecting the second urine sample, roughly according to the following schedule:

08.00 hours . . . . tablet(s)
16.00 hours . . . . tablet(s)
24.00 hours . . . . tablet(s)

Hence the last (third) morning urine sample will be collected about 8 hours after administering the last tablet(s). The tablets can be given with or without food (e.g., in a small piece of meat). It is likely that the dog will drink more and urinate more than usual for about a day after the tablets have been given.

University Clinic for Companion Animals
Yalelaan 8, P.O. Box 80.154
3508 TD UTRECHT

For cats the procedure is similar but the collection of urine may pose specific problems. The owner is advised to replace at night the usual litter box by a litter box containing washed (tap water) and dried aquarium gravel. The next morning the urine is collected with a syringe or a pipet. The urine is poured into the tubes through a gauze.

Addendum to section 13.3

At the time of the reading of the proof prints the first reports were presented on the development of immunoassays for the measurement of canine TSH.[32,33,34] The results are promising, but need further evaluation.

14. Treatment protocols

In the previous pages diagnostic procedures and treatments have been discussed for the endocrine disturbances known to occur in dogs and cats. In this chapter attention is given to the management of endocrine emergencies. The outcome of an emergency case is highly dependent upon prompt recognition and quick institution of appropriate treatment. Therefore some diagnostic and therapeutic aspects of endocrine emergencies are summarized here as a quick reference.

At the end of this chapter there is an addendum with instructions for owners on the treatment of hyperadrenocorticism with o,p'-DDD. These instructions have proven to be very useful for owners in the completion of this somewhat complicated protocol.

14.1 Acute adrenocortical insufficiency (Addison crisis)

History. Lethargy, weakness, anorexia, vomiting and (finally) colic symptoms with diarrhea characterized by dark colored feces.

Presentation. Severe depression, hypovolemia and often bradycardia.

Laboratory examinations. Immediately: Na (often < 130 mmol/l), K (often > 6.0 mmol/l), urea and creatinine (often indicating prerenal azotemia), eventually hematocrit and total protein (as a measure of dehydration), glucose and calcium. After stabilization: ACTH-stimulation test for definite diagnosis (Section 13.4.1).

Principles of treatment. The signs and symptoms are first of all the result of a lack of mineralocorticoids. Therefore the first and often life saving step should be the correction of the water- and electrolyte disturbances by fluid therapy (dehydration usually 10–15% of body weight!!).

Treatment protocol:
1. NaCl 0.9% iv: 10–15% of body weight during the first 4–8 h; thereafter 100 ml/kg/24 h. Monitoring of urine production and central venous pressure.
2. Glucocorticoids: To the first infusion bottle is added 5 mg hydrocortisone acetate[a]/kg, or 1 mg prednisolone succinate[b]/kg or 0.2 mg dexamethasone phosphate[c]/kg. Thereafter every 6 h subcutaneous administration of 1 mg hydrocortisone[a]/kg or 0.2 mg prednisolone[b]/kg body weight.
3. Mineralocorticoids (alternatives):
   - Desoxycorticosterone(DOCA) pivalate[d]; 2 mg/kg as a subcutaneous depot for ≥ 20 days.
   - DOCA in oil[e]; once daily 0.1 mg/kg subcutaneously.

When none of these alternatives can be used, and for glucocorticoid replacement hydrocortisone is available, one may double the dose of this drug and rely upon its intrinsic mineralocorticoid activity. As soon as possible this should be followed by oral substitution with fludrocortisone[f] and supplementation of salt (Section 4.2.1).

---

[a] Solu Cortef®, Upjohn
[b] Solu-Medrol®, Upjohn
[c] Dexadreson®, Intervet
[d] Percorten-V®, Ciba-Geigy
[e] Veterinary Pharmacy, Faculty of Veterinary Medicine, Yalelaan 6, 3584 CM Utrecht, The Netherlands. Fax: 31–30–532065
[f] Florinef®, Squibb (0.1 mg/tablet) or Kombivet bv (0.0625 mg/tablet)

213

A. Rijnberk (ed.), Clinical Endocrinology of Dogs and Cats, 213–218.
© 1996 *Kluwer Academic Publishers.*

14.2 Diabetic ketoacidosis

History. Vomiting, polyuria/polydipsia, weakness and weight loss.

Presentation. Dehydration/hypovolemia, depression varying from lethargy to coma.

Laboratory examinations. Immediately: Blood glucose, urine ketone bodies (strips, tablets). Next: Blood glucose, sodium, potassium, urea, creatinine, hematocrit, differential leucocyte count, and if possible acid-base status and/or anion gap.

Principles of treatment. The fluid loss via osmotic diuresis, vomiting and hyperventilation usually amounts 10–12% of body weight. The lack of insulin contributes to the loss of intracellular potassium, which is aggravated by vomiting, osmotic diuresis and secondary hyperaldosteronism due to the hypovolemia.

Treatment protocol:[1]
1. Rehydration by intravenous infusion of lactated Ringer's solution to which 5 mmol KCl/500 ml is added: 20 ml/kg during the first hour, 10 ml/kg/h during the next 2–3 h and thereafter 4 ml/kg/h (= 100 ml/kg/24 h). When there are no longer signs of prerenal azotemia, the infusion rate can be reduced to 2 ml/kg/h.
2. Insulin administration is based upon frequent glucose measurements in blood (strip and reflectometer). Glucose < 15 mmol/l: no insulin is given. Glucose > 15 mmol/l: 2 units regular insulin[g] intramuscularly (im) for cats and for dogs of 10 kg or less; 0.25 unit/kg for dogs over 10 kg. Check blood glucose every hour and repeat im administration of regular insulin every hour: 1 unit per dose for cats and for dogs < 10 kg, and 0.1 unit/kg for dogs > 10 kg. When plasma glucose has been lowered to the range of 8–13 mmol/l (usually after 4 h) the fluid therapy can be changed from lactated Ringer's solution to 5% glucose with 5 mmol of KCl added to each bottle of 500 ml. Then also regular insulin therapy is changed as follows: glucose < 8 mmol/l, no insulin; 8–13 mmol/l,

0.5 unit/kg subcutaneously every 6 h. Further adjustments (by 1–2 units) can be based upon glucose checks at 2–3 h after each injection.
It is practical to administer the last dose of regular insulin at about 03.00 h and then check glucose again the next morning (e.g., 08.00 h) and begin administration of IZS-P insulin[h] as described in Section 5.2.1.
3. Although not a very accurate measure for intracellular K loss, plasma K concentration is used to calculate the K deficit, i.e., the difference between the patient's plasma K value and 4.4 (= approximately the middle of the reference range). Then the dose in mmol (in most preparations 1 ml = 1 mmol) is: deficit × body weight × 0.6. The dose is added to the infusion fluid and the rate of administration should not exceed 0.5 mmol/kg/h. Such a calculated dose can be repeated as needed.
4. Bicarbonate is administered only in very severe acidosis and the administration should be stopped when pH reaches about 7.2 (see Section 5.2.1).

14.3 Hypoglycemia

History. Episodes of weakness, incoordination and tetany.

Presentation. May be presented in a coma, with or following convulsions. When not reversed rapidly, there may be irreversible brain damage.

Diagnosis. Signs of hypoglycemia are to be expected when plasma glucose < 3 mmol/l.

Principles of treatment. Convulsions are treated by administering substrate for the brain (glucose) and an anti-epileptic drug if needed. Further therapeutic measures are dependent upon the primary cause (insulinoma or excess of exogenous insulin).

Treatment protocol:
1. Glucose 50% (or 20%) intravenously: small dogs 3–5 ml (6–12) and large dogs 10–15 ml

---

[g] Actrapid® (Novo) or Humulin Regular® (Lilly), both in a concentration of 100 U/ml

[h] Caninsulin®, Intervet (40 units/ml)

(20–35). If the convulsions do not stop immediately, a total dose of 5–10 mg diazepam[i] can be administered by slow intravenous injection. The dose can be repeated after 3–5 min until the effect is satisfactory. As an alternative propofol[j] may be used. This non-barbiturate hypnotic does not cumulate and the animals rapidly awake following cessation of administration. It is given iv as a bolus of 2–6 mg/kg, followed by infusion at a rate of 2–4 mg/kg/h depending on the effect.

2. Suspicion of insulinoma: Intravenous infusion of glucose 20% at a rate of 1 ml/min and monitored by frequent plasma glucose measurements. Oral administration of diazoxide[k]: 2 capsules (100 mg) as a start, followed by 1 capsule every 8 h during the first two days and thereafter 1 capsule per day and 4–5 small meals per day.

So far experience is limited but the somatostatin analogue octreotide[l] may be more effective for immediate lowering of the insulin release. Dose rates of 1 µg/kg 3–4 times per day subcutaneously may be effective (see also Section 5.3.1).

3. In case of hypoglycemia due to insulin administration, glucose 5% (1 ml/min) is infused until a plasma glucose concentration of 5–10 mmol/l is reached. Initially plasma glucose concentration is checked every 20 min and later every hour. Usually within 18 h the plasma glucose concentrations begin to rise and the infusion can be stopped.

14.4 Hypocalcemic tetany

History. Signs of tetany and/or a recent neck surgery.

Presentation. Muscle twitching, rear limb cramping, generalized muscle spasms and eventually convulsions.

---

[i] Valium®, Roche or Stesolid®, Dumex (10 mg diazepam/ampoule)
[j] Diprivan®, ICI
[k] Proglicem®, Schering-Plough, 100 mg diazoxide/capsule
[l] Sandostatin®, Sandoz

Diagnosis. Plasma calcium concentration < 1.8 mmol/l, but treatment is usually needed before the laboratory result is available.

Treatment protocol. Slow (5–10 min) intravenous injection of calcium in a dose of 0.5–1.0 mmol Ca per kg body weight (= 20–40 mg Ca^{++}/kg) as calcium gluconate (a 20% solution contains about 0.4 mmol/ml), preferably with ECG monitoring. Once the signs of hypocalcemia are controlled, the calcium gluconate can be administered subcutaneously (diluted 1:2 with NaCl 0.9%) every 6 h until oral medication can be started (Section 9.2).

14.5 Hypercalcemic crisis

History. Inappetence, nausea, vomiting, polyuria, lethargy and weakness.

Presentation. Depressed animal with signs of dehydration/hypovolemia.

Laboratory examinations. Plasma Ca concentrations usually > 4.0 mmol/l. Plasma phosphate concentration can be low, but may be normal or high in the presence of renal insufficiency.

Principles of treatment. The first step in the treatment of hypercalcemia is to restore normal hydration as the hypovolemia decreases glomerular filtration and thus calcium clearance. Secondly measures should be taken to decrease bone resorption.

Treatment protocol:
1. NaCl 0.9% intravenously: 10–15% of body weight is administered over a period of about 6 h. Thereafter the rate of administration is gradually reduced to 2 ml/kg/h, while plasma concentrations of Ca and K are monitored. Furosemide[m] may be added to the infusion so that it is administered at a rate of 1 mg/kg/h. However, this drug should not be given until rehydration is complete, because it may further reduce the glomerular filtration rate and thereby reduce the filtered load of calcium.

---

[m] Lasix®, Hoechst-Roussel or Dimazon®, Hoechst Veterinär

2. Prednisone acetate: 2 mg/kg once daily sub-cutaneously. Glucocorticoids are primarily used to reduce bone resorption from malignant lymphomas.
3. Mithramycin[n]: 25 µg/kg intravenously. A single administration inhibits osteoclastic bone resorption in a predictable and impressive fashion for two days or longer.[2]

In principle also diphosphonates such as pamidronate[o] can be used. These drugs act by blocking bone resorption without affecting bone formation. However, as yet the experience with their use in dogs and cats is very limited.

---

[n] Mithracin®, Pfizer

[o] Aredia®, Ciba-Geigy

Client information for o,p′-DDD therapy in dogs (after Rijnberk and Belshaw, 1992[3])

The adrenal cortices of your dog produce excessive amounts of the hormone cortisol. The treatment with o,p′-DDD aims at complete destruction of the cortex of both adrenal glands. The requirement for the hormones they normally produce is then provided by lifelong administration of replacement hormone tablets. It is very important that the instructions for the replacement hormone be followed carefully and completely, for deficiency of these hormones can result in a life-threatening crisis.

The initial treatment of your dog consists of:
. . . tablets of o,p′-DDD (= Lysodren) . . . times daily for 25 days.

For good absorption and to prevent vomiting, the tablets should always be given with food. For the first 2 days only the o,p′-DDD is given. On the third day the replacement of the adrenocortical hormones is begun, with the administration of cortisone, fludrocortisone, and ordinary salt. To allow a more gradual change from the excessive hormone production, the dose of cortisone is kept higher than the normal requirement until 1 week after the end of the o,p′-DDD therapy.

During the first month your dog receives as replacement therapy:
Cortisone acetate: . . . × daily . . . tablets of . . . mg
Fludrocortisone acetate: . . . × daily . . . tablets of . . . mg
NaCl: . . . × daily . . . gram

Follow-up. The first follow-up examination is carried out 1 month after the beginning of the o,p′-DDD therapy. At this time the dose of cortisone is usually reduced by one-half. Results of blood examination will be used to determine whether the doses of fludrocortisone and salt need to be adjusted. After this, follow-up examinations are usually made once every 6 months. Their purpose is to be certain that the replacement doses of fludrocortisone and salt are correct. Sometimes, in spite of the destructive action of o,p′-DDD on the adrenal cortices, signs of the disease reappear. This can occur after several months or even after 4 to 5 years. It is then necessary to repeat the treatment with o,p′-DDD.

The first signs of recovery often already appear during the o,p′-DDD therapy. The excessive thirst and hunger disappear and the dog's endurance returns. The recovery of the coat takes longer, but once this begins, after about 2 months, a very thick coat usually develops. The recovery of the skin and coat may be preceded by a short period of excessive scaling and some itching. This can be relieved by a thorough shower with shampoo once or twice a week.

Complications. With the above treatment instructions, most dogs recover without complications. There can be complications associated with the o,p′-DDD or the replacement therapy. If you notify the veterinarian in time, problems can usually be resolved without difficulty.

In the beginning of treatment there may be mild side effects from o,p′-DDD, such as nausea, incoordination, or slight disorientation. These signs usually disappear if administration is continued but spread more over the day. If the dog refuses to eat or eats almost nothing, stop the o,p′-DDD completely, but be sure to continue the replacement medications, and notify the veterinarian.

A deficiency in replacement medications can lead to a life-threatening crisis and emergency treatment may be required. It is far better to contact the veterinarian before a crisis occurs. The first warning is often loss of appetite. Many dogs with the disease have an excessive appetite, and a decrease in appetite is an expected sign of recovery. However, an almost complete refusal to eat should be recognized as a warning. You should stop o,p′-DDD immediately, continue the replacement medications, and obtain the veterinarian's advice promptly.

Special circumstances in replacement therapy. It is extremely important to give the replacement medications without interruption. Yet there may be situations in which your dog cannot or will not take anything orally or cannot retain the medications because of vomiting. If for any reason your dog cannot take or retain the tablets and salt for two times in succession, injectable medications should be started. This applies, for example, when your dog is brought to the veterinarian for a treatment that requires anesthesia. Then:
- The cortisone tablets are replaced by sub-

218

cutaneous injections of hydrocortisone acetate (50 mg/ml) in a dose of . . . ml twice daily. The hydrocortisone injections are continued until the dog can again swallow and retain the cortisone tablets.

- The fludrocortisone tablets and salt are replaced by subcutaneous injections of DOCA (1 mg/ml) in a dose of . . . ml once daily, or DOCP (= depot for ≥ 20 days). In countries where DOC is unavailable, it is advised to administer double the dose of hydrocortisone. The salt is not needed when DOC injections are used. The DOCA injections are continued until the dog can again swallow and also retain the fludrocortisone and salt.

If you take your dog on vacation or on a trip away from home for more than 1 or 2 days, also take the injectable medications, syringes, and needles, and this instruction sheet, for not all veterinarians may have these medications at hand. If you leave the dog in the care of someone else, also make provision for the possible need for the injections, even if you have not yet had to use them yourself.

In cases of anesthesia, severe physical stress, or injury, the dose of cortisone should be doubled for 1 or 2 days. With these exceptions, the dose of cortisone remains unchanged for life, while the dose of fludrocortisone and salt may have to be adjusted by the veterinarian.

15. Algorithms

15.1 Introduction

In these step-by-step procedures for problem solving there is emphasis on possible associated signs and symptoms that may point to an endocrine disturbance. History and physical examination are directed to the detection of endocrine disease, for which a form may be helpful.[1] When the suspicion of an endocrine disturbance arises, such a hypothesis can be tested by specific examinations.

In case history and physical examination do not present clues for an endocrine disturbance, the next step will be laboratory examinations of blood and urine. If these routine laboratory examinations reveal no abnormal values, work-up at specialist level may be required.

15.2 Alopecia

Endocrine disturbance may cause atrophy of skin an adnexa. The atrophy of hair follicles results in slow, abnormal (dull) or absent hair growth. Depending upon the severity and the duration of the endocrine disturbance, alopecia will develop. In the dog the classical causes of alopecia are hypothyroidism, hyperadrenocorticism and hyperestrogenism (Sections 3.3, 4.3, 6.4). Also growth hormone deficiency may be cause of alopecia, although the alopecias that have been ascribed to acquired growth hormone deficiency may not all fit into that category (Section 2.2.2).

15.3 Polyuria/polydipsia

In the first part of this algorithm the problem polyuria/polydipsia (pu/pd) is based upon the information from history. As a second step urinalysis has been introduced as it my happen that an animal presented with a seemingly convincing history of pu/pd, has only pd because the owner has changed the food to dry food.

Apart from kidney disease, hepatic failure may also cause polyuria, especially when associated with hepato-encephalopathy (HE). There is evidence that in this condition abnormal metabolism of amino acids may give rise to "false" neurotransmitters, which may lead to elevated ACTH secretion and consequently hyperadrenocorticism.[2, 3] As parathyroid tumors are usually very small and a malignacy causing hypercalcemia may not have been detected by physical examination, measurements of plasma concentrations of calcium and phosphate should always be included in the laboratory profile (Chapters 9–11).

15.4 Weight loss (despite good appetite)

This algorithm can be used when the animal looses weight without any evidence of other problems such as pu/pd, fever, or diarrhea. The first step should be a careful history on food intake. Some owners feed strictly according to the recommendations of the manufacturer or seller of the food, thereby not always taking into account the energy expenditure.

In principle, large or widespread malignancies such lymphomas may be associated with an increased energy demand. This also holds true for highly insufficient cardiac action. However, only very rarely are such cases presented for weight loss as the primary problem.

A. Rijnberk (ed.), Clinical Endocrinology of Dogs and Cats, 219–222.
© 1996 *Kluwer Academic Publishers.*

220

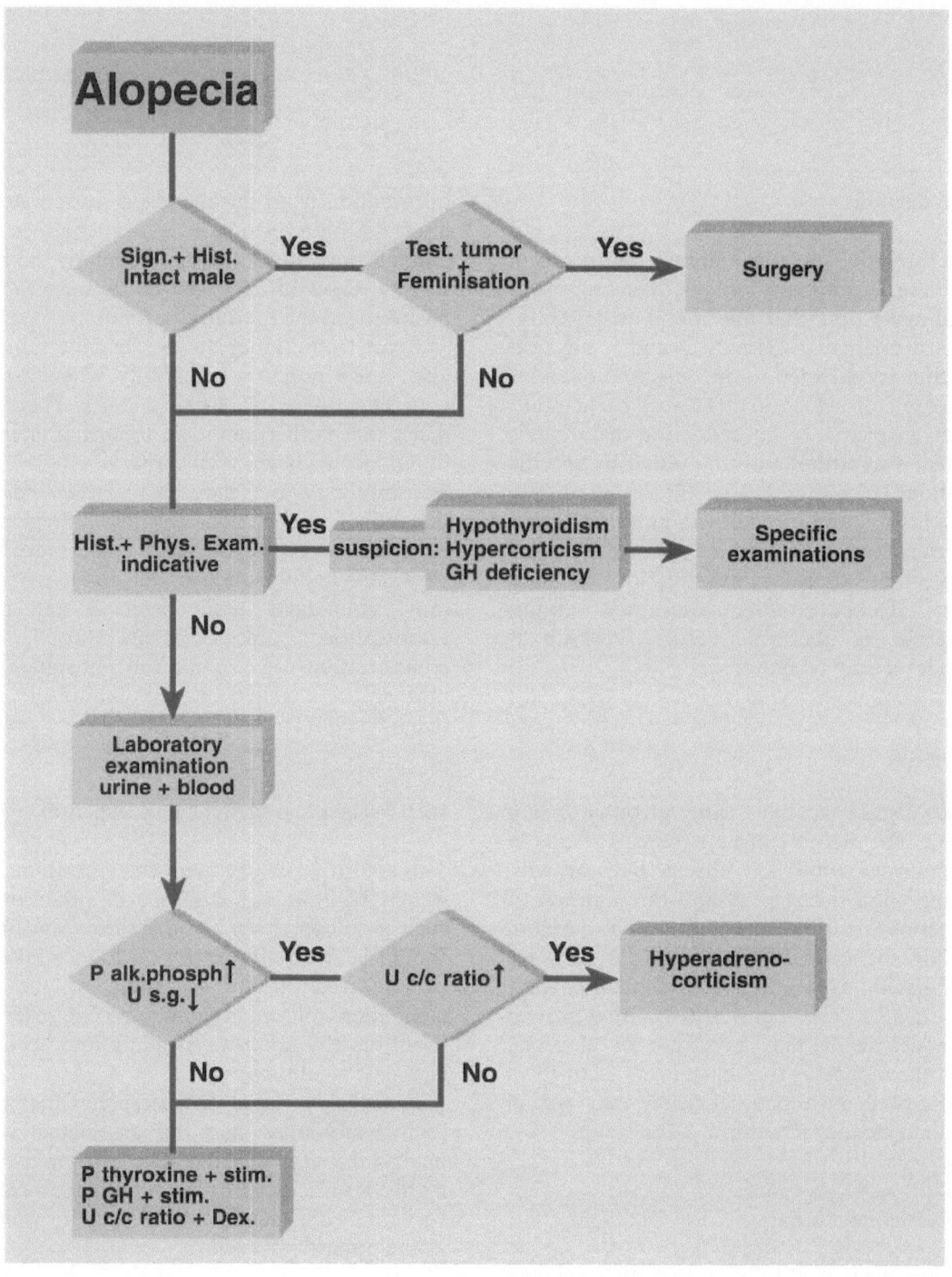

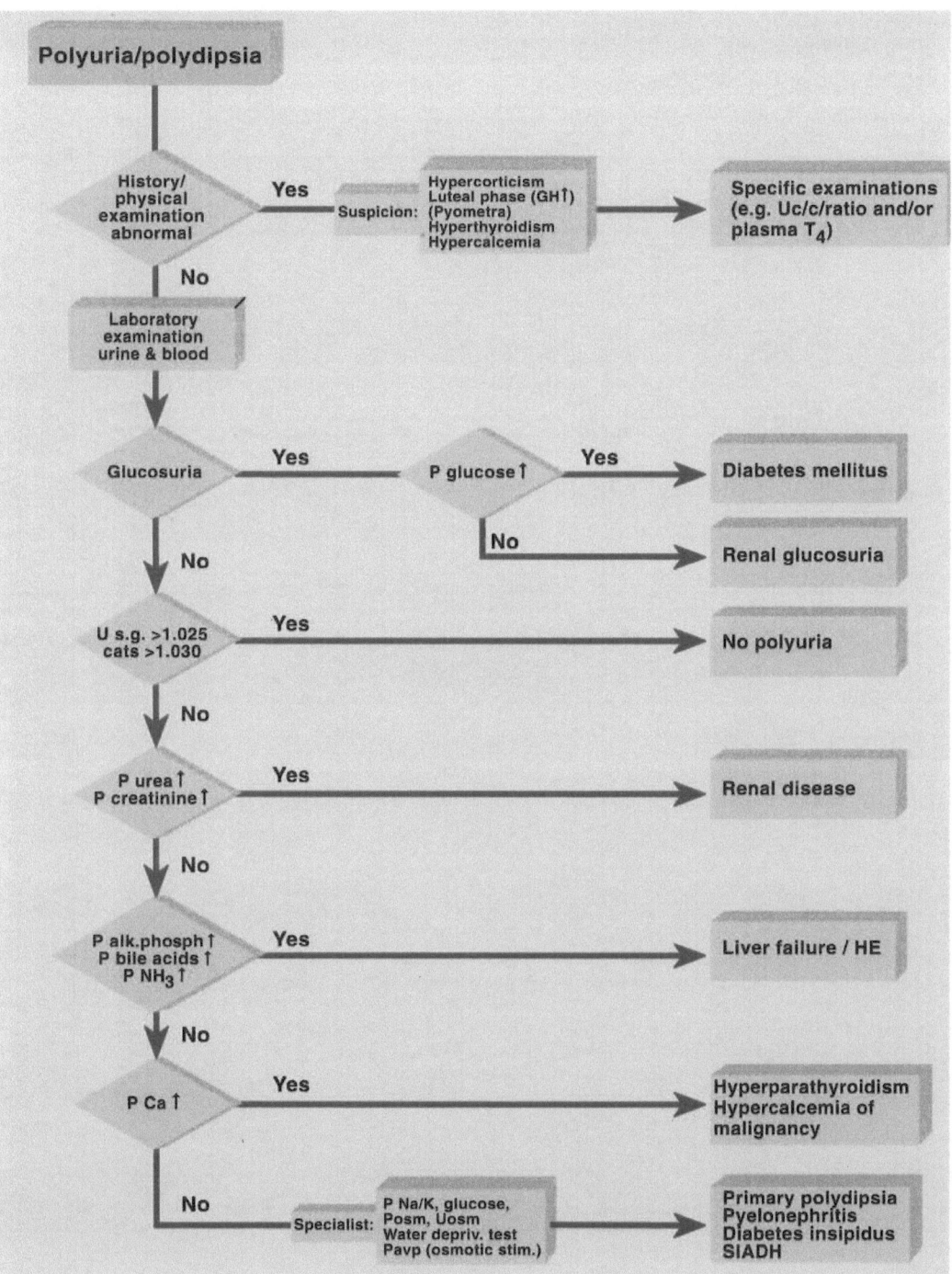

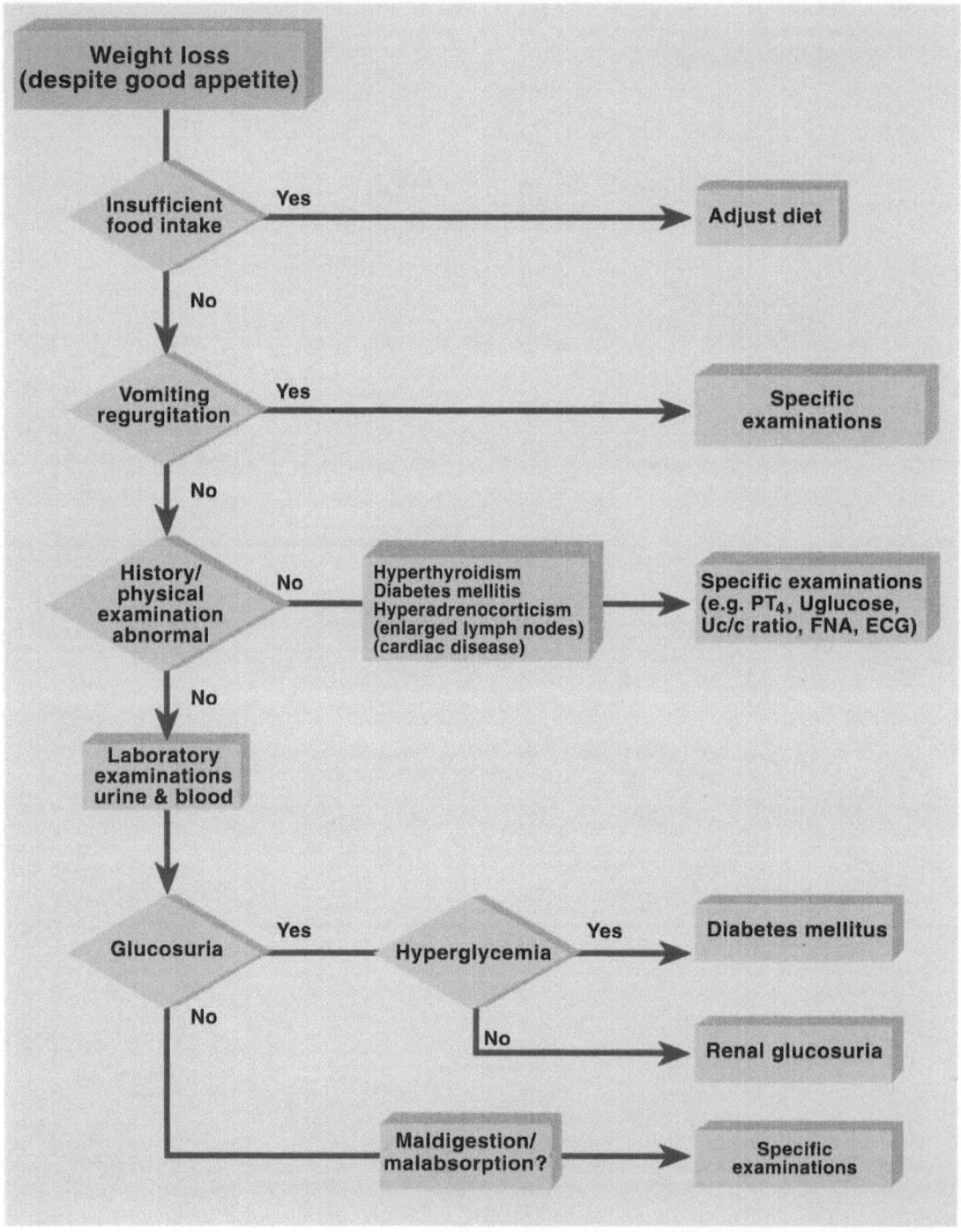

References

Chapter 1: Introduction

1. Granner DE. Hormonal action. General features of hormone systems and historical perspective. In: Becker KL, ed. *Principles and Practice of Endocrinology and Metabolism.* Philadelphia: J.B. Lippincott, 1990:25–37.
2. LeRoith D, Roberts Jr CT, Wilson G-L, Delahunty G, Roth J. Evolutionary origins of intercellular communication: Implications for mammalian endocrinology. In: Piva F, Bardin CW, Forti G, Motta M, eds. *Cell to Cell Communication in Endocrinology. Serono Symposia Publications* 49. New York: Raven Press, 1988:1–9.
3. Rijnberk A, Belshaw BE. Endocrine Glands. In: Rijnberk A, de Vries HW eds. *Medical History and Physical Examination in Companion Animals.* Dordrecht, Boston, London: Kluwer Academic Publishers, 1995:263–71

Chapter 2: Hypothalamus-pituitary system

1. Mol JA, Rijnberk A. Pituitary function. In: Kaneko JJ ed., *Clinical Biochemistry of Domestic Animals, Fourth Edition.* San Diego: Academic Press, 1989:576–609.
2. Ben-Jonathan N, Laudon M, Garris PA. Novel aspects of posterior pituitary function: Regulation of Prolactin secretion. *Front Neuroendocrinol* 1991;12:231–77.
2a. Ascacio-Martinez, JA, Barrera-Saldana. A dog growth hormone cDNA codes for a mature protein identical to pig growth hormone. *Gene* 1994;277–80.
2b. Mol JA, van Garderen E, Selman PJ, Wolfswinkel J, Rijnberk A, Rutteman GR. Growth hormone mRNA in mammary gland tumors of dogs and cats. *J. Clin Invest* 1955;95: 2028–34.
3. Eigenmann JE. Insulin-like growth factor I in the dog. *Front Horm Res* 1987;161–172.
4. Nap RC. *Nutritional Influences on Growth and Skeletal Development in the Dog.* Thesis, Utrecht University, 1993, pp 45–56.
5. Andresen E, Willeberg P. Pituitary dwarfism in German Shepherd dogs: Additional evidence of simple autosomal recessive inheritance. *Nord Vet Med* 1976;28:481–6.
6. Müller-Peddinghaus R, El Etreby MF, Siefert J, Ranke M. Hypophysärer Zwergwuchs beim Deutschen Schäferhund. *Vet Path* 1980;17:406–21.
7. Rijnberk A, Van Herpen H, Mol JA, Rutteman GR. Disturbed release of growth hormone in mature dogs: a comparison with congenital growth hormone deficiency. *Vet Rec 1993*;133:542–5.
8. Van Herpen H, Rijnberk A, Mol JA. Production of antibodies to biosynthetic human growth hormone in the dog. *Vet Rec* 1994;134:171.
9. Lothrop CD. Pathophysiology of canine growth hormone-responsive alopecia. *Comp Contin Educ Pract Vet* 1988; 10:1346–9.
10. Schmeitzel LP, Lothrop CD. Hormonal abnormalities in Pomeranians with normal coat and in Pomeranians with growth hormone-responsive dermatosis. *J Am Vet Med Assoc* 1990;197:1333–41.
11. Peterson ME, Altszuler N. Suppression of growth hormone secretion in spontaneous canine hyperadrenocorticism and its reversal after treatment. *Am J Vet Res 1981*;42:1881–3.
12. Eigenmann JE, Eigenmann RY, Rijnberk A, Van der Gaag I, Zapf J, Froesch ER. Progesterone-controlled growth hormone overproduction and naturally occurring canine diabetes and acromegaly. *Acta Endocrinol* 1983;104: 167–76.
13. Selman PJ, Mol JA, Rutteman GR, Van Garderen E, Rijnberk A. Progestin-induced growth hormone excess in the dog originates in the mammary gland. *Endocrinology* 1994;134:287–92.
14. Peterson ME, Randolph JF. Endocrine diseases. In: Sherding RG, ed. The Cat: Diseases and Clinical Management. New York: Churchill Livingstone, 1989:1095–161.
15. Peterson ME. Effects of megestrol acetate on glucose tolerance and growth hormone secretion in the cat. *Res Vet Sci* 1987;42:354–7.
16. Selman PJ, Mol JA, Rutteman GR, Rijnberk A. Progestin treatment in the dog. II. Effects on the hypothalamic-pituitary-adrenocortical axis. *Eur J Endocrinol* 1994;131: 422–30.
17. Watson ADJ, Rutteman GR, Rijnberk A, Mol JA. Effect of Somatostatin Analogue SMS 201–995 and Anti-progestin Agent RU 486 in canine acromegaly. *Front Horm Res* 1987;17:193–8.
18. Nelson RW, Ihle SL, Feldman EC. Pituitary macroadenomas and macroadenocarcinomas in dogs treated with mitotane for pituitary-dependent hyperadrenocorticism: 13 cases (1981–1986). *J Am Vet Med Assoc* 1989;194:1612–7.
19. Sarfaty D, Carillo JM, Peterson ME. Neurologic, endocrinologic, and pathologic findings associated with large

A. Rijnberk (ed.), Clinical Endocrinology of Dogs and Cats, 223–237.
© 1996 *Kluwer Academic Publishers.*

pituitary tumors in dogs: Eight cases (1976–1984). *J Am Vet Med Assoc* 1988;193:854–6.

20. Dow SW, LeCouteur RA. Radiation therapy for canine ACTH-secreting pituitary tumors. In: Kirk RW, ed. *Current Veterinary Therapy X*. Philadephia: WB Saunders Co, 1989:1031–4.

21. Biewenga WJ, Rijnberk A, Mol JA. Osmoregulation of systemic vasopressin release during long-term gluco-corticoid excess: A study in dogs with hyperadreno-corticism. *Acta Endocrinol* 1991;124:583–8.

22. Papanek PE, Raff H. Physiological increases in cortisol inhibit basal vasopressin release in conscious dogs. *Am J Physiol* 1994;266:R1744–51.

23. Biewenga WJ, Rijnberk A, Mol JA. Persistent polyuria in two dogs following adrenocorticolysis for pituitary-dependent hyperadrenocorticism. *Vet Quart* 1989;11:193–7.

24. Perrin IV, Bestetti GE, Zanesco SA, Sterchi HP. Diabetes insipidus centralis durch Larva migrans visceralis in der Neuro-Hypophyse beim Hund. *Schweiz Arch Tierheilk* 1986;128:483–6.

25. Post K, McNeill JRJ, Clark EG, Digneau MA, Olynyk GP. Congenital central diabetes insipidus in two sibling Afghan Hound pups. *J Am Vet Med Assoc* 1989;194:1086–8.

26. DiBartola SP, Johnson SE, Johnson GC, Robertson GL. Hypodipsic hypernatremia in a dog with defective osmo-regulation of antidiuretic hormone. *J Am Vet Med Ass* 1994;204:922–5.

27. Luzius H, Jans DA, Grünbaum E-G, Moritz A, Rascher W, Fahrenholz F. A low affinity vasopressin V_2-receptor in inherited nephrogenic diabetes insipidus. *J Receptor Res* 1992;12:351–68.

28. Zerbe RL, Robertson GL. A comparison of plasma vaso-pressin measurments with a standard indirect test in the differential diagnosis of polyuria. *New Engl J Med 1981*; 305:1639–46.

29. Moses AM, Clayton B. Impairment of osmotically stim-ulated AVP release in patients with primary polydipsia. *Am J Physiol* 1993;265:R1247–52.

30. Rijnberk A, Biewenga WJ, Mol JA. Inappropriate vaso-pressin secretion in two dogs. *Acta Endocrinol* 1988; 117:59–64.

31. Houston DM, Allen DG, Kruth SA, Pook H, Spinato MT, Keough L. Syndrome of inappropriate antidiuretic hor-mone secretion in a dog. *Can Vet J* 1989;30:423–5.

32. Van Oosterhout ICAM, Rijnberk A, Mol JA. Effect of the aquaretic vasopressin antagonists d(CH_2)$_5$[D-Tyr(ET)^2-Val^4]AVP and d(CH_2)$_5$[D-Phe^2-Phe^4]AVP on urine pro-duction in healthy dogs. *Horm Metab Res* 1992;24:244–5.

33. Stolp R, Steinbusch HWM, Rijnberk A, Croughs RJM. Organization of ovine corticotrophin-releasing factor immunoreactive neurons in the canine hypothalamo-pituitary system. *Neurosci Lett* 1987;74:337–42.

34. Miller MA, Dunstan RW. Seasonal flank alopecia in Boxers and Airdale Terriers: 24 cases (1985–1992). *J Am Vet Med Ass* 1993;203:1567–72.

35. Hullinger RL. The Endocrine System. In: Evans HE, Christensen GC, eds. *Miller's Anatomy of the Dog*. Philadelphia: WB Saunders Co, 1979:602–31.

36. Mol JA, Van Wolferen M, Kwant M, Meloen R. Predicted primary and antigenic structure of canine corticotropin releasing hormone. *Neuropeptides* 1994;27:7–13.

Chapter 3: Thyroids

1. St.Germain DL. Iodothyronine deiodinases. *Trends Endocrinol Metab* 1994;5:36–42.

2. Saunders MH, Jezyk PK. The radiographic appearance of canine congenital hypothyroidism: Skeletal changes with delayed treatment. *Vet Radiol* 1991;32:171–7.

3. Tanase H, Kudo K, Horikoshi H, Mizushima H, Okazaki T, Ogata E. Inherited primary hypothyroidsim with thyrotrophin resistance in Japanese cats. *J Endocrinol* 1991;129:245–51.

4. Peterson ME, Randolph JF. Endocrine diseases. In: Sherd-ing RG, ed. *The Cat: Diseases and Clinical Management*. New York: Churchill Livingstone, 1989:1095–161.

5. Sjollema BE, Den Hartog MT, De Vijlder JJM, Van Dijk JE, Rijnberk A. Congenital hypothyroidism in two cats due to defective organification: data suggesting loosely anchored thyroperoxidase. *Acta Endocrinol* 1991;125:435–40.

5a. Jones BR, Gruffydd-Jones TJ, Sparkes AH, Lucke VM. Preliminary studies on congenital hypothyroidism in a family of Abyssinian cats. *Vet Rec* 1992;131:145–8.

6. Eigenmann JE, Van der Haage MH, Rijnberk A. Poly-endocrinopathy in two canine littermates: Simultaneous occurrence of carbohydrate intolerance and hypo-thyroidism. *J Am Anim Hosp Assoc* 1984;20:143–8.

7. Kooistra HS, Rijnberk A, Van den Ingh ThSGAM. Polyglandular deficiency syndrome in a Boxer dog: thyroid hormone and glucorticoid deficiency. *Vet Quart* 1995:17:59–63.

8. Young DW, Haines DM, Kemppainen RJ. The relation-ship between autoantibodies to triiodothyronine (T3) and thyroglobulin (Tg) in the dog. *Autoimmunity* 1991;9:41–6.

9. Gaschen F, Thompson J, Beale K, Keisling K. Recognition of triiodothyronine-containing epitopes in canine thyro-globulin by circulating thyroglobulin autoantibodies. *Am J Vet Res* 1993;54:244–7.

10. Rand JS, Levine J, Best SJ, Parker W. Spontaneous adult-onset hypothyroidism in a cat. *J Vet Int Med* 1993;7:272–6.

11. Chastain CB. Unusual manifestations of hypothyroidism in dogs. In: Kirk RW, Bonagura JD, eds. *Current Veterinary Therapy XI*. Philadelphia: WB Saunders Co, 1992:330–4.

12. Towell TL, Shell LC. Endocrinopathies that affect peri-pheral nerves of cats and dogs. *Comp Cont Educ Pract Vet* 1994;16:157–62.

13. Kaptein EM, Moore GE, Ferguson DC, Hoenig M. Effects of prednisone on thyroxine and 3,53′-triiodo-thyronine metabolism in normal dogs. *Endocrinology* 1992;130:1669–79.

14. Nelson RW, Ihle SL, Feldman EC, Bottoms GD. Serum free thyroxine concentration in healthy dogs, dogs with hypothyroidism, and euthyroid dogs with concurrent illness. *J Am Vet Med Ass* 1991;198:1401–7.

15. Ferguson DC, Peterson ME. Serum free and total

iodothyronine concentrations in dogs with hyperadreno-corticism. *Am J Vet Res* 1992;53:1636–40.

16. Kaptein EM, Moore GE, Ferguson DC, Hoenig M. Thyroxine and triiodothyronine distribution and metabolism in thyroxine-replaced athyreotic dogs and normal humans. *Am J Physiol* 1993;264:E90–100.

17. Nachreiner RF, Refsal KR, Ravis WR, Hauptman J, Rosser EJ, Pedersoli WM. Pharmacokinetics of L-thyroxine after its oral administration in dogs. *Am J Vet Res* 1993;54:2091–8.

18. Cook SM, Daniel GB, Walker MA, Maddux JM, Jenkins CC, Klebanow ER, Bouley DM, Dean DF, Petersen MG. Radiographic and scintigraphic evidence of focal pulmonary neoplasia in three cats with hyperthyroidism: Diagnostic and therapeutic considerations. *J Vet Int Med* 1993;7:303–8.

19. Peter HJ, Gerber H, Studer H, Becker DV, Peterson ME. Autonomy of growth and of iodine metabolism in hyperthyroid feline goiters transplanted onto nude mice. *J Clin Invest* 1987;80:491–8.

20. Thoday KL, Mooney CT. Historical, clinical and laboratory features of 126 hyperthyroid cats. *Vet Rec* 1992;131:257–64.

21. Peterson ME, Graves TK, Gamble DA. Triiodothyronine (T3) suppression test: An aid in the diagnosis of mild hyperthyroidism in cats. *J Vet Int Med* 1990;4:233–8.

22. Sjollema BE, Pollak YWEA, Van den Brom WE, Rijnberk A. Thyroidal radioiodine uptake in hyperthyroid cats. *Vet Quart* 1989;11:165–70.

23. Nap AMP, Pollak YWEA, Van den Brom WE, Rijnberk A. Quantitative aspects of thyroid scintigraphy with pertechnetate (^{99m}TcO$_4^-$) in cats. *J Vet Int Med* 1994;8:302–3.

24. Peeters ME. Thyroidectomy. In: Van Sluijs FJ, ed. *Atlas of Small Animal Surgery*. New York: Churchill Livingstone, 1992:20–2 (and personal communications).

25. Meric SM, Rubin SI. Serum thyroxine concentrations following fixed-dose radioactive iodine treatment in hyperthyroid cats: 62 cases (1986–1989). *J Am Vet Med Ass* 1990;197:621–3.

26. Peterson ME, Kintzer PP, Hurvitz AI. Methimazole treatment of 262 cats with hyperthyroidism. *J Vet Int Med* 1988;2:150–7.

27. Verschueren CP, Selman PJ, Mol JA, Vos JH, Van Dijk JE, Sjollema BE, De Vijlder JJM. Circulating thyroglobulin measurements by homologous radioimmunoassay in dogs with thyroid carcinoma. *Acta Endocrinol* 1991; 125:291–8.

28. Verschueren CP, Rutteman GR, Vos JH, Van Dijk JE, De Bruin TWA. Thyrotropin receptors in normal and neoplastic (primary and metastatic) canine thyroid tissue. *J Endocrinol* 1992;132:461–8.

29. Verschueren CP, Rutteman GR, Kuipers-Dijkshoorn NJ, Sjollema BE, Vos JH, Van Dijk JE, Cornelisse CJ. Flow-cytometric DNA ploidy analysis in primary and metastatic canine thyroid carcinomas. *Anticancer Res* 1991;11: 1755–62.

30. Wynford-Thomas D. Molecular genetics of thyroid cancer. *Trend Endocrinol Metab* 1993;4:224–31.

31. Leav I, Schiller AL, Rijnberk A, Legg MA, Der Kinderen PJ. Adenomas and carcinomas of the canine and feline thyroid. *Am J Path* 1976;83:61–93.

32. Lantz GC, Salisbury SK. Surgical excision of ectopic thyroid carcinoma involving the base of the tongue in dogs: Three cases (1980–1987). *J Am Vet Med Ass* 1989; 195:1606–8.

33. Peterson ME, Kintzer PP, Hurley JR, Becker DV. Radioactive iodine treatment of a functional thyroid carcinoma producing hyperthyroidism in a dog. *J Vet Int Med* 1989;3:20–5.

34. Ware WA, Merkley DF, Riedesel DH. Intracardiac thyroid tumor in a dog: Diagnosis and surgical removal. *J Amer Anim Hosp Ass* 1994;30:20–3.

35. Verschueren CP, Rutteman GR, Van Dijk JE, Vos, JH, Franken HCM. Evaluation of some prognostic factors in surgically-treated canine thyroid cancer. In: Verschueren CP. *Clinico-Pathological and Endocrine Aspects of Canine Thyroid Cancer*. Thesis, Utrecht University, 1992:11–25.

36. Clark OH, Duh Q-Y. Thyroid cancer. In: Greer MA, ed. *The Thyroid Gland*. New York: Raven Press, Ltd, 1990: 537–72.

37. Rijnberk A, Der Kinderen PJ, Thijssen JHH. Canine Cuhing's syndrome. *Zbl Vet Med A* 1969;16:13–28.

38. Rijnberk A. *Iodine Metabolism and Thyroid Disease in the Dog*. Utrecht: Drukkerij Elinkwijk, 1971:32–40.

Chapter 4: Adrenals

1. IUPAC Commission on the Nomenclature of Organic Chemistry and IUPAC-IUB Commission on Biochemical Nomenclature. *Biochim Biophys Acta* 1968;164:453–86.

2. Rijnberk A, Mol JA. Adrenocortical function. In: Kaneko JJ, ed. *Clinical Biochemistry of Domestic Animals, 4th edition*. San Diego: Academic Press, Inc., 1989:610–29.

3. Meyer HP, Rothuizen J. Determination of the percentage of free cortisol in plasma in the dog by ultrafiltration/dialysis. *Domest Anim Endocrinol* 1993;10:45–53.

4. Kemppainen RJ, Peterson ME, Sartin JL. Plasma free cortisol concentrations in dogs with hyperadrenocorticism. *Am J Vet Res* 1991;52:682–6.

5. Bamberg-Thalén B, Nyberg L, Fackler L, Edqvist LE. Cortisol binding capacity of corticosteroid binding globulin in hyperadrenocorticoid and healthy dogs. *Res Vet Sci* 1992;52:363–6.

6. Jansson J-O, Oscarsson J, Mode A, Ritzén EM. Plasma growth hormone pattern and androgens influence the levels of corticosteroid-binding globulin in rat serum. *J Endocrinol* 1989;122:725–32.

7. Mol JA, Van Mansfeld DM, Kwant MM, Van Wolferen M, Rothuizen J. The gene encoding proopiomelanocortin in the dog. *Acta Endocrinol* 1991;125(Suppl 1):77–83.

8. Halmi NS, Peterson ME, Colurso GJ, Liotta AS, Krieger DT. Pituitary intermediate lobe in dog: Two cell types and high bioactive adrenocorticotropin content. *Science* 1981;211:72–4.

9. Buckingham JC, Smith T, Loxley HD. The control of ACTH secretion. In: James VHT, ed. *The Adrenal Gland, 2nd edition*. New York: Raven Press, Ltd, 1992:131–58.

10. Kemppainen RJ, Sartin JL. Evidence for episodic but not

226

circadian activity in plasma concentrations of adreno-corticotrophin, cortisol and thyroxine in dogs. *J Endocrinol* 1984;103:219–26.

11. Peterson ME, Randolph JF. Endocrine diseases. In: Sherding RG, ed. *The Cat – Diseases and Clinical Management*. New York: Churchill Livingstone, 1989:1095–161.

12. Meijer JC, De Bruijne JJ, Rijnberk A, Croughs RJM. Biochemical characterization of pituitary-dependent hyperadrenocorticism in the dog. *J Endocrinol* 1978;77: 111–8.

13. Kemppainen RJ, Sartin JL. Differential regulation of peptide release by the canine pars distalis and pars intermedia. *Front Horm Res* 1987;17:18–27.

14. Knol BW, Dieleman SJ, Bevers MM. The responses of plasma luteinizing hormone, testosterone, and cortisol during social stress and immobilization in dominant and subordinate male dogs. Chapter VII. In: Knol BW. Thesis, Utrecht University, 1989.

15. Willemse T, Vroom MW, Mol JA, Rijnberk A. Changes in plasma cortisol, corticotropin, and α-melanocyte-stimulating hormone concentrations in cats before and after physical restraint and intradermal testing. *Am J Vet Res* 1993;54:69–72.

16. Reul JMHM, De Kloet ER, Van Sluijs FJ, Rijnberk A, Rothuizen J. Binding characteristics of mineralocorticoid and glucocorticoid receptors in dog brain and pituitary. *Endocrinology* 1990;127:907–15.

17. Rothuizen J, Reul JMHM, Van Sluijs FJ, Mol JA, Rijnberk A, De Kloet ER. Increased neuroendocrine reactivity and decreased brain mineralocorticoid receptor-binding capacity in aged dogs. *Endocrinology* 1993;132: 161–8.

18. Berkenbosch F, Van Oers J, Del Rey A, Tilders F, Besedovsky H. Corticotropin-releasing factor-producing neurons in the rat activated by interleukin-1. *Science* 1987, 238:524–6.

19. Funder JW, Pearce PT, Smith R, Smith AI. Mineralocorticoid action: Target tissue specificity is enzyme, not receptor, mediated. *Science* 1988;242:583–5.

20. Wolfsheimer KJ, Peterson ME. Erythrocyte insulin receptors in dogs with spontaneous hyperadrenocorticism. *Am J Vet Res* 1991;52:917–21.

21. Winqvist O, Karlsson FA, Kämpe O. 21-Hydroxylase, a major autoantigen in idiopathic Addison's disease. *Lancet* 1992;i:1559–62.

22. Shaker E, Hurvitz AI, Peterson ME. Hypoadrenocorticism in a family of Standard Poodles. *J Am Vet Med Ass* 1988;192:1091–2.

23. Ahlgren M, Bamberg-Thalén B. Hypoadrenocorticism in the dog. *Eur J Comp Anim Pract* 1993;3:62–8.

24. Peterson ME, Greco DS, Orth DN. Primary hypoadrenocorticism in ten cats. *J Vet Int Med* 1989; 3:55–8.

25. Lynn RC, Feldman EC, Nelson RW. Efficacy of microcrystalline desoxycorticosterone pivalate for treatment of hypoadrenocorticism in dogs. *J Am Vet Med Ass* 1993; 202:392–6.

26. Nelson RW. Endocrine disorders. In: Nelson RW, Couto CG, eds. *Essentials of Small Animal Internal Medicine*. St. Louis: Mosby-Year Book, 1992:525–607.

27. Sauter NP, Toni R, McLaughlin CD, Deyss EM, Kritzman J, Lechan RM. Isolated adrenocorticotropin deficiency associated with an autoantibody to a corticotroph antigen that is not adrenocorticotropin or other proopiomelanocortin-derived peptides. *J Clin Endocrinol Metab* 1990;70:1391–7.

28. Kooistra HS, Rijnberk A, Van den Ingh ThSGAM. Polyglandular deficiency syndrome in a Boxer dog: Thyroid hormone and glucocorticoid defiency. *Vet Quart* 1995;17:59–63.

29. Peterson ME, Kemppainen RJ, Orth DN. Effects of ovine corticotropin-releasing hormone on plasma concentrations of immunoreactive adrenocorticotropin, alph-melanocyte-stimulating hormone, and cortisol in dogs with naturally acquired adrenocortical insufficiency. *Am J Vet Res* 1992;53:421–5.

30. Appleby EC, Sohrabi-Haghdoost I. Cortical hyperplasia of the adrenal gland in the dog. *Res Vet Sci* 1980;29:190–7.

31. Van Sluijs FJ, Sjollema BE, Voorhout G, Van den Ingh TSGAM, Rijnberk A. Results of adrenalectomy in 36 dogs with hyperadrenocorticism caused by adrenocortical tumour. *Vet Quart* 1995; 17:113–6.

31a. Nothelfer HB, Weinhold K. Formale Pathogenese, Durchschnittsalter und Rassenverteilung im Vergleich 61 Lysodren-behandelter und 36 unbehandelter Fälle von caninem Hyperadrenokortizismus, die in den Jahren 1975 bis 1991 am Institut für Veterinär-Pathologie der Freien Universität Berlin seziert wurden. *Berl Münch Tierärztl Wschr* 1992; 105:305–11.

32. Peterson ME, Krieger DT, Drucker WD, Halmi NS. Immunocytochemical study of the hypophysis in 25 dogs with pituitary-dependent hyperadrenocorticism. *Acta Endocrinol* 1982;101:15–24.

33. Middleton DJ, Rijnberk A, Bevers MM, Goos HJTh, Beeftink EA, Thijssen JHH, Croughs RJM. Some functional and morphologic aspects of canine corticotrophs. *Front Horm Res* 1987;17:10–7.

34. Boujon CE, Ritz U, Rossi GL, Bestetti GE. A clinicopathological study of canine Cushing's disease caused by a pituitary carcinoma. *J Comp Path* 1991;105:353–65.

35. Davis JRE, Hoggard N. Towards the pathogenesis of human pituitary tumors. *J Endocrinol* 1993;136:3–6.

36. Scholten-Sloof BE, Knol BW, Rijnberk A, Mol JA, Middleton DJ, Ubbink G. Pituitary-dependent hyperadrenocorticism in a family of Dandie Dinmont terriers. *J Endocrinol* 1992;135:535–42.

37. Van Wijk PA, Rijnberk A, Croughs RJM, Voorhout G, Sprang EPM, Mol JA. Corticotropin-releasing hormone and adrenocorticotropic hormone concentrations in cerebrospinal fluid of dogs with pituitary-dependent hyperadrenocorticism. *Endocrinology* 1992;131:2659–62.

38. Peterson ME, Orth DN, Halmi NS, Zielinski AC, Davis DR, Chavez FT, Drucker WD. Plasma immunoreactive proopiomelanocortin peptides and cortisol in normal dogs and dogs with Addison's disease and Cushing's syndrome: Basal concentrations. *Endocrinology* 1986;119:720–30.

39. Kemppainen RJ, Sartin JL. Differential regulation of peptide release by the canine pars distalis and pars intermedia. *Front Horm Res* 1987;17:18–27.

40. Orth DN, Peterson ME, Drucker WD. Plasma immuno-

reactive proopiomelanocortin peptides and cortisol in normal dogs and dogs with Cushing's syndrome: Diurnal rhythm and responses to various stimuli. *Endocrinology* 1988;122:1250–62.

41. Rijnberk A, Mol JA, Kwant MM, Croughs RJM. Effects of bromocriptine on corticotrophin, melanotrophin and corticosteroid secretion in dogs with pituitary-dependent hyperadrenocorticism. *J Endocrinol* 1988;118:271–7.

42. Biewenga WJ, Rijnberk A, Mol JA. Osmoregulation of systemic vasopressin release during long-term glucocorticoid excess: A study in dogs with hyperadrenocorticism. *Acta Endocrinol* 1991;124:583–8.

43. Daley CA, Zerbe CA, Schick RO, Powers RD. Use of metyrapone to treat pituitary-dependent hyperadrenocorticism in a cat with large cutaneous wounds. *J Am Vet Med Ass* 1993;202:956–60.

44. Teske E, Rothuizen J, De Bruijne JJ, Mol JA. Corticosteroid-induced alkaline phosphatase isoenzyme in the diagnosis of canine hypercorticism. *Vet Rec* 1989;125:12–4.

45. Jones CA, Refsal KR, Lippert AC, Nachreiner RF, Schwacha MM. Changes in adrenal cortisol secretion as reflected in the urinary cortisol/creatinine ratio in dogs. *Domest Anim Endocrinol* 1990;7:559–72.

46. Rijnberk A, Voorhout G, Mol JA. Corticoid production by four dogs with hyperfunctioning adrenocortical tumours during treatment with mitotane (o,p'-DDD). *Vet Rec* 1992;131:484–7.

47. Van Wijk PA, Rijnberk A, Croughs RJM, Wolfswinkel J, Selman PJ, Mol JA. Responsiveness to corticotropin-releasing hormone and vasopressin in canine Cushing's syndrome. *Eur J Endocrinol* 1994;130:410–6.

48. Rijnberk A, Der Kinderen PJ, Thijssen JHH. Spontaneous hyperadrenocorticism in the dog. *J Endocrinol* 1968;41: 397–406.

49. Lubberink AAME. Therapy for spontaneous hyperadrenocorticism. In: Kirk RW, ed. *Current Veterinary Therapy VII*. Philadelphia: WB Saunders Co, 1980:979–83.

50. Eigenmann JE, Lubberink AAME. The pituitary. In: Slatter DH, ed. *Textbook of Small Animal Surgery*. Philadelphia: WB Saunders Co, 1985:1840–51.

51. Niebauer GW. Hypophysectomy. In: Slatter DH, ed. *Textbook of Small Animal Surgery, 2nd edition*. Philadelphia: WB Saunders Co, 1992:1496–1510.

52. Feldman EC, Vaden S. Adrenalectomy for treatment of feline hyperadrenocorticism. *ACVIM Abstract 7. J Vet Int Med* 1993;7:113.

53. Kintzer PP, Peterson ME. Mitotane (o,p'-DDD) treatment of 200 dogs with pituitary-dependent hyperadrenocorticism. *J Vet Int Med* 1991;5:182–90.

54. Rijnberk A, Belshaw BE. O,p'-DDD treatment of canine hyperadrenocorticism: an alternative protocol. In: Kirk RW, Bonagura JD, eds. *Current Veterinary Therapy XI*. Philadelphia: WB Saunders Co, 1992:345–9.

55. VandenBossche H, De Coster R, Amery WK. Pharmacology and clinical uses of ketoconazole. In: Furr BJA, Wakeling AE, eds. *Pharmacology and Clinical Uses of Inhibitors of Hormone Secretion and Action*. London: Baillière Tindall, 1987:288–307.

56. Feldman EC, Nelson RW. Use of ketoconazole for control of canine hyperdrenocorticism. In: Kirk RW, Bonagura JD, eds. *Current Veterinary Therapy XI*. Philadelphia: WB Saunders Co, 1992:349–52.

57. Dow SW, LeCouteur A, Rosychuk RAW, Powers BE, Kemppainen RJ, Gillette EL. Response of dogs with functional pituitary macroadenomas and macrocarcinomas to radiation. *J Small Anim Pract* 1990;31:287–94.

58. Mackedanz R, Struckmann B. Bericht über einen Fall von Hypercortisolismus bei einer Katze. *Kleintierpraxis* 1992; 37:843–6.

59. Immink WFGA, Van Toor AJ, Vos JH, Van der Linde-Sipman JS, Lubberink AAME. Hyperadrenocorticism in four cats. *Vet Quart* 1992;14:81–5.

60. Ford SL, Feldman EC, Nelson RW. Hyperadrenocorticism caused by bilateral adrenocortical neoplasia in dogs: Four cases (1983–1988). *J Am Vet Med Ass* 1993;202:789–92.

61. Evans K, Hosgood G, Boon GD, Kowalewich N. Hemoperitoneum secondary to traumatic rupture of an adrenal tumor in a dog. *J Am Vet Med Ass* 1991;198: 278–80.

62. Vandenbergh AGGD, Voorhout G, Van Sluijs FJ, Rijnberk A, Van den Ingh TSGAM. Haemorrhage from a canine adrenocortical tumour: a clinical emergency. *Vet Rec* 1992;131: 539–40.

63. Voorhout G, Stolp R, Rijnberk A, Van Waes PFGM. Assessment of survey radiography and comparison with x-ray computed tomography for detection of hyperfunctioning adrenocortical tumors in dogs. *J Am Vet Med Ass* 1990;196:1799–1803.

64. Voorhout G, Rijnberk A, Sjollema BE, Van den Ingh TSGAM. Nephrotomography and ultrasonography for the localization of hyperfunctioning adrenocortical tumors in dogs. *Am J Vet Res* 1990;51:1280–5.

65. Reusch CE, Feldman EC. Canine hyperadrenocorticism due to adrenocortical neoplasia. *J Vet Int Med* 1991; 5:3–10.

66. Axelrod L. Corticosteroid therapy. In: Becker KL, ed. *Principles and Practice of Endocrinology and Metabolism*. Philadelphia: Lippincott, 1990:613–23.

67. Compton MM, Cidlowski JA. Thymocyte Apoptosis. A model of programmed cell death. *Trends Endocrinol Metab* 1992;3:17–23.

68. Jeffers JG, Shanley KJ, Schick RO. Diabetes mellitus induced in a dog after administration of corticosteroids and methylprednisolone pulse therapy. *J Am Vet Med Ass* 1991;199:77–80.

69. Bellah JR, Lothrop CD, Helman RG. Fatal iatrogenic Cushing's syndrome in a dog. *J Am Anim Hosp Assoc* 1989;25:673–6.

70. Toombs JP, Collins LG, Graves GM, Crowe DT, Caywood DD. Colonic perforation in corticosteroid-treated dogs. *J Am Vet Med Ass* 1986;188:145–50.

71. Zenoble RD, Kemppainen RJ. Adrenocortical suppression by topically applied corticosteroids in healthy dogs. *J Am Vet Med Ass* 1987;191:685–8.

72. Moriello KA, Fehrer-Sawyer SL, Meyer DJ, Feder B. Adrenocortical suppression associated with topical otic administration of glucocorticoids in dogs. *J Am Vet Med Ass* 1988;193:329–31.

73. Glaze MB, Crawford MA, Nachreiner RF, Casey HW,

Nafe LA, Kearney MT. Ophthalmic corticosteroid therapy: Systemic effects in the dog. *J Am Vet Med Ass* 1988;192:73–5.

74. Moore GE, Hoenig M. Duration of pituitary and adreno-cortical suppression after long-term administration of anti-inflammatory doses of prednisone in dogs. *Am J Vet Res* 1992;53:716–20.

75. Selman PJ, Mol JA, Rutteman GR, Rijnberk A. Progestin treatment in the dog. II. Effects on the hypothalamic-pituitary-adrenocortical axis. *Eur J Endocrinol* 1994;131:422–30.

76. Middleton DJ, Watson ADJ, Howe CJ, Caterson ID. Suppression of cortisol responses to exogenous adreno-corticotrophic hormone, and the occurrence of side effects attributable to glucocorticoid excess, in cats during therapy with megestrol acetate and prednisolone. *Can J Vet Res* 1987;51:60–5.

77. Brigell DF, Fang VS, Rosenfield RL. Recovery of responses to ovine corticotropin-releasing hormone after withdrawal of a short course of glucocorticoid. *J Clin Endocrinol Metab* 1992;74:1036–9.

78. Frey FJ, Frey BM. Pharmacology of Synthetic Gluco-corticoids. Alternate-day glucocorticoid therapy: 30 years later. In: James VHT, ed. *The Adrenal Gland, 2nd edition.* New York: Raven Press, Ltd, 1992:441–50.

79. Cryer PE. The adrenal medullae. In: James VHT, ed. *The Adrenal Gland, 2nd edition.* New York: Raven Press, Ltd, 1992:465–89.

80. Connolly CC, Steiner KE, Stevenson RW, Neal, DW, Williams PE, Alberti KGMM, Cherrington AD. Regulation of glucose metabolism by norepinephrine in conscious dogs. *Am J Physiol* 1991;261:E764–72.

81. Patnaik AK, Erlandson RA, Lieberman PH, Welches CD, Marretta SM. Extra-adrenal pheochromocytoma (para-ganglioma) in a cat. *J Am Vet Med Ass* 1990;197:104–6.

82. Bouayad H, Feeney DA, Caywood DD, Hayden DW. Pheochromocytoma in dogs: 13 cases (1980–1985). *J Am Vet Med Ass* 1987;191:1610–5.

83. Gilson SD, Withrow SJ, Wheeler SL, Twedt DC. Pheo-chromocytoma in 50 dogs. *J Vet Int Med* 1994;8:228–32.

84. Young WF. Pheochromocytoma: 1926–1993. *Trends Endocrinol Metab* 1993;4:122–7.

85. D'Alesandro MM, Gruber DF, Reed HL, O'Halloran KP, Robertson R. Effects of collection methods and storage on the in vitro stability of canine plasm catecholamines. *Am J Vet Res* 1990;51:257–9.

86. Gilson SD, Withrow SJ, Orton EC. Surgical treatment of pheochromocytoma: Technique, complications and results in six dogs. *Vet Surg* 1994;23:195–200.

87. Henry CJ, Brewer WG, Montgomery RD, Groth AH, Cartee RE, Griffin KS. Adrenal pheochromocytoma. *J Vet Int Med* 1993;7:199–201.

88. Lenestour E, Abecassis JP, Bertagna X, Bonnin A, Luton JP. Silent necrosis of a pituitary corticotroph adenoma revealed by timely magnetic resonance imaging: A cause of spontaneous remission of Cushing's disease. *Eur J Endo-crinol* 1994;130:469–71.

89. Watson ADJ, Rijnberk A, Moolenaar AJ. Systemic availability of o,p'-DDD in normal dogs, fasted and fed, and in dogs with hyperadrenocorticism. *Res Vet Sci* 1987;43:160–5.

Chapter 5: Endocrine pancreas

1. Bonner-Weir S. Morphology of the endocrine pancreas. In: Becker KL, ed. *Principles and Practice of Endocrinology and Metabolism.* Philadelphia: JB Lippincott Co, 1990:1064–8.

2. Halldén G, Gafvelin G, Mutt V, Jörnvall H. Character-ization of cat insulin. *Arch Biochem Biophys* 1986;247:20–7.

3. Halban PA, Weir GC. Islet cell hormones: Production and degradation. In: Becker KL, ed. *Principles and Practice of Endocrinology and Metabolism.* Philadelphia: JB Lip-pincott Co, 1990:1068–73.

4. Chastain CB, Ganjam VK. *Clinical Endocrinology of Companion Animals.* Philadelphia: Lea & Febiger, 1986:257–302.

5. Feldman EC, Nelson RW. *Canine and Feline Endo-crinology and Reproduction.* Philadelphia: WB Saunders Co, 1987:229–73.

6. Unger RH, Foster DW. Diabetes mellitus. In: Wilson JD, Foster DW, eds. *Williams Textbook of Endocrinology, 8th edition.* Philadelphia: WB Saunders Co, 1992:1255–1333.

7. Nelson RW. Disorders of the endocrine pancreas. In: Nelson RW, Couto CG, eds. *Essentials of Small Animal Internal Medicine.* St. Louis: Mosby-Year Book Inc, 1992:561–86.

8. Hoenig M, Ferguson DC. Impairment of glucose tolerance in hyperthyroid cats. *J Endocrinol* 1989;121:249–51.

9. Mattheeuws D, Rottiers R, Baeyens D, Vermeulen A. Glucose tolerance and insulin response in obese dogs. *J Am Anim Hosp Assoc* 1984;20:287–93.

10. Nelson RW, Himsel CA, Feldman EC, Bottoms GD. Glucose tolerance and insulin response in normal-weight and obese cats. *Am J Vet Res* 1990;51:1357–62.

11. Kahn CR, Smith RJ, Chin WW. Mechanism of action of hormones that act at the cell surface. In: Wilson JD, Foster DW, eds. *Williams Textbook of Endocrinology, 8th edition.* Philadelphia: WB Saunders Co, 1992:91–134.

12. Adams LG, Hardy RM, Weiss DJ, Bartges JW. Hypo-phosphatemia and hemolytic anemia associated with dia-betes mellitus and hepatic lipidosis in cats. *J Vet Int Med* 1993;7:266–71.

13. Grooters AM, Sherding RG, Biller DS, Johnson SE. Hepatic abscesses associated with diabetes mellitus in two dogs. *J Vet Int Med* 1994;8:203–6.

14. Eigenmann JE, Van der Haage MH, Rijnberk A. Poly-endocrinopathy in two canine littermates: simultaneous occurrence of carbohydrate intolerance and hypo-thyroidism. *J Am Anim Hosp Assoc* 1984;20:143–8.

15. Hoenig M, Dawe DL. A qualitative assay for beta cell antibodies. Preliminary results in dogs with diabetes mellitus. *Vet Immunol Immunopath* 1992;32:195–203.

16. Kramer JW, Klaassen JK, Baskin DG, Prieur DJ, Rantanen NW, Robinette JD, Graber WR, Rashti L. Inheritance of diabetes mellitus in Keeshond dogs. *Am J Vet Res* 1988;49:428–31.

17. Ogawa A, Johnson JH, Ohneda M, McAllister CT, Inman L, Alam T, Unger RH. Roles of insulin resistance and β-cell dysfunction in dexamethasone-induced diabetes. *J Clin Invest* 1992;90:497–504.

18. Eigenmann JE, Eigenmann RY, Rijnberk A, Van der Gaag I, Zapf J, Froesch E. Progesterone-controlled growth hormone overproduction and naturally occurring canine diabetes and acromegaly. *Acta Endocrinol* 1983;104: 167–76.

19. Bovee KC, Anderson T, Brown S, Goldschmidt MH, Segal S. Renal tubular defects of spontaneous Fanconi syndrome in dogs. In: Desnick RJ, Patterson DF, Scarpelli DG, eds. *Animal Models of Inherited Metabolic Diseases.* New York: Alan R. Liss, Inc, 1982:435–47.

20. Goeders LA, Esposito LA, Peterson ME. Absorption kinetics of regular and isophane (NPH) insulin in the normal dog. *Domest Anim Endocrinol* 1987;4:43–50.

21. Lorenzen FH. The use of isophane insulin for the control of diabetes mellitus in dogs. *Acta Vet Scand* 1992;33: 219–27.

22. Graham PA, Nash AS, McKellar QA. Pharmacokinetics of a highly purified porcine insulin zinc suspension (IZS-P) in dogs with naturally-occurring diabetes mellitus. Submitted for publication.

23. Belshaw BE. *Endocrinology Lecture Notes.* Department of Clinical Sciences of Companion Animals, Utrecht University, 1994.

24. Holste LC, Nelson RW, Feldman EC, Bottoms GD. Effect of dry, soft moist, and canned dog food on postprandial blood glucose and insulin concentrations in healthy dogs. *Am J Vet Res* 1989;50:984–9.

25. Nelson RW, Ihle SL, Lewis LD, Salisbury SK, Miller T, Bergdall V, Bottoms GD. Effects of dietary fiber supplementation on glycemic control in dogs with alloxan-induced diabetes mellitus. *Am J Vet Res* 1991;52:2060–6.

26. DeFronzo RA, Alvestrand A, Smith D, Hendler A, Hendler E, Wahren J. Insulin resistance in uremia. *J Clin Invest* 1981;67:563–8.

27. Ford SL, Nelson RW, Feldman EC, Niwa D. Insulin resistance in three dogs with hypothyroidism and diabetes mellitus. *J Am Vet Med Assoc* 1993;202:1478–80.

28. Reusch CE, Liehs MR, Hoyer M, Vochezer R. Fructosamine. A new parameter for diagnosis and metabolic control in diabetic dogs and cats. *J Vet Int Med* 1993;7: 177–82. (and communication at 40th Annual Conference FKDVG, Dresden, 1994).

28a. Jensen AL. Serum fructosamine as a screening test for diabetes mellitus in non-healthy middle-aged to older dogs. *J Vet Med A* 1994;41:480–484.

29. Macintire DK. Treatment of diabetic ketoacidosis in dogs by continuous low-dose intravenous infusion of insulin. *J Am Vet Med Assoc* 1993;202:1266–72.

30. Curtis R, Barnett KC, Leon A. Diseases of the canine posterior segment. In: Gelatt KN, ed. *Veterinary Ophthalmology, 2nd edition.* Philadeplhia: Lea & Febiger, 1991:461–525.

31. Westermark P, Wernstedt C, O'Brien TD, Hayden DW, Johnson KH. Islet amyloid in type 2 human diabetes mellitus and adult diabetic cats contains a novel putative polypeptide hormone. *Amer J Path* 1987;127:414–7.

32. Bretherton-Watt D, Bloom SR. Islet amyloid polypeptide. The cause of type-2 diabetes? *Trends Endocrinol Metab* 1991;2:203–6.

33. Clark A. Islet Amyloid: An enigma of type 2 diabetes.

Diab/Metab Rev 1992;8:117–32.

34. Kirk CA, Feldman EC, Nelson RW. Diagnosis of naturally acquired type-I and type-II diabetes mellitus in cats. *Am J Vet Res* 1993;54:463–7.

35. Panciera DL, Thomas CB, Eicker SW, Atkins CE. Epizootiologic patterns of diabetes mellitus in cats: 333 cases (1980–1986). *J Am Vet Med Assoc* 1990;197:1504–8.

36. Nelson RW, Feldman EC, Ford SL, Roemer OP. Effect of an orally administered sulfonylurea, glipizide, for treatment of diabetes mellitus in cats. *J Am Vet Med Assoc* 1993;203:821–7.

37. Peterson ME, Randolph JF. Endocrine diseases. In: Sherding RG, ed. *The Cat. Diseases and Clinical Management.* New York: Churchill Livingstone, 1989:1095–1161.

38. Gand OP, Weir GC. Oral hypoglycemic agents. In: Becker KL, ed. *Principles and Practice of Endocrinology and Metabolism.* Philadelphia: JB Lippincott Co, 1990: 1099–1102.

39. De Bruijne JJ, Altszuler N, Hampshire J, Visser TJ, Hackeng WHL. Fat mobilization and plasma hormone levels in fasted dogs. *Metabolism* 1981;30:190–4.

40. De Bruijne JJ, De Koster P. Glycogenolysis in the fasting dog. *Comp Biochem Physiol* 1983;75B:553–5.

41. Strauss G, Christensen L, Zapf J. Tumor-induced hypoglycemia due to "big" IGF-II. *J Int Med* 1994; 236:97–9.

42. Bestetti G, Rossi GL. Islet cell carcinomas in dogs. *Virchows Arch [Pathol Anat]* 1985;405:203–14.

43. Hawkins KL, Summers BA, Kuhajda FP, Smith CA. Immunocytochemistry of normal pancreatic islets and spontaneous islet cell tumors in dogs. *Vet Pathol* 1987;24: 170–9.

44. O'Brien TD, Westermark P, Johnson KH. Islet amyloid polypeptide and calcitonin gene-related peptide immunoreactivity in amyloid and tumor cells of canine pancreatic endocrine tumors. *Vet Pathol* 1990;27:194–8.

45. Caywood DD, Klausner JS, O'Leary TP, Withrow SJ, Richardson RC, Harvey HJ, Norris AM, Henderson RA, Johnston SD. Pancreatic insulin-secreting neoplasms: Clinical, diagnostic, and prognostic features in 73 dogs. *J Am Anim Hosp Assoc* 1988;24:577–84.

46. O'Brien TD, Norton F, Turner TM, Johnson KH. Pancreatic endocrine tumor in a cat: Clinical, pathological and immunohistochemical evaluation. *J Am Anim Hosp Assoc* 1990;26:453–7.

47. Dunn JK, Heath MF, Herrtage ME, Jackson KF, Walker MJ. Diagnosis of insulinoma in the dog: A study of 11 cases. *J Small Anim Pract* 1992;33:514–20.

48. Krenning EP, Kwekkeboom DJ, Bakker WH, Breeman WAP, Kooij PPM, Oei HY, Van Hagen M, Postema PTE, De Jong M, Reubi JC, Visser TJ, Reijs AEM, Hofland LJ, Koper JW, Lamberts SWJ. Somatostatin receptor scintigraphy with [^{111}In-DTPA-D-Phe^1]- and [^{123}I-Tyr^3]-octreotide: the Rotterdam experience with more than 1000 patients. *Eur J Nucl Med* 1993;20:716–31.

49. Van Sluijs FJ. Pancreatectomy. In: Van Sluijs FJ, ed. *Atlas of Small Animal Surgery.* New York: Churchill Livingstone, 1992:70–4.

50. Van Toor AJ, Van der Linde-Sipman JS, Van den Ingh TSGAM, Wensing Th, Mol JA. Experimental induction of

fasting hypoglycemia and fatty liver syndrome in three Yorkshire Terrier pups. *Vet Quart* 1991;13:16–23.

51. Vroom MW, Slappendel RJ. Transient juvenile hypoglycemia in a Yorkshire Terrier and a Chihuahua. *Vet Quart* 1987;9:172–6.

52. Happé RP, Van der Gaag I, Lamers CBHW, Van Toorenburg J, Rehfeld JF, Larsson LI. Zollinger-Ellison syndrome in three dogs. *Vet Pathol* 1980;17:177–86.

53. Zerbe CA. Islet cell tumors secreting insulin, pancreatic polypeptide, gastrin, or glucagon. In: Kirk RW, Bonagura JD, eds. *Kirk's Current Veterinary Therapy XI*. Philadelphia: WB Saunders Co, 1992:368–75.

Chapter 6: Testes

1. Hart Elcock L, Schoning P. Age-related changes in the cat testis and epididymis. *Am J Vet Res* 1984;45:2380–4.

2. Lowseth LA, Gerlach RF, Gillett NA, Muggenburg BA. Age-related changes in the prostate and testes of the beagle dog. *Vet Pathol* 1990;27:347–53.

3. Jégou B. The Sertoli cell. In: The Testes. De Kretser DM, ed. *Clinical Endocrinology and Metabolism* 1992;6:273–311.

4. Pescovitz OH, Srivasta CH, Breyer PR, Monts BA. Paracrine control of spermatogenesis. *Trends Endocrinol Metab* 1994;5:126–31.

5. De Kretser DM, McLachlan RI, Robertson DM, Wreford NG. Control of spermatogenesis by follicle stimulating hormone and testosterone. In: De Kretser DM, ed. *The Testes. Clinical Endocrinology and Metabolism* 1992;6: 335–54.

6. Rommerts FFG, Van der Molen HJ. Testicular steroidogenesis. In: Burger H, De Kretser D, eds. *The Testis, 2nd ed*. New York: Raven Press, 1989:303–28.

7. Günzel-Apel AR, Brinckmann HG, Hoppe HO. Dynamik der LH- und Testosteron-Sekretion bei Beagle-Rüden verschiedener Altersgruppen. *Reprod Domest Anim* 1990; 25:78–86.

8. Knol BW, Dieleman SJ, Bevers, MM, Van den Brom WE. Diurnal and seasonal variations in plasma levels of luteinizing hormone and testosterone in the male dog. *Proceedings 12th Int. Congress on Animal Reproduction*, The Hague, 1992:1788–90.

9. Brabant G, Prank K, Schöfl C. Pulsatile patterns in hormone secretion. *Trends Endocrinol Metab* 1992;3: 18,3–90.

10. Verhoeven G. Local control systems within the testis. In: De Kretser DM, ed. *The Testes. Clinical Endocrinology and Metabolism* 1992;6:313–33.

11. König H, Schärer V, Küpfer U, Tschudi P. Hodenhypoplasie (Fehlen von Spermiogonien) und linksseitige Nebenhodenhypoplasie bei einem dreifarbigen Kater vom 39/xxy-Karyotyp. *Dtsch Tierärtzl Wschr* 1983;90:341–3.

12. Kemppainen RJ, Thompson FN, Lorenz MD, Munnell JF, Chakraborty PK. Effects of prednisone on thyroid and gonadal endocrine function in dogs. *J Endocrinol* 1983;96:293–302.

13. Hart BL. Behavioral Effects of Castration. Canine Practice. June 1976:10–21.

14. Woodall PF, Johnstone IP. Dimensions and allometry of testes, epididymides and spermatozoa in the domestic dog (Canis familiaris). *J Reprod Fert* 1988;82:603–9.

15. Kawakami E, Tsutsui T, Yamada Y, Yamauchi M. Cryptorchidism in the dog: occurrence of cryptorchidism and semen quality in the cryptorchid dog. *Jpn J Vet Sci* 1984;46:303–8.

16. Reif JS, Brodey RS. The relationship between cryptorchidism and canine testicular neoplasia. *J Am Vet Med Assoc* 1969;155:2005–10.

17. Romagnoli SE. Canine cryptorchidism. *Vet Clin North Amer Small Anim Pract* 1991:21:533–44.

18. Hayes HM Jr, Wilson GP, Pendergrass TW, Cox VS. Canine cryptorchidism and subsequent testicular neoplasia: case-control study with epidemiological update. *Teratology* 1976;32:51–6.

19. Millis DL, Hauptman JG, Johnson CA. Cryptorchidism and monorchism in cats: 25 cases (1980–1989). *J Am Vet Med Assoc* 1992;200:1128–30.

20. Richardson EF, Mullen H. Cryptorchidism in cats. *Comp Contin Ed Vet Pract Small Anim Pract* 1993;15:1342–69.

21. Baumans V, Dijkstra G, Wensing CJG. The effect of orchidectomy on gubernacular outgrowth and regression in the dog. *Int J Androl* 1982;5:387–401.

22. Baumans V, Dijkstra G, Wensing CJG. The role of a non androgenic testicular factor in the process of testicular descent. *Int J Androl* 1983;6:541–52.

23. Fentener van Vlissingen JM, Van Zoelen EJJ, Ursem PJF, Wensing CJG. In vitro model of the first phase of testicular descent: identification of a low molecular weight factor from fetal testis involved in proliferation of gubernaculum testis cells and distinct from specified polypeptide growth factors and fetal gonadal hormones. *Endocrinology* 1988;123:2868–77.

24. Mattheeuws D, Comhaire FH. Concentrations of estradiol and testosterone in peripheral and spermatic venous blood of dogs with unilateral cryptorchidism. *Domest Anim Endocrinol* 1989;6:203–6.

25. Baumans V, Dijkstra G, Wensing CJG. Testicular descent in the dog. *Zbl Vet Med C; Anat Hist Embryol* 1981;10: 97–110.

26. Cox VS, Wallace LJ, Jessen CR. An anatomic and genetic study of canine cryptorchidism. *Teratology* 1978;18: 233–40.

27. Dunn ML, Foster WJ, Goddard KM. Cryptorchidism in dogs: A clinical survey. *J Am Anim Hosp Assoc* 1968;4: 180–2.

28. Burke TJ. Anatomical abnormalities. In: Burke TJ, ed. *Small Animal Reproduction and Infertility*. Philadelphia: Lea & Febiger, 1986:227–44.

29. Feldman EC, Nelson RW. Disorders of the canine male reproductive tract. In: Feldman EC, Nelson RW, eds. *Canine and Feline Endocrinology and Reproduction*. Philadelphia: WB Saunders Co, 1987:481–524.

30. Rhoades JD, Foley CW. Cryptorchidism and intersexuality. *Vet Clin North Am* 1977;7:789–94.

31. Kawakami E, Tsutsui T, Yamada Y, Ogasa A, Yamauchi M. Spermatogenic function in cryptorchid dogs after orchiopexy. *Jpn J Vet Sci* 1989;50:227–35.

32. Kawakami E, Tsutsui T, Yamada Y, Ogasa A, Yamauchi

M. Spermatogenic function in unilateral cryptorchid dogs after orchiopexy and unilateral castration. *Jpn J Vet Sci* 1988;50:754–62.

33. Bosch AG, Van Sluijs FJ, Van Nes JJ. Medische besliskunde in de veterinaire praktijk. *Tijdschr Diergeneesk* 1989;114:369–75.

34. Theilen GH, Madewell BR. Tumors of the urogenital tract. In: Theilen GH, ed. *Veterinary Cancer Medicine*. Philadelphia: Lea & Febiger, 1979:375–81.

35. Dorn CR, Taylor DON, Schneider R, Hibbard HH, Klauber MR. Survey of animal neoplasms in Alameda and Costa counties, California. II Cancer morbidity in dogs and cats from Alameda county. *J Int Canc* 1962;40:307–18.

36. Hayes HM, Pendergrass TW. Canine testicular tumours: epidemiologic features of 410 dogs. *Int J Cancer* 1976;18:482–7.

37. Nielsen SW, Lein DH. Tumours of the testis. *Bull WHO* 1974;50:71–8.

38. Prange H, Katenkamp D, Baumann G, Falk Junge G, Kosmehl H. Die Pathologie der Hodentumoren des Hundes. 1. Epidemiologie und vergleichend-epidemiologische Aspekte. *Arch Exp Vet* 1986;40:555–65.

39. Nieto JM, Pizarro M, Fontaine JJ. Testicular neoplasms in dogs. Epidemiological and pathological aspects. *Recueil Med Vet* 1989;165:149–53.

40. Patnaik AK, Liu SK. Leiomyoma of the tunica vaginalis in a dog. *Cornell Vet* 1975;65:228–31.

41. Rothwell TLW, Papadimitriou JM, Xu FN, Middleton DJ. Schwannoma in the testis of a dog. *Vet Pathol* 1986;23:629–31.

42. Turk JR, Turk MAM, Gallina AM. A canine testicular tumor resembling gonadoblastoma. *Vet Pathol* 1981;18:201–7.

43. Rosen DK, Carpenter JL. Functional ectopic interstitial cell tumor in a castrated male cat. *J Am Vet Med Assoc* 1993;202:1865–6.

44. Lipowitz AJ, Schwartz A, Wilson GP, Ebert JW. Testicular neoplasms and concomitant clinical changes in the dog. *J Am Vet Med Assoc* 1973;143:1364–8.

45. Weaver AD. Survey with follow-up of 67 dogs with testicular sertoli cell tumours. *Vet Rec* 1983;113:105–7.

46. Reifinger M. Statistische Untersuchungen zum Vorkommen von Hodentumoren bei Haussäugetieren. *J Vet Med* 1988:A35:63–72.

47. Kasbohm C, Saar C. Östrogenbedingte Knochenmarkschäden bei Hunden mit Hodenneoplasien. *Tierärtzl Praxis* 1975;3:225–9.

48. Edwards DF Bone marrow hypoplasia in a feminized dog with a Sertoli cell tumor. *J Am Vet Med Assoc* 1981;178:494–6.

49. Sherding RG, Wilson GP, Kociba GJ. Bone marrow hypoplasia in eight dogs with Sertoli cell tumor. *J Am Vet Med Assoc* 1981;178:497–501.

50. Morgan RV. Blood dyscrasias associated with testicular tumours in the dog. *J Am Anim Hosp Assóc* 1982;18:970–5.

51. Morris BJ. Fatal bone marrow depression as a result of Sertoli cell tumor (in a dog). *Vet Med Small Anim Clin* 1983;78:1070–2.

52. Chastain CB. Feminizing testicular tumor. *Comp Cont Educ Pract Vet Small Anim Pract* 1993;15:197–201,245.

53. Grootenhuis AJ, Van Sluijs FJ, Klaij IA, Steenbergen J, Timmerman MA, Bevers MM, Dieleman SJ, De Jong FH. Inhibin, gonadotropins and sex steroids in dogs with Sertoli cell tumours. *J Endocrinol* 1990;127:235–42.

54. Mattheeuws DRG, Comhaire FH. Tumors of the testes. In: Kirk RW, ed. *Current Veterinary Therapy VI*. Philadelphia: Saunders Co, 1977;1054–8.

55. Wallace MS. Infertility in the male dog. *Problems Vet Med* 1992;4:531–44.

56. Ellington JE. Diagnosis, treatment, and management of poor fertility in the stud dog. *Sem Vet Med Surg (Small Anim)* 1994;9:46–53.

57. Root MV, Johnston SD. Basics for a complete reproductive examination of the male dog. *Sem Vet Med Surg (Small Anim)* 1994;9:41–5.

58. James RW, Heywood R, Fowler DJ. Serial percutaneous testicular biopsy in the Beagle dog. *J Small Anim Pract* 1979;20:219–28.

59. Lopate C, Threlfall WR, Rosol TJ. Histopathologic and gross effects of testicular biopsy in the dog. *Theriogenology* 1989;32:585–602.

60. Mickelsen WD, Memon MA, Anderson PB, Freeman DA. The relationship of semen quality to pregnancy rate in and litter size following artificial insemination in the bitch. *Theriogenology* 1993;41:553–60.

61. Belchetz PE. The testis. In: Besser GM, Cudworth AG, eds. *Clinical Endocrinology*. London: Chapman and Hall, 1987:10.1–18.

62. Wensing CJG. Developmental anomalies, including cryptorchidism. In: Morrow DA, ed. *Current Therapy in Theriogenology: Diagnosis, Treatment and Prevention of Reproductive Diseases in Animals*. Philadelphia: WB Saunders Co, 1980:583–9.

Chapter 7: Ovaries

1. Evans HE and Christensen GC. The urogenital system. In: Evans HE, ed. *Miller's Anatomy of the dog,* 3rd edition. Philadelphia: WB Saunders Co, 1993:531–40.

2. Olson PN, Bowen RA, Behrendt M, Olson JD, Nett TM. Concentrations of reproductive hormones in canine serum throughout late anestrus, proestrus and estrus. *Biol Reprod* 1982;27:1196–1206.

3. Okkens AC, Dieleman SJ, Bevers MM, Willemse AH. Evidence for the non-involvement of the uterus in the lifespan of the corpus luteum in the cyclc dog. *Vet Quart* 1985;7:169–73.

4. Okkens AC, Bevers MM, Dieleman SJ, Willemse AH. Evidence for prolactin as the main luteotrophic factor in the cyclic dog. *Vet Quart* 1990;12:193–201.

5. Okkens AC, Dieleman SJ, Bevers MM, Lubberink AAME, Willemse AH. Influence of hypophysectomy on the lifespan of the corpus luteum in the cyclic dog. *J Reprod Fert* 1986;77:187–92.

6. Van Haaften B, Bevers MM, Van de Brom WE, Okkens AC, Van Sluijs FJ, Willemse AH, Dieleman SJ. Increasing

232

sensitivity of the pituitary to GnRH from early to late anoestrus in the beagle bitch. *J Reprod Fert* 1994;101: 221–5.

7. Concannon PW. Biology of gonadotrophin secretion in adult and prepubertal female dogs. *J Reprod Fert Suppl* 1993;47:3–27.

8. Okkens AC, Bevers MM, Dieleman SJ, Willemse AH. Shortening of the interoestrous interval and the lifespan of the corpus luteum of the cyclic dog by bromocriptine treatment. *Vet Quart* 1985;7:173–6.

9. Naaktgeboren C. *De Geboorte van de Hond en zijn Wilde Verwanten. Third revised edition*. Naarden (NL): Strengholt, 1987:31–5.

10. Concannon P, Whaley S, Lein D, Wissler R. Canine gestation length: Variation related to time of mating and fertile life of sperm. *Am J Vet Res* 1983;44:1819–21.

11. Okkens AC, Hekerman TWM, De Vogel JWA. Infuence of litter size and breed on the variation in length of gestation in the dog. *Vet Quart* 1993;15:160–1.

12. Van der Weyden GC, Taverne MAM, Dieleman SJ, Wurth Y, Bevers MM, Van Oord HA. Physiological aspects of pregnancy and parturition in dogs. *J Reprod Fert Suppl* 1989;39:211–24.

13. Concannon PW, Isaman L, Frank DA, Michel FJ, Currie WB. Elevated concentrations of 13,14-dihydro-15-keto-prostaglandin F-$_2\alpha$ in maternal plasma during prepartum luteolysis and parturition in dogs (Canis familiaris). *J Reprod Fert* 1988;84:71–7.

14. Concannon PW, Butler WR, Hansel W, Knight PJ, Hamilton JM. Parturition and lactation in the bitch: serum progesterone, cortisol and prolactin. *Biol Reprod* 1978; 19: 1113–8.

15. Verhage HG, Beamer NB, Brenner RM. Plasma levels of estradiol and progesterone in the cat during poly-estrus, pregnancy and pseudo-pregnancy. *Biol Reprod* 1976; 14:579–85.

16. Concannon PW, Hogson B, Lein D. Reflex LH release in estrous cats following single and multiple copulations. *Biol Reprod* 1980;23:111–7.

17. Leyva H, Addiego L, Stabenfeldt G. The effect of different photoperiods on plasma concentrations of melatonin, prolactin and cortisol in the domestic cat. *Endocrinology* 1984;115:1729–36.

18. Leyva H, Madley T, Stabenfeldt GH. Effect of light manipulation on ovarian activity and melatonin and prolactin secretion in the domestic cat. *J Reprod Fert Suppl* 1989; 39:125–33.

19. Verstegen JP, Onclin K, Silva LDM, Wouters-Balman P, Delahaut P, Ectors F. Regulation of progesterone during pregnancy in the cat: studies on the roles of corpora lutea, placenta and prolactin secretion. *J Reprod Fert Suppl* 1993;47:165–73.

20. Banks DH, Paape SR, Stabenfeldt GH. Prolactin in the cat: I Pseudopregnancy, pregnancy and lactation. *Biol Reprod* 1983;28:923–32.

21. Lawler DF, Evans RH, Reimers TJ, Colby ED, Monti KL. Histologic features, environmental factors, and serum estrogen, progesterone, and prolactin values associated with ovarian phase and inflammatory uterine disease in cats. *Am J Vet Res* 1991;52:1747–53.

22. Åsheim Å. Pathogenesis of renal damage and polydipsia in dogs with pyometra. *J Am Vet Med Assoc* 1965;147: 736–45.

23. Olson PN, Wrigley RH, Husted PW, Bowen RA, Nett TM. Persistent estrus in the bitch. In: Ettinger SJ, ed. *Textbook of Veterinary Internal Medicine, 3rd* edition. Philadelphia: WB Saunders Co, 1989:1793–6.

24. Van Haaften B, Dieleman SJ, Okkens AC, Willemse AH. Timing the mating of dogs on the basis of blood progesterone concentration. *Vet Rec* 1989;125:524–6.

25. Kemppainen RJ, Thompson FN, Lorenz MD, Munnell JF. Chakraborty PK. Effects of prednisone on thyroid and gonadal endocrine function in dogs. *J Endocrinol* 1983;96: 293–302.

26. Van der Weyden GC, De Schepper J. Female genital tract. In: Rijnberk A, De Vries HW, eds. *Medical History and Physical Examination in Companion Animals*. Dordrecht/ Boston: Kluwer Academic Publishers, 1995;139–49.

27. Johnston SD. Clinical approach to infertility in bitches with primary anestrus. *Vet Clin of North Am Small Animal Practice* 1991;21:421–5.

28. Vanderlip, SL, Wing AE, Felt P, Linkie D, Rivier J, Concannon PW, Lasley BL. Ovulation induction in anestrous bitches by pulsatile administration of gonadotropin-releasing hormone. *Lab Anim Sci* 1987;37:459–64.

29. Cain JL, Lasley BL, Cain GR, Feldman EC, Stabenfeldt GH. Induction of ovulation in bitches with pulsatile or continuous infusion of GnRH. *J Reprod Fert Suppl* 1989; 39:143–7.

30. Verstegen JP, Onclin K, Silva LDM, Concannon PW. Early termination of anestrus and induction of fertile estrus in dogs by the dopamine super-agonist cabergoline. *Biol Reprod Suppl* 1994;50:Abstr 410.

31. Okkens AC, Bevers MM, Dieleman SJ, Willemse AH. Shortening of the interoestrous interval of the cyclic dog by bromocriptine treatment. *Proc Voorjaarsdagen Royal Netherlands Vet Assoc*, 1985:28.

32. Van Haaften B, Dieleman SJ, Okkens AC, Bevers MM, Willemse AH. Induction of oestrus and ovulation in dogs by treatment with PMSG and/or bromocriptine. *J Reprod Fert Suppl* 1989;39:330–1.

33. Soules MR. Luteal dysfunction. In: Adashi EY, Leung PCK, eds. *The Ovary*. New York: Raven Press, Ltd, 1993: 607–27.

34. Nickel RF, Okkens AC, Van der Gaag I, Van Haaften B. Oophoritis in a dog with abnormal corpus luteum function. *Vet Rec* 1991;128:333–4.

35. Post K, Van Haaften B, Okkens AC. Vaginal hyperplasia in the bitch; Literature review and commentary. *Can Vet J* 1991;32:35–7.

36. Carmichael LE. Canine brucellosis. In: Burke ThJ, ed. *Small Animal Reproduction and Infertility*. Philadelphia: Lea and Febiger, 1986:269–75.

37. Misdorp W. Progestagens and mammary tumours in dogs and cats. *Acta Endocrinol* 1991;125(Suppl 1):27–31.

38. Rutteman GR, Blankenstein MA, Minke J, Misdorp W. Steroid receptors in mammary tumours of the cat. *Acta Endocrinol* 1991;125(Suppl 1):32–7.

39. Vickery BH, McRae GI, Goodpasture JC, Sanders LM. Use of potent LHRH analogues for chronic contraception

and pregnancy termination in dogs. *J Reprod Fert* 1989; 39:175–87.

40. McCann JP, Altszuler N, Hampshire J, Concannon PW. Growth hormone, insulin, glucose, cortisol, luteinizing hormone, and diabetes in beagle bitches treated with medroxyprogesterone acetate. *Acta Endocrinol* 1987;116: 73–80.

41. Colon J, Kimball M, Hansen B, Concannon PW. Effects of contraceptive doses of the progestagen megestrol acetate on luteinizing hormone and follicle-stimulating hormone secretion in female dogs. *J Reprod Fert* (Suppl) 1993; 47:519–21.

42. Middleton DJ, Watson ADJ, Howe CJ, Caterson ID. Suppression of cortisol responses to exogenous adrenocorticotrophic hormone, and the occurrence of side effects attributable to glucocorticoid excess, in cats during therapy with megestrol acetate and prednisolone. *Can J Vet Res* 1987;51:60–5.

43. Middleton DJ, Watson ADJ. Glucose intolerance in cats given short-term therapies of prednisolone and megestrol acetate. *Am J Vet Res* 1985;46:2623–5.

44. Selman PJ, Mol JA, Rutteman GR, Rijnberk A. Progestin treatment in the dog: II. Effects on the hypothalamic-pituitary-adrenocortical axis. *Eur J Endocrinol* 1994;131: 422–30.

45. Russo IH, Russo J. Progestagens and mammary gland development: Differentiation versus carcinogenesis. *Acta Endocrinol* 1991;125(Suppl 1):7–12.

46. Hayden DW, Johnson KH. Feline mammary hypertrophy-fibroadenoma complex. In: Kirk RW, ed. *Current Veterinary Therapy IX*. Philadelphia: WB Saunders Co, 1986: 477–80.

Chapter 8: Disorders of sexual differentiation

1. Peters H. Migration of gonocytes in the mammalian gonad and their differentiation. *Phil Trans R Soc Lond* 1970;259: 91–101.

2. O'Rahilly R. The development of the vagina in the human. In: Blandau RJ, Bergsma D, eds. *Morphogenesis and Malformation of the Genital System*. New York: Alan Liss, 1977:123–36.

3. Josso N. Differentiation of the genital tract: Stimulators and inhibitors. In: Austin GR, Edwards RG, eds. *Mechanisms of Sex Differentiation in Animals and Man*. London: Academic Press, 1981:165–203.

4. Meyers-Wallen VN, Manganaro FF, Kuroda T, Concannon PW, MacLaughlin DT, Donahoe PK. The critical period for Mullerian duct regression in the dog embryo. *Biol Reprod* 1991;45:623–33.

5. Wilson JD, Griffin JE, George FW. Sexual differentiation: Early hormone synthesis and action. *Biol Reprod* 1980; 22:9–18.

6. Meyers-Wallen VN, Patterson DF. Disorders of sexual development in dogs and cats. In: Kirk, RW, ed. *Current Veterinary Therapy Vol X*. Philadelphia: WB Saunders Co, 1989:1261–9.

7. Löfstedt RM, Buoen LC, Weber AF, Johnston SD,

Huntington A, Concannon PW. Prolonged proestrus in a bitch with X-chromosomal monosomy (77:XO). *J Am Vet Med Assoc* 1992;200:1104–6.

8. Norby DE, Hegreberg GA, Thuline HC. An XO-cat. *Cytogenet Cell Genet* 1974;13:448–53.

9. Simpson JC. *Disorders of Sexual Differentiation*. New York: Academic Press, 1976:303–37.

10. Meyers-Wallen VN, Patterson DF. Disorders of sexual development in the dog. In: Morrow, DA, ed. *Current Therapy in Theriogenology*, 2nd ed. Philadelphia: WB Saunders Co, 1986:564–7.

11. König H, Schärer V, Küpper U, Tschudi P. Hodenhypoplasie (Fehlen von Spermiogonien) und linksseitige Nebenhodenaplasie bei einem dreifarbigen Kater vom 39/XXY-Karyotyp. *Dtsch Tierärztl Wschr* 1983;90:341–84.

12. Rogge UW. Dreifarbiger Kater. *Dtsch Tierärztl Wschr* 1978;6:499–500.

13. Johnston SD, Buoen LC, Weber AF, Madl JE. X trisomy in an Airedale bitch with ovarian dysplasia and primary anestrus. *Theriogenology* 1985;24:597.

14. Selden JR, Moorhead PS, Koo GC, Wachtel SS, Haskins ME, Patterson DF. XX sex reversal in the Cocker Spaniel dog. *Hum Genet* 1984;67:62–9.

15. Selden JR, Wachtel SS, Koo GC, Haskins ME, Patterson DF. Genetic basis of XX male syndrome and XX true hermaphroditism: Evidence in the dog. *Science* 1978; 201:644–6.

16. Meyers-Wallen VN, Donahoe PK, Manganaro TF, Patterson DF. Mullerian Inhibiting Substance in sex-reversed dogs. *Biol Reprod* 1987;37:1015–22.

17. Hare WCD. Intersexuality in the dog. *Can Vet J* 1976; 17:7–15.

18. Wentink GH, Breeuwsma AJ, Goedegebeure SA, Teunissen GHB, Aalfs RHG. Three cases of intersexuality in the dog. *Tijdschr Diergeneesk* 1973; 98;437–45.

19. Biewenga WJ, Okkens AC, Wensing CJG. Anabolics are a hazard in some cases. *Tijdschr Diergeneesk* 1975;100:391–2.

20. Rothuizen J, Voorhout G, Okkens AC, Biewenga WJ. Urovagina associated with female pseudohermaphroditism in four bitches from one litter. *Tijdschr Diergeneesk* 1978; 103:1109–13.

21. Peter AT, Markvelder D, Asem EK. Phenotypic feminisation in a genetic male dog caused by non-functional androgen receptors. *Theriogenology* 1993;40:1093–105.

22. Meyers-Wallen VN, Wilson JD, Griffin JE, Fisher S, Moorhead PH, Goldschmidt MH, Haskins ME, Patterson DF. Testicular feminisation in a cat. *J Am Vet Med Assoc* 1989;195:631–4.

23. Meyers-Wallen VN, Donahoe PK, Ueno S, Manganaro TF, Patterson DF. Mullerian Inhibiting Substance is present in testes of dogs with Persistent Mullerian Duct Syndrome. *Biol Reprod* 1989;41:881–8.

24. Nickel RF, Ubbink G, Van Der Gaag I, Van Sluijs FJ. Persistent Mullerian Duct Syndrome in the Bassethound. *Tijdschr Diergeneesk* 1992;117:31S.

25. Marshall LS, Oehlert ML, Haskins ME, Selden JR, Patterson DF. Persistent Mullerian duct syndrome in Miniature Schnauzers. *J Am Vet Med Assoc* 1982; 181:798–801.

234

Chapter 9: Parathyroids

1. Peterson ME, James KM, Wallace M, Timothy SD, Joseph RJ. Idiopathic hypoparathyroidism in five cats. *J Vet Int Med* 1991;5:47–51.
2. Bruyette DS, Feldman EC. Primary hypoparathyroidism in the dog. Report of 15 cases and review of 13 previously reported cases. *J Vet Int Med* 1988;2:7–14.
3. Forbes S, Nelson RW, Guptill L. Primary hypoparathyroidism in a cat. *J Am Vet Med Assoc* 1990;196:1285–7.
4. Aurbach GD, Marx SJ, Spiegel AM. Parathyroid hormone, calcitonin, and the calciferols. In: Wilson JD, Foster DW, eds. *Williams Textbook of Endocrinology, 8th edition*. Philadelphia: WB Saunders Co, 1992:1397–476.
5. Reusch C, Münster M. Hypoparathyreoidismus bei einem Mittelschauzer. *Kleintierpraxis* 1988;33:299–302.
6. Torrance AG, Nachreiner R. Human-parathormone assay for use in dogs: Validation, sample handling studies, and parathyroid function testing. *Am J Vet Res* 1989;50:1123–7.
7. Flanders JA, Reimers TJ. Radioimmunoassay of parathyroid hormone in cats. *Am J Vet Res* 1991;52:422–5.
8. Berger B, Feldman EC. Primary hyperparathyroidism in dogs: 21 cases (1976–1986). *J Am Vet Med Assoc* 1987;191:350–6.
9. Kallet AJ, Richter KP, Feldman EC, Brum DE. Primary hyperparathyroidism in cats: Seven cases (1984–1989). *J Am Vet Med Assoc* 1991;199:1767–71.
10. DeVries SE, Feldman EC, Nelson RW, Kennedy PC. Primary parathyroid gland hyperplasia in dogs: Six cases (1982–1991). *J Am Vet Med Assoc* 1993;202:1132–6.
11. Nelson RW. Disorders of the parathyroid gland. In: Nelson RW, Couto CG, eds. *Essentials of Small Animal Internal Medicine*. St. Louis: Mosby-Year Book Inc, 1992:537–43.
12. Martin KJ, Slatopolsky E. Renal osteodystrophy. In: Becker KL, ed. *Principles and Practice of Endocrinology and Metabolism*. Philadelphia: JB Lippincott Co, 1990:457–63.
13. Finco DR, Brown SA, Crowell WA, Duncan RJ, Barsanti JA, Bennett SE. Effects of dietary phosphorus and protein in dogs with chronic renal failure. *Am J Vet Res* 1992;53:2264–71.
14. Finco DR, Brown SA, Cooper T, Crowell WA, Hoenig M, Barsanti JA. Effects of parathyroid hormone depletion in dogs with induced renal failure. *Am J Vet Res* 1994;55:867–73.
15. Dzanis DA, Corbellini CN, Krook L, Kallfelz FA. Effects of 1,25-dihydroxycholecalciferol and 24,25-dihydroxycholecalciferol in dogs with impaired renal function. *J Nutr* 1991;121:S70–2.

Chapter 10: Calciotropic hormones and bone metabolism

1. Recker RR. Embryology, anatomy, and microstructure of bone. In: Coe FL, Favus MJ, eds. *Disorders of Bone and Mineral Metabolism*. New York: Raven Press, 1992:219–40.
2. Nap RC, Hazewinkel HAW. Growth and skeletal development in the dog in relation to nutrition: a review. *Vet Quart* 1994;16:50–9.
3. Howell DS, Dean DD. The biology, chemistry, and biochemistry of the mammalian growth plate. In: Coe FL, Favus MJ, eds. *Disorders of Bone and Mineral Metabolism*. New York: Raven Press, 1992:313–53.
4. Chesnut CH. Bone imaging technique. In: Becker KL, ed. *Principles and Practice of Endocrinology and Metabolism*. Philadelphia: JB Lippincott, 1990:480–4.
5. Marcus R. Endocrine control of bone and mineral metabolism. In: Manolagas SC, Olefsky JM, eds. *Metabolic Bone Disease and Mineral Disorders*. London: Churchill Livingstone, 1988:13–31.
6. Dempster DW. Bone remodeling. In: Coe FL, Favus MJ, eds. *Disorders of Bone and Mineral Metabolism*. New York: Raven Press, 1992:355–80.
7. Hazewinkel HAW. Skeletal diseases. In: Wills JM, Simpson KW, eds. *The Waltham Book of Clinical Nutrition of the Dog and Cat*. Oxford: Pergamon, 1994:395–425.
8. How KL, Hazewinkel HAW, Mol JA. Dietary vitamin D dependence of cat and dog due to inadequate cutaneous photosynthesis of vitamin D. *Gen Comp Endocrinol* 1994;96:12–8.
9. Fletch SM, Smart ME, Pennock PW, Subden RE. Clinical and pathological features of chondrodysplasia (dwarfism) in the Alaskan Malamute. *J Amer Vet Med Assoc* 1973;162:357–61.
10. Chew DJ, Carothers MA. Hypercalcemia. *Vet Clin North Am/Small Anim Pract* 1989;19:265–87.
11. Azria M. *The Calcitonins, Physiology and Pharmacology*. Basel: Karger, 1989.
12. Mol JA, Kwant MM, Arnold ICJ, Hazewinkel HAW. Elucidation of sequence of canine (pro-)calcitonin. A molecular biological and protein chemical approach. *Reg Peptides* 1991; 35:189–95.
13. Hazewinkel HAW, Hackeng WHL, Bosch R, Goedegebuure SA, Voorhout G, van den Brom WE, Bevers MM. Influences of different calcium intakes on calciotropic hormones and skeletal development in young growing dogs. *Front Horm Res* 1987;17:221–32.
14. Chrisman CL. *Problems in Small Animal Neurology, 2nd edition*. Philadelphia: Lea & Febiger, 1991.
15. Olsson SE. Pathophysiology, morphology, and clinical signs of osteochondrosis in the dog. In: Bojrab MJ, Smeak DD, Bloomberg MS, eds. *Disease Mechanisms in Small Animal Surgery*. Philadelphia: Lea & Febiger, 1993:777–96.
16. Voorhout G, Nap RC, Hazewinkel HAW. A radiographic study on the development of the antebrachium in Great Dane pups, raised under standardized conditions. *Vet Radiol Ultrasound* 1994;35:271–6.
17. Slater MR, Scarlett, JM, Donoghue S, Kaderley RE, Bonnett BN, Cockshutt J, Holis N. Diet and exercise as potential risk factors for osteochondritis dissecans in dogs. *Am J Vet Res* 1992;53:2119–24.
18. Saunders MH, Jezyk PK. The radiographic appearance of canine congenital hypothyroidism: skeletal changes with delayed treatment. *Vet Radiol* 1991;32:171–7.

19. Salmeri KR, Bloomberg MS, Scruggs SL, Shille V. Gonadectomy in immature dogs: effects on skeletal, physical and behavioral development. *J Am Vet Med Assoc* 1991;198:1193–203.
20. Fuagere M-C, Friedler RM, Fanti P, Malluche HH. Bone changes occurring early after cessation of ovarian function in Beagle dogs: A histomorphometric study employing sequential biopsies. *J Bone Min Res* 1990;5:263–72.
21. Ross AC. Overview of retinoid metabolism. *J Nutr* 1993;123:346–50.
22. Linney E. Retinoid acid receptors: Transcription factors modulating gene regulation, development, and differentiation. In: Pedersen RA, ed. *Current Topics in Developmental Biology, Vol 27.* San Diego: Academic Press Inc, 1992:309–50.
23. Nap RC. *Nutritional Influences on Growth and Skeletal Development in the Dog.* Thesis, Utrecht University, 1993.

Chapter 11: Tissue hormones and hormonal manifestations of cancer

1. Nylén ES, Becker KL. The diffuse neuroendocrine system. In: Becker KL, ed. *Principles and Practice of Endocrinology and Metabolism.* Philadelphia: JB Lippincott Co, 1990: 1276–83.
2. Odell WD, Appleton WS. Humoral manifestations of cancer. In: Wilson JD, Foster DW, eds. *Williams Textbook of Endocrinology, 8th edition.* Philadelphia: WB Saunders Co, 1992:1599–617.
3. Samson WK. Natriuretic peptides. A family of hormones. *Trends Endocrinol Metab* 1992;3:86–90.
4. Vollmar AM, Reusch C, Kraft W, Schulz R. Atrial natriuretic peptide concentration in dogs with congestive heart failure, chronic renal failure, and hyperadrenocorticism. *Am J Vet Res* 1991;52:1831–4.
5. Häggström J, Hansson K, Karlberg BE, Kvart C, Olsson K. Plasma concentration of atrial natriuretic peptide in relation to severity of mitral regurgitation in Cavalier King Charles Spaniels. *Am J Vet Res* 1994;55:698–703.
6. Spivak JL. The mechanism of action of erythropoietin. *Int J Cell Cloning* 1986;4:139–66.
7. King LG, Giger U, Diserens D, Nagode LA. Anemia of chronic renal failure in dogs. *J Vet Int Med* 1992;6:264–70.
8. Meyer HP, Slappendel RJ, Greydanus-van der Putten SWM. Polycythaemia vera in a dog treated by repeated phlebotomies. *Vet Quart* 1993;15:108–11.
9. Cook SM, Lothrop CD. Serum erythropoietin concentrations measured by radioimmunoassay in normal, polycythemic, and anemic dogs and cats. *J Vet Int Med* 1994;8:18–25.
10. Berk PD. Erythrocytosis and polycythemia. In: Wyngaarden JB, Smith LH, Bennett JC, eds. *Cecil Textbook of Medicine, 19th ed.* Philadelphia: WB Saunders Co, 1992:920–9.
11. Cowgill LD. Erythropoietin: Its use in the treatment of chronic renal failure in dogs and cats. In: *Proc Waltham/OSU Symposium for the Treatment of Small Animal Diseases,* Vernon, CA: Kal Kan Foods Inc, 1992:65–71.
12. De Papp AE, Stewart F. Parathyroid hormone-related protein. A peptide of diverse physiologic funtions. *Trends Endocrinol Metab* 1993;4:181–7.
13. Holt EH, Lu C, Dreyer BE, Dannies PS. Broadus AE. Regulation of parathyroid hormone-related peptide gene expression by estrogen in GH_4C_1 rat pituitary cells has the pattern of a primary response gene. *J Neurochem* 1994;62: 1239–46.
14. Osborne CA, Stevens JB. Pseudohyperparathyroidism in the dog. *J Am Vet Med Assoc* 1973;162:125–35.
15. Chew DJ, Schaer M, Liu S, Owens J. Pseudohyperparathyroidism in a cat. *J Am Anim Hosp Assoc* 1975;11:46–52.
16. Rijnberk A, Elsinghorst ThAM, Koeman JP, Hackeng WHL, Lequin RM. Pseudohyperparathyroidism associated with perirectal adenocarcinomas in elderly female dogs. *Tijdschr Diergeneesk* 1978;103:1069–75.
17. Meuten DJ, Kociba GJ, Capen CC, Chew DJ, Segre GV, Levine L, Tashjian AH, Voelkel EF, Nagode LA. Hypercalcemia in dogs with lymphosarcoma. Biochemical, ultrastructural and histomorphometric investigations. *Lab Invest* 1983;49:553–62.
18. Rosol TJ, Nagode LA, Couto CG, Hammer AS, Chew DJ, Peterson JL, Ayl RD, Steinmeyer CL, Capen CC. Parathyroid hormone (PTH)-related protein, PTH, and 1,25-dihydroxyvitamin D in dogs with cancer-associated hypercalcemia. *Endocrinology* 1992;131:1157–64.
19. Teske E. Canine malignant lymphoma: a review and comparison with human non-Hodgkin's lymphoma. *Vet Quart* 1994;16:209–19.
20. Meuten DJ, Cooper BJ, Capen CC, Chew DJ, Kociba GJ. Hypercalcemia associated with an adenocarcinoma derived from the apocrine glands of the anal sac. *Vet Pathol* 1981; 18:454–71.
21. Teske E, van Heerde P, Rutteman GR, Kurzman ID, Moore PF, MacEwen EG. Prognostic factors for treatment of malignant lymphoma in dogs. *J Am Vet Med Ass* 1994;205:1722–8.
22. Atwater SW, Powers BE, Park RD, Straw RC, Ogilvie GK, Withrow SJ. Thymoma in dogs: 23 cases (1980–1991). *J Am Vet Med Assoc* 1994;205:1007–13.
23. Stokhof AA, Overduin LM, Mol JA, Rijnberk A. Effect of pericardiocentesis on circulating concentrations of atrial natriuretic hormone and arginine vasopressin in dogs with spontaneous pericardial effusion. *Eur J Endocrinol* 1994;130:357–60.

Chapter 12: Obesity

1. Markwell PJ, Butterwick RF. Obesity. In: Wills JM, Simpson KW, eds. *The Waltham Book of Clinical Nutrition of the Dog & Cat.* Oxford: Elsevier Science Ltd, 1994:131–48.
2. Houpt KA, Coren B, Hintz HF, Hilderbrant JE. Effect of sex and reproductive status on sucrose preference, food intake and body weight of dogs. *J Am Vet Med Assoc* 1979;174:1083–5.
3. Wilkinson MJA, McEwan NA. Use of ultrasound in the measurement of subcutaneous fat and prediction of total

body fat in dogs. *J Nutr* 1991;121:S47–50.

4. De Bruijne JJ, Lubberink AAME. Obesity. In: Kirk RW, ed. *Current Veterinary Therapy VI*. Philadelphia: WB Saunders Co, 1977:1068–70.

5. Belshaw BE. *Endocrinology Lecture Notes*. Department of Clinical Sciences of Companion Animals, Utrecht University, 1994.

6. Kurzman ID, MacEwen EG, Haffa ALM. Reduction in body weight and cholesterol in spontaneously obese dogs by dehydropiandrosterone. *Int J Obes* 1990;14:95–104.

7. MacEwen EG, Kurzman ID. Obesity in the dog: role of the adrenal steroid dehydroepiandrosterone (DHEA). *J Nutr* 1991;121:S51–5.

8. Butterwick RF, Wills JM, Sloth C, Markwell PJ. A study of obese cats on a calorie-controlled weight reduction programme. *Vet Rec* 134:372–7.

9. Biourge VC, Massat B, Groff JM, Morris JG, Rogers QR. Effects of protein, lipid, or carbohydrate supplementation on hepatic lipid accumulation during rapid weight loss in obese cats. *Am J Vet Res* 1994;55:1406–15.

Chapter 13: Protocols for functions tests

1. Kemppainen RJ, Zerbe CA. Common endocrine diagnostic tests: normal values and interpretation. In: Kirk RW, ed. *Current Veterinary Therapy X*. Philadelphia: WB Saunders Co, 1989:961–73.

2. Van Wijk PA, Rijnberk A, Croughs RJM, Wolfswinkel J, Selman PJ, Mol JA. Responsiveness to corticotropin-releasing hormone and vasopressin in canine Cushing's syndrome. *Eur J Endocrinol* 1994;130:410–6.

3. Selman PJ, Mol JA, Rutteman GR, Rijnberk A. Progestin treatment in the dog. II. Effects on the hypothalamic-pituitary-adrenocortical axis. *Eur J Endocrinol* 1994;131:422–30.

4. Meij BP, Mol JA, Hazewinkel HAW, Bevers MM, Rijnberk A. Assessment of a combined anterior pituitary function test in Beagle dogs: rapid sequential intravenous administration of four hypothalamic releasing hormones *Domest Anim Endocrinol* (accepted).

5. Selman PJ, Mol JA, Rutteman GR, Rijnberk A. Progestin treatment in the dog. I. Effects on growth hormone, insulin-like growth factor I and glucose homeostasis. *Eur J Endocrinol* 1994;131:413–21.

6. Peterson ME, Altszuler N. Suppression of growth hormone secretion in spontaneous hyperadrenocorticism and its reversal after treatment. *Am J Vet Res* 1981;42:1881–3.

7. Mulnix JA, Rijnberk A, Hendriks HJ. Evaluation of a modified water-deprivation test for diagnosis of polyuric disorders in dogs. *J Am Vet Med Assoc* 1976;169:1327–30.

8. Biewenga WJ, Van den Brom WE, Mol JA. Vasopressin in polyuric syndromes in the dog. *Front Horm Res* 1987;17:139–48.

9. Burkhard A, Kraft W. Untersuchungen zum Thyrotropin-Releasing Hormon-(TRH) Test beim Hund: Injektion oder Infusion? *Tierärztl Praxis* 1994;22:159–64.

9a. Sparkes AH, Jones BR, Gruffydd-Jones TJ, Walker MJ. Thyroid function in the cat: Assessment by the TRH response test and the thyrorophin stimulation test *J Small Anim Pract* 1992;32:59–63.

10. Rijnberk A, Van Wees A, Mol JA. Assessment of two tests for the diagnosis of canine hyperadrenocorticism. *Vet Rec* 1988;122:178–80.

11. Meijer JC, De Bruijne JJ, Rijnberk A, Croughs RJM. Biochemical characterization of pituitary-dependent hyperadrenocorticism in the dog. *J Endocrinol* 1978;77:111–8.

12. Nickel R. Zur Diagnostik und Therapie beim Cushing-Syndrom des Hundes. *Kleintierpraxis* 1990;35:224–34.

13. Cayzer J, Jones BR. Canine hyperadrenocorticism. *N Z Vet J* 1993;41:53–68.

14. Feldman EC, Mack ME. Urine cortisol:creatinine ratio as a screening test for hyperadrenocorticism in dogs. *J Am Vet Med Assoc* 1992;200:1637–41.

15. Smiley LE, Peterson ME. Evaluation of a urine cortisol:creatinine ratio as a screening test for hyperadrenocorticism in dogs. *J Vet Int Med* 1993;7:163–8.

16. Goossens MMC, Meyer HP, Voorhout G, Sprang EPM. Urinary glucocorticoid excretion in the diagnosis of feline hyperadrenocorticism. *Domest Anim Endocrinol* (in press)..

17. Jones CA, Refsal KR, Lippert AC, Nachreiner RF, Schwacha MM. Changes in adrenal cortisol secretion as reflected in the urinary cortisol/creatinine ratio in dogs. *Domest Anim Endocrinol* 1990;7:559–72.

18. Rijnberk A, Voorhout G, Mol JA. Corticoid production by four dogs with hyperfunctioning adrenocortical tumors during treatment with mitotane (o,p′-DDD). *Vet Rec* 1992;131:484–7.

19. Van Haaften B, Bevers MM, Van den Brom WE, Okkens AC, Van Sluijs FJ, Willemse AH, Dieleman SJ. Increasing sensitivity of the pituitary to GnRH from early to late anoestrus in the beagle bitch. *J Reprod Fert* 1994;101:221–5.

20. Knol BW, Dieleman SJ, Bevers MM, Van den Brom WE. GnRH in the male dog: dose-response relationships with LH and testosterone. *J Reprod Fert* 1993;159–61.

21. Memon MA, Ganjam VK, Pavletic MM, Schelling SH. Use of human chorionic gonadotropin stimulation test to detect a retained testis in a cat. *J Am Vet Med Assoc* 1992;201:1602.

22. England GCW, Allen E, Porter DJ. Evaluation of the testosterone response to hCG and the identification of a presumed anorchid dog. *J Small Anim Pract* 1989;30:441–3.

23. Tremblay Y, Belanger A. Changes in plasma steroid levels after single administration of hCG or LHRH agonist analogue in dog and rat. *J Steroid Biochem* 1985;22:315–20.

24. Greve T, Anderson NV. The high-dose, intravenous glucose tolerance test (H-IVGTT) in dogs. *Nordisk Vet Med* 1973;25:436–45.

25. Hoenig M, Ferguson DC. Glucose tolerance and insulin secretion in spontaneously hyperthyroid cats. *Res Vet Sci* 1992;53:338–41.

26. Church DB. A comparison of intravenous and oral glucose tolerance tests in the dog. *Res Vet Sci* 1980;29:353–9.

27. Kaneko JJ, Mattheeuws D, Rottiers RP, Vermeulen A.

Glucose tolerance and insulin response in diabetes mellitus of dogs. *J Small Anim Pract* 1977;18:85–94.

28. Altszuler N, Morrison A, Gottlieb B, Bjerknes C, Rathgeb I, Steele R. Alteration by fasting of the effects of methylprednisolone on carbohydrate metabolsim in the normal dog. *Metabolism* 1974;23:369–74.
29. Belo PS, Romsos DR, Leveille GA. Influence of diet on glucose tolerance, on the rate of glucose utilization and on gluconeogenic enzyme activities in the dog. *J Nutr* 1976;106:1465–74.
30. Mattheeuws D, Rottiers R, Kaneko JJ, Vermeulen A. Effects of anaesthesia and atropine on the intravenous glucose tolerance test in normal dogs. *J Small Animal Pract* 1981;22:779–86.
31. Hsu WH, Hembrough FB. Intravenous glucose tolerance test in cats: Influenced by acetylpromazine, ketamine, morphine, thiopental, and xylazine. *Am J Vet Res* 1982;43:2060–1.
32. Nachreiner RF, Forsberg M, Johnson CA, Refsal KR. Validation of an assay for canine TSH (cTSH). Abstract 17 of the 13th Annual ACVIM Forum. *J Vet Int Med* 1995; 9:184.
33. Williams DA, Scott-Moncrieff JC, Bruner J, Sustarsic D, Panosian-Sahakian N, Unver E, El Shami AS. Canine serum thyroid-stimulating hormone following induction of hypothyroidism. Abstract 18 of the 13th Annual ACVIM Forum *J Vet Int Med* 1995;9:184.
34. Su X. Katakam P, Yang X, Grosse WM, Li OW, McGraw RA, Ferguson DC. Cloning, expression, and development of monoclonal antibodies against the beta subunit of canine thyrotropin. Abstract 21 of the 13th Annual ACVIM Forum. *J Vet Int Med* 1995;9:185.

Chapter 14: Treatment protocols

1. Belshaw BE. *Endocrinology Lecture Notes.* Department of Clinical Sciences of Companion Animals, Utrecht University, 1994.
2. Rosol TJ, Chew DJ, Hammer AS, Ward H, Peterson JL, Carothers MA, Couto CG. Effect of Mithramycin on hypercalcemia in dogs. *J Am Anim Hosp Assoc* 1994; 30:244–50.
3. Rijnberk A, Belshaw BE. O,p'-DDD treatment of canine hyperadrenocorticism: an alternative protocol. In: Kirk RW, Bonagura JD, eds. *Current Veterinary Therapy XI.* Philadelphia: WB Saunders Co, 1992:345–9.

Chapter 15: Algorithms

1. Rijnberk A, Belshaw BE. Endocrine glands. In: Rijnberk A, De Vries HW, eds. *Medical History and Physical Examination of Companion Animals.* Dordrecht/Boston: Kluwer Academic Publishers, 1995:263–71.
2. Rothuizen J, Mol JA. The pituitary-adrenocortical system in canine hepato-encephalopathy. *Front Horm Res* 1987; 17:28–36.
3. Rothuizen J, Biewenga WJ, Mol JA. Chronic glucocorticoid excess and impaired osmoregulation of vasopressin release in dogs with hepatic encephalopathy. Domest Anim Endocrinol 1995; 12:13–24.

Index